Fundamentals of Radiation Biology

nova science publishers
www.novapublishers.com

Radiation Oncology: Clinical, Translational and Laboratory Research Series

Frontiers in Intensity-Modulated Radiotherapy Research
Sibel Karaca, PhD (Editor)
ISBN: 979-8-88697-252-8
eBook ISBN: 979-8-88697-264-1

Stereotactic Radiosurgery (SRS): Procedure, Results and Risks (2 Volume Set)
Antonio Meola, MD, PhD
and Steven D. Chang, MD (Editors)
ISBN: 978-1-53617-679-7
eBook ISBN: 978-1-53617-680-3

More information about this series can be found at
https://novapublishers.com/product-category/series/radiation-oncology-clinical-translational-and-laboratory-research/

Anurag Luharia
Ashish Uke
Gaurav Mishra
Sanjay Dhoble
Editors

Fundamentals of Radiation Biology

nova
science publishers
www.novapublishers.com

DOI: https://doi.org/10.52305/NHBI1476

Library of Congress Cataloging-in-Publication Data

ISBN: 979-8-89530-806-6 (Hardcover)
ISBN: 979-8-89530-905-6 (eBook)

Published by Nova Science Publishers, Inc. † New York

To all the students, teachers, mentors and practitioners who devote their minds and hearts to the responsible use of radiation in science and medicine. And to every patient whose courage inspires our commitment to safety, compassion, and progress.

Contents

Foreword

It is indeed very heartening and equally gratifying that *Dr. Anurag A. Luharia,* Head Radiophysicist & Radiological Safety officer (Radiology, Therapy, Nuclear Medicine) of Jawaharlal Nehru Medical College, Sawangi Meghe, Wardha and Secretary / Convener Radiation Safety Committee Datta Meghe Institute of Higher Education & Research (Deemed to be University) along with *Dr. Gaurav Mishra, Hon. Pro-Vice Chancellor DMIHER (DU), Dr. Ashish Uke, Consultant Radiation Oncologist and Dr. Sanjay Dhoble, Sr. Professor Department of Physics Rashtrasant Tukdoji Maharaj, Nagpur University,* have ventured in bringing out a creative magnificent creation in the form of this Book titled *'Fundamentals of Radiation Biology'* for various academic programmes in the domain of medical education technology.

It is pertinent to note that the healthcare delivery system in terms of the Global charter is required to be not only evidence based but has to be *'Best Evidence Based'.* This mandates diligent conduct of research resulting in generation of credible and cogent levels of evidence to be availed for invocation of the practice and the protocol in terms of best evidence invoked.

In this context it is worth noting that best *'Evidence Based Healthcare'* delivery system cannot be invoked by the medical education in vogue which is the mother repository for the same. It is a matter of common knowledge that the entire gamut of structuring, operation, use and utilization of any and every model of medical education is *'experience based'* and not *'Evidence based'* in the classical sense as it ought to be which is primarily attributable to non-existence or negligible evidence in the public domain because of paucity or near absence of the same with reference to the arena of 'Radiation Biology' undertaken by the all concerned.

This huge and wide gap, which has remained unfilled is the precursor and genuine in nature and realistic in character for the authors to have undertaken the onus and bring out this creative manifestation which has come in its best form specially in the hitherto untouched domain of 'Radiation Biology' on which the relevant readable material in the context of diagnostics in the domain of Modern medicine for learners in the form of a handy text book is wanting. It is this *'want on gap,'* which has been sincerely aimed at bridging it to its score by the author along with his co-authors, which definitely would go a long way in catering to the required cause of learners in a big way in the said domain and also trainers and teachers associated thereto providing a genuine, cogent and credible road-map for the handy and easy decipherability of the intricacies, niceties and nuances in the difficult terrain of Radiation Biology per se. it is a very valiant attempt on part of the collective authorship to unfold these vita aspects for a learner to handily pick them up for the purposes of equipping himself / herself with the required clarity and understanding resulting in better conceptualization and therefore, its consequential applicability.

The topics compiled in the book under Chapters are vital and significant in 'general' as a whole, but the significant aspect is the emphasis that is worked out in the embodied chapters is significantly facilitatory in nature for the purposes of required invocation of 'Doability, Demonstrability and Deliverability' in the arena of Radiation Biology.

The depiction in various chapters covering the entire spectrum of Radiation Biology in a kaleidoscopic manner brings out the expertise of the author along with his co-authors in an emphatic and self-speaking vociferous manner. He has poured the life long experience of his in this Book to make any and every reader decipher the scope, the meaning and the ambit of what is designated as 'Radiation Biology' including the manifestations that are expected out of it for the purposes of its translational accomplishments in larger educational and societal interests. This opens genuine and wide vistas of focused understanding in the otherwise non decipherable domain of Radiation Biology in a big way.

Speaking for the special feature of the book from beginning to end, the only expression at my disposal is that it is a handy 'treatise' on 'Radiation Biology', which is easy, handy, free-flowing decipherable and usable by one and all independent of the status of the level of the user. As such, the creative writing that has been invoked by the author is bound to be of immense use to every user from the point of view of clarity of understanding, utility and purpose fulfillment but it is bound to fill in a huge void that remained unfilled all these years for wide and varied reasons.

I would be failing in my duty if I do not wholeheartedly salute the diligent effort of the author and co-authors whom I have known for well substantial period of time including their commitment and passion unending in nature and open ended in character to cater to the cause of academics in a big way, which they have catered to in an addon manner in the form of this novel useful book on Radiation Biology. I unhesitatingly and candidly state that 'this craftsmanship generated out of this treasure on Radiation Biology entitles them to a state of 'immortality' which otherwise is the most toughest and difficult of the attainments in human life.

Dr. Vedprakash Mishra
Pro-Chancellor,
Datta Meghe Institute of Higher Education and Research
(Deemed to be University)

Date: 12.07.2025

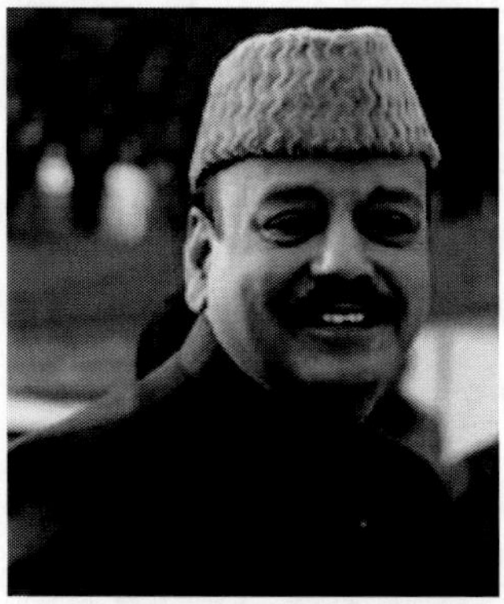

Dr. Vedprakash Mishra
Professor of Excellence, Professor of Eminence,
Professor Emeritus and Distinguished Professor,
Dr. B. C. Roy National Awardee,
D.Sc. (Honoris Causa) by Eight Universities
Secretary General, International Council of Global Network for Medical,
Health Professions & Bioethics Education,
President, Association of Medical Educators of India (AMEI)
International Co-Chair Global Network of Medical and Health Professions Education
Melbourne Australia
Head of the Medical and Health Professions Schools of the Indian program of
the ICB-UNESCO Chair
Chairperson, National Task Force on Medical Education constituted by NAMS,
Government of India
National Head of the Academic Programme of Indian Programme UNESCO Chair
in Bio-Ethics Haifa & Member of the International Committee for Bioethics
for Asia Pacific Region
Chief Advisor to Hon'ble Chancellor and Krishna Vishwa Vidyapeeth
(Deemed to be University), Karad
Chief Advisor, Datta Meghe Institute of Higher Education and Research
(Deemed to be University), Nagpur
Advisor, Human Ethics Committees Association (HECA), Bangalore
Dean, Academic and Accreditation Board, National Indian Medical Association,
New Delhi
Honorary Professor, Indian Medical Association
Honorary Director, Centre for Health Sciences Education Policy and Planning,
DMIHER (DU), Nagpur
Former Pro-Chancellor, Datta Meghe Institute of Higher Education & Research
(Deemed to be University), Nagpur
Former Vice Chancellor, Datta Meghe Institute of Medical Sciences
(Deemed University), Nagpur
Former Chairman, Postgraduate Medical Education Committee,
Medical Council of India, New Delhi
Former Chairman, Academic Council, Medical Council of India, New Delhi

Preface

Radiation biology stands at the crossroads of physics, chemistry, and life sciences. As medical imaging, radiotherapy, and nuclear technologies become increasingly central to healthcare and industry, understanding the biological consequences of radiation exposure has never been more critical.

Fundamentals of Radiation Biology has been designed to provide an in-depth yet accessible resource for students, clinicians, scientists, and radiation safety professionals seeking a comprehensive understanding of this field. This book brings together foundational principles, evolving concepts, and practical applications across thirteen carefully curated chapters.

Chapter 1 introduces the historical evolution of radiobiology and the fundamental concepts that underpin the discipline. Chapters 2 and 3 build on this base with detailed explorations of radiation physics, units, and measurement techniques critical for quantifying radiation exposure and interpreting its effects.

Chapters 4 and 5 delve into radiation detection technologies and the unique chemical interactions of ionizing radiation with biological molecules, emphasizing how these processes translate into cellular damage. The next chapters (6 to 9) explore the cellular and molecular consequences of radiation exposure, from DNA damage and chromosomal aberrations to cell survival mechanisms, normal tissue responses, and radiation toxicity.

Chapters 10 and 11 shift the focus to late radiation effects, syndromes associated with chronic exposure, and the complex factors influencing radiosensitivity and radioresistance, including genetic determinants and tumor microenvironment.

Chapter 12 highlights the role of hyperthermia as an adjunct to radiotherapy and explains time-dose fractionation concepts essential for optimizing therapeutic outcomes.

Finally, Chapter 13 outlines the principles of radiation safety, the regulatory framework governing radiation use, and the ethical responsibility of protecting workers, patients, and the public.

Across all chapters, the book balances theoretical rigor with clinical relevance, integrating recent advances, established guidelines from bodies such as the ICRP and NCRP, and evidence-based practices in radiation protection and therapy.

We have endeavoured to present this content in a clear, structured format, supplemented with equations, practical examples, and references to guide further learning. Whether you are a student embarking on your first study of radiation biology or a practitioner refining your expertise, we hope this book will serve as a reliable foundation and a catalyst for curiosity.

Fundamentals of Radiation Biology aspires to contribute to the safe and effective use of radiation, informed by sound science, thoughtful application, and a commitment to improving human health.

Acknowledgments

This book would not have been possible without the collective efforts of many individuals and institutions whose expertise, encouragement, and guidance shaped its development.

We express our sincere gratitude to our colleagues and mentors in the Departments of Radiophysics, Radiobiology, Radiation safety, Radiation Oncology, and Medical Physics across institutions in India and abroad for their insightful discussions and invaluable feedback. Your shared commitment to advancing knowledge in this field has been a constant source of motivation.

We extend special thanks to the International Commission on Radiological Protection (ICRP) and the National Council on Radiation Protection and Measurements (NCRP) for their foundational contributions to the principles and standards presented here.

All the reference articles and dedicated books which has been used to craft this book hold a special place and we thoroughly acknowledge them from bottom of our heart.

We also wish to acknowledge our students Mr Prashik Dube, Mr Aqeeb Sheikh, Ms. Sneha Shrungare and Ms Vedanti Chirde whose questions and curiosity challenged us to refine and clarify these concepts, and whose dedication to learning inspired the writing of this text.

Finally, we thank our families and loved ones for their unwavering support, patience, and understanding throughout the long hours dedicated to this work.

Chapter 1

Introduction

Gaurav Mishra[1,*], MD, PhD
Ashish Uke[1], MD
Anurag Luharia[2], PhD
and Ignatius Komakech[3], PhD

[1]Department of Radiodiagnosis, Datta Meghe Institute of Higher Education and Research, Wardha, India
[2]Department of Radio physics and Radio safety, Datta Meghe Institute of Higher Education and Research, Wardha, India
[3]Department of Oncology, Uganda Cancer Institute, Kampala, Uganda

Abstract

Radiobiology is a field of biology that studies the biological impacts of ionizing radiation on cells and tissues. It encompasses a wide range of fields, including physics, genetics, biochemistry, and medicine. Understanding the basic concepts of radiobiology is critical for radiation protection, radiation treatment, nuclear medicine, and determining the dangers associated with radiation exposure. The sources of ionizing radiation, interactions of radiation with live cells, the impact of radiation on DNA and cells, mechanisms for radiation-induced damage and repair, and biological reactions to radiation are all covered in this thorough overview, which serves as an introduction to radiobiology. It entails examining how radiation affects individual cells, tissues, organs, and entire organisms. The goal of radiobiologists is to comprehend the mechanisms of radiation-induced cellular damage, as well as the long-term effects on human health. Radiation protection, radiation therapy, nuclear medicine, environmental radiation assessment, and radiation-related research are all included in the field of radiobiology. The effects of ionizing radiation, which include X-rays, gamma rays, alpha particles, beta particles, and neutrons, are studied by radiobiologists. These radiation types have enough energy to free securely bonded electrons from atoms, which can cause biological harm by producing charged particles (ions). Ionizing radiation can come from both natural (like cosmic rays and radioactive isotopes) and man-made (like industrial machinery, nuclear reactors, and medical X-rays) sources.

Keywords: deoxyribose nuclide acid, radiobiology, radiosensitivity, radiophysics, X-ray

---

* Corresponding Author's Email: drgvmishra@gmail.com

In: Fundamentals of Radiation Biology
Editors: Anurag Luharia, Ashish Uke, Gaurav Mishra et al.
ISBN: 979-8-89530-806-6

1.1. Introduction and Historical Overview of Radiobiology

Radiobiology has a rich history that dates to the discovery of X-rays by Wilhelm Conrad Roentgen in 1895. Since then, many developments and discoveries have changed how we currently understand radiation biology. The historical overview of radiobiology provides an overview of major advancements and contributions. Wilhelm Conrad Roentgen unintentionally discovered X-rays in 1895 while dealing with cathode rays. He saw that a fluorescent screen continued to glow even when protected from direct cathode rays, which led him to discover new kinds of penetrating radiation. Roentgen's discovery laid the foundation for the field of radiobiology [1]. The discovery and isolation of radioactive materials like polonium and radium by Marie and Pierre Curie (1896) contributed to our understanding of radiation. Marie Curie won two Nobel Prizes for her groundbreaking study on radioactivity, which also established the way for later radiobiology research. Early Research on Radiation Impacts in the early 20th century, researchers started looking into the impact of radiation on living organisms. Photographic plates were damaged by radiation, as noted by the French physicist Antoine Becquerel, and long-term exposure to X-rays resulted in injuries, as noted by the British radiologist John Hall-Edwards. Wilhelm Roentgen made important studies about the biological impacts of X-rays in the early 20th century. He saw tissue damage and skin burns in people who had endured protracted exposure to a high dose of X-rays. Roentgen's findings highlighted the necessity of radiation safety precautions [2].

Ernest Rutherford's experiments with alpha particles in the 20th century provided insights into the highly ionizing nature of these particles. He provided evidence that alpha particles might seriously harm tissues and organs. Bergonié and Tribondeau's Law, which was established in 1906 by radiobiologists G. Bergonié and L. Tribondeau, said that cells are more at risk to radiation if they are highly proliferative, undifferentiated, and have a lengthy mitosis cycle. The study of tissue and cellular radiosensitivity was made possible by this law [3]. The genetic consequences of radiation were proven by Hermann Muller's fruit fly research during the 1920s and 1930s. His research established a connection between radiation and DNA damage by demonstrating that X-rays can cause mutations and inherited alterations. Early in the 20th century, radiation therapy as a clinical practice started to take shape for the treatment of cancer. Early pioneers, including Emil Grubbe and Marie Curie, investigated radiation's therapeutic potential in the treatment of tumours.

During World War II, the nuclear bombings of Hiroshima and Nagasaki tragically demonstrated the adverse impact of radiation on human health. These occurrences led to extensive investigation into the long-term impacts of radiation exposure as well as assisted in the creation of radiation safety recommendations [4].

Mid-20th-century technological developments sparked the creation of more advanced radiobiology research methodologies. This included improvements in radiation dosimetry, cell culture research, and the use of animal models. Radiation research and molecular biology.

Radiation research was transformed in the late 20th century by the development of molecular biology [5]. To better understand how cells react react to radiation, researchers started looking into the molecular mechanisms of radiation-induced DNA damage and even repair. In the 20th-century radiation safety and radioprotection were made in creating radiation safety rules and protection measures and at the same time, radiobiology made advances. To establish standards and recommendations for radiation protection, international organizations like the International Commission on Radiological Protection (ICRP) were created [6].

1.2. Radiophysics

Physics plays a crucial role in radiobiology, providing the fundamental principles and tools necessary to understand the interactions of ionizing radiation with living organisms. Physics is used in radiobiology to clarify radiation properties, dose calculations, interactions of radiation with matter, and the execution of radiation for therapeutic purposes. The main physics concepts in radiobiology are examined in this section, along with topics like radiation properties, dosimetry, radiation therapy, and radiation safety. Physics aids in describing and characterizing the properties of ionizing radiation. Ionizing radiation has enough energy to expel an atom's electrons, resulting in the formation of ion pairs. Based on their energy and mass, various radiation types, including X-rays, gamma rays, alpha particles, beta particles, and neutrons, have different penetrating powers [7]. Ionizing radiation deposits energy in matter, resulting in the formation of ion pairs and subsequent biological effects. Relative Biological Effectiveness (RBE), linear energy transfer (LET), and the spread of energy deposition along a radiation path are all terms used to describe the type and specific properties of ionizing radiation.

Dosimetry, which determines the amount of energy deposited by radiation in a particular material or tissue, is the measurement as well as the calculation of the absorbed dose. The following physics concepts and methods are available for precise radiation dosimetry:

1. *Radiation Units:* To measure the absorbed dose as well as the biological effect of radiation, physics established radiation measurement units like grey (Gy) and the sievert (Sv).
2. *Dosimeters:* Dosimeters, or instruments used to measure radiation dose, include thermoluminescent dosimeters (TLDs), ionization chambers, film badges, and electronic dosimeters. Physics contributes to their development and calibration.
3. *Monte Carlo Simulations*: Based on mathematical models as well as statistical techniques, Monte Carlo simulations enable physicists to simulate the behaviour of radiation within various materials and precisely estimate radiation doses [8].
4. *Radiation Therapy*: Radiation therapy, which is also referred to as radiotherapy, is used to treat cancerous tumours by using ionizing radiation. Radiation therapy relies heavily on physics [9].
5. *Treatment Planning*: For each patient, the best radiation dose, beam energy, beam shape, and therapeutic methods are determined by physicists in collaboration with radiation oncologists and dosimetrists.
6. *Delivery of Treatment*: Physics is used to ensure that radiation is delivered precisely during treatment sessions, accurately targeting the tumour while minimizing radiation to nearby healthy tissues.
7. *Quality Assurance*: To ensure precise and secure treatment delivery, physicists oversee the quality assurance procedure for radiation therapy, which includes machine calibration, dose examination, and observation of treatment parameters [10].

1.3. Radiation Protection

Radiation protection is aimed at reducing radiation exposure and assuring people's safety in public and work environments. By providing a framework for designing shielding materials as well as structures to attenuate and absorb ionizing radiation, physics helps to protect people and the environment from radiation exposure [11].

1. *Radiation Monitoring*: Physics is used in the design and calibration of radiation monitoring instruments, for example, Geiger-Muller counters or scintillation detectors, that are used to measure and keep track of radiation levels in both occupational and environmental settings.
2. *Dose Limits and Regulations*: To ensure that radiation doses stay within acceptable ranges, physics plays a role in the development of radiation protection rules and regulations, such as occupational exposure standards and dose restrictions.
3. *Radiation Biology Research*: Radiobiological research uses physics methods and equipment to examine the biological impacts of radiation. Physics gives researchers the tools they need to precisely irradiate cell cultures, administer radiation doses, and examine the cellular reactions and mechanisms that radiation causes [12].
4. *Imaging Techniques*: Physics plays a role in the development of imaging techniques like X-ray imaging, computed tomography (CT), magnetic resonance imaging (MRI), and positron emission tomography (PET) that are used in radiobiology research to visualize biological structures and radiation-induced changes.

1.4. General Radiation Chemistry

Radiation chemistry is a fascinating branch of science that explores the chemical changes and reactions that occur when materials are exposed to various forms of radiation. Its main goal is to understand how radiation affects matter at both the molecular and atomic levels, resulting in the emergence of new chemical species as well as the modification of existing compounds [13]. Ionizing radiation has the energy for loosening tightly bound electrons from atoms and molecules, producing the highly reactive species known as free radicals in the process. These free radicals are essential to radiation-induced chemistry because they set off a chain reaction that can have a significant impact on the material being exposed to radiation.

Applications for radiation chemistry research can be found in a variety of fields. As an example, radiation is used in industrial processes to start or alter chemical reactions, like polymerization or even the synthesis of specialized materials. Coatings, adhesives, and composites are all made using radiation curing, which causes polymer chains to cross-link because of radiation exposure [14]. Radiation chemistry is essential in medicine for comprehending how radiation affects biological systems. Focused radiation is used in radiation therapy to treat cancer; Radiation therapy works by selectively destroying cancerous cells while causing the least amount of harm to healthy tissue. For bettering treatment effectiveness and reducing side effects, it is crucial to understand the underlying chemical processes. Studies of the environment use radiation chemistry as well. It aids in the analysis of radiation effects on pollutants like pesticides or contaminants within water, enabling the development of more potent remediation techniques. It also assists in determining the long-term behaviour and stability of materials used in the management of radioactive waste [15].

1.5. Cellular and Molecular Radiobiology

Since the discovery that exposure to ionizing radiation had biological effects almost 90 years ago, the field of cellular radiobiology has grown considerably. Since then, a wealth of knowledge has been gathered from research involving radiation-exposed animals and plants, as well as studies of the effects on cellular, physical, and chemical levels, particularly over the past 50 years. Both our understanding of the physical and chemical processes that contribute to the induction of the radiation effects and our knowing of the responses seen in entire organisms have benefited greatly from molecular and cellular radiobiology [16]. The successful operation of a cell as well as the faithful transmission to its offspring of the genetic material contained therein, depend on each deoxyribonucleic acid (DNA) molecule maintaining its structural integrity. The transcription or replication of the cellular genome can be hampered by modifications to the bases or sugars that make changes to the double helix of the DNA, changes to the nucleotide sequence.

The primary source of radiobiological effects (cell death, loss of reproductive ability, mutation) is damage to DNA molecules. Therefore, mechanisms for repairing broken DNA molecules are crucial. Repair procedures may result in complete restoration or improper repair with potentially serious practical repercussions (such as carcinogenesis). It is possible to predict the effects of irradiation by looking at the lesions in chromosomes, also known as chromosomal aberrations, which are a good indicator for the lesions within a population of cells [17].

Genes are supported by chromosomes. An intriguing illustration of the morphological phenomena brought on by irradiation is the effect of radiation on chromosomes. 22 pairs of autosomal chromosomes and 1 pair of sex chromosome (XX or XY) make up a human cell, except for germinal cells. Each pair has one chromosome that is paternal origin and the other that is maternal. There are at least 50, 000 genes per human cell, and they are distributed along the chromosomes. The chromosomes' diameter during interphase is 50 nm. At the start of mitosis, they produce long filaments that roll over on them, thickening considerably. At the beginning of metaphase, the chromosomes in the nucleus are visible under an optical microscope after fixation and the appropriate staining. Under a microscope, abnormalities of number or structure (clastogenic effects) are discernible among the chromosomal alterations brought on by ionizing radiation. Additionally, there are modifications that cannot be seen under the microscope, but which can still have detrimental functional effects (gene mutations) [18].

1.6. Impact of Radiation in Biological System

The irreversible loss of a cell's ability to reproduce (reproductive death that occurs at the next or subsequent mitosis) is referred to as cell death. All cellular processes come to an end after being exposed to several hundred grey of radiation, which is known as immediate cell death or death in interphase. A portion of the cells lose their ability to divide or proliferate when lower doses of a few grays are administered to dividing or still able to divide cells (like bone marrow, skin, or intestinal crypts cell lines) [19].

Consequently, a non-viable damaged cell that morphologically appears intact in tissue may still be able to synthesis proteins or DNA and may even be able to undergo one or a few mitoses; however, this cell is killed in the sense defined above if it has lost the ability to divide indefinitely and if its descendants are destined to perish. A clonogenic cell, on the other hand, is a surviving or viable cell because it has retained its ability to proliferate and can therefore give rise to a colony or clone. Only a small portion of the cells *in vivo*, whether in tumors or normal tissues, are clonogenic, and their number decreases after radiation [20]. This definition is pertinent to radiotherapy as a tumour is locally controlled if all its cells, even those that are still present, have lost their capacity for unrestricted proliferation and, consequently, for local invasion or distant metastasis. Like this, loss of cellular viability accounts for most radiation's acute and late effects on normal tissues. This definition of cell death is appropriate for radiation protection when interpreting the immediate effects of radiation. When radiation damages a tissue, its ability to regenerate depends on the quantity of stem cells that have endured and the health of their ability for proliferating; it is these surviving cells that, by proliferating quickly, restore the damaged tissue. Differentiated cells, such as nerve, muscle, and secretory cells, that can carry out a specialized function but that do not normally divide, are obviously not included in that idea of reproductive death. These cells are naturally very resistant to radiation, but in the tissue to which they belong, harm to interstitial or vascular cells, which are crucial to their survival and function, can kill them indirectly [21].

1.6.1. Method of Measuring the Proportion of Surviving Cells

The field of quantitative cellular radiobiology was introduced by the work of Puck and Marcus, who also obtained the first survival curves for mammalian cells. The curves were created through *in vitro* cloning using methods that are comparable to, but more delicate than, those utilized in microbiology to count the number of yeast or bacterial cells. These methods are now widely utilized after the initial practical issues were gradually resolved. The procedure is reasonably quick, repeatable, and inexpensive [22]. It is challenging to determine how closely the behaviour of cells that are cultured in vino corresponds to how they behave *in vivo*, though.

A. *Cell Survival Curves:* As the dose (D) rises, the percentage of surviving cells (S) decreases. The survival curve, which graphically depicts this relationship, is created by drawing a smooth curve by means of the experimental points while accounting for each point's level of uncertainty. Typically, it is displayed as a logarithmic coordinate plot (log S as a function of D). This kind of plot highlights the extremely low values of S at high doses, but it might be challenging to understand survival after low doses [23]. It is simple to represent curves by mathematical functions when comparing them. These are based on speculative, commonly referred to as models, mechanisms of cell lethality.

B. *Intrinsic Cellular Radiosensitivity:* The cellular species has a significant impact on survival curves. Several physical or chemical factors, the effects of which will be explored later, can also alter them. By contrasting survival curves acquired with the same radiation according to optimal oxygenation, nutrient, and temperature conditions, one can understand differences in radiosensitivity related to biological characteristics. Viruses are biological structures that are extremely radioresistant. The mass for the virus has a nearly inverse relationship with the mean lethal dose. Target theory has its roots in this straightforward relation. In contrast, eukaryotic cells are extremely radiosensitive, while bacteria exhibit a range of radiosensitivity. We have observed that the amount of nucleic acid in a biological structure correlates with an increase in radiosensitivity. Ploidy affects the survival curve's shape, with yeast (Saccharomyces cerevisiae), Learjet has demonstrated that survival curves for haploid cells are exponential but have a shoulder to diploid or hyper diploid cells [24]. This can be understood by assuming that the total number of the targets that must be harmed to kill a cell rises with the the number of chromosome copies. Bacterial mutants reveal the impact of reconstruction on survival curves. Mutants lacking a repair system for a particular cellular species, like E. coli, are more sensitive compared with the wild type, and the survival curve lacks a shoulder. For several hereditary diseases connected to deficiencies in the cellular repair system, an analogous phenomenon is observed in humans. The survival curve's shape is influenced by the *in vitro* culture conditions, particularly the medium's composition.

1.7. Effects on Normal Tissue

The cells that make up normal tissues are not separate from one another; instead, they work together to form a complex structure. Birth and death maintain a delicate balance under typical circumstances. This is made possible by regulatory mechanisms that keep the tissue organization and cell count constant. When tissue is damaged, it is important to consider both the actual cell death and the reaction the death of the cells caused in the tissue [25]. Understanding the structure and dynamics of the tissue is necessary for this. These two factors can account for significant variations in timing and intensity of reactions between two tissues made up of radiosensitive cells.

1.7.1. Acute and Delayed Effects in Radiation

The two main categories of radiation exposure effects in radiobiology are acute and delayed effects. These words describe the biological reactions to radiation in terms of their timing and intensity.

Acute effects are the immediate biological reactions that happen soon after receiving a significant dose of radiation. Usually, these results show up days, weeks, or hours after exposure. The radiation dose as well as the sensitivity for the exposed organs and tissues determine how severe the acute effects will be. Radiation sickness, nausea, vomiting, burns to the skin, and harm to the gastrointestinal tract and bone marrow are a few examples of acute effects [26]. With high-dose radiation exposures, like those received during a nuclear accident or as a high-dose radiation therapy session, acute effects are more likely to manifest.

Long-lasting side effects that appear months, years, or weeks after radiation exposure are known as delayed effects. Most of the time, lower radiation doses, like those received during occupational exposure or low-dose radiation therapy, are linked to these effects. The accumulative effect of genetic mutations and long-term harm to cells and tissues are two factors that frequently contribute to delayed effects. Increased chances for cancer (such as leukemia, thyroid cancer, or solid tumours), radiation-induced fibrosis, dysfunction of the organs, and secondary malignancies are a few examples of delayed effects. These consequences can take years or even decades to manifest, depending on the radiation dose, radiation type, and individual susceptibility. It is crucial to remember that there can occasionally be an overlap between the acute and delayed effects, making the distinction between them difficult to make. Some immediate effects could linger or change over time into delayed effects [27]. In addition, factors like the dose rate, duration of exposure, radiation type (such as gamma rays, X-rays, and alpha particles), as well as personal characteristics like age, general health, and genetic predisposition, can affect the severity and occurring of both acute and delayed effects.

1.8. Radiosensitivity and Radioresistivity

The extent of tumour regression, the speed of the response, and the persistence of the response are all indicators of radiosensitivity, which is the tumor's response to radiation. A lot of variables affect radiosensitivity. The capacity for repairing damage, hypoxia, cell cycle position, and growth fraction are a few of these variables. Additionally, it has been shown that the ability to remove tumours is influenced by the size of the initial tumour. It is crucial to realize that radiosensitivity and radio curability do not mean the same thing. High-dose local radiation therapy may cure relatively radioresistant tumours, but it can only control radiosensitive tumours that have spread widely. Cervical squamous cell carcinoma is a prime example of a relatively radioresistant tumour, but it is also one of the most treatable cancers in humans due to its susceptibility to high-dose radiation and the relatively radioresistant characteristics of the normal tissues it is hosted in (such as the cervix and vagina) [28]. The secret to success is being able to juxtapose radium or cesium to the malignancy at doses that are safe for the nearby healthy tissue.

1.9. Hyperthermia in Radiotherapy

To treat cancer with radiotherapy, a therapeutic strategy called hyperthermia involves increasing the temperature of certain target tissues. It is based upon the idea that heat can make radiation more effective at killing cancer cells. To enhance the effects of radiotherapy, hyperthermia can be used either locally or regionally to heat up tumour sites and surrounding areas. Despite the benefits of hyperthermia in radiotherapy, it is important to remember that only certain cancer cases are candidates for this treatment. The characteristics of the tumour, the patient's health, and the treatment objectives all play a role in treatment decisions. The appropriateness and possible advantages for hyperthermia as part of an individual treatment plan must be determined in consultation with a medical expert skilled in hyperthermia as well as radiation therapy.

1.10. Radiation Safety

To safeguard researchers, employees, patients, and the environment from the potential risks associated with ionizing radiation, radiation safety is crucial in the field of radiobiology. The study of radiation effects on biological systems is a part of radiobiology, and responsible research and experimentation require the use of safe procedures. Evaluation of potential risks related to radiation exposure is a component of the radiation risk assessment. This includes determining the possibility and severity of health effects depending on the kind of radiation used, the dose received, the length of exposure, and the radiation use. Risk assessment influences decisions about radiation protection and aids in the development of protective measures. The abbreviation ALARA means "As Low as Reasonably Achievable." This principle emphasizes the significance of minimizing radiation exposures and doses while considering a variety of elements, including the type of work, the technology available, and financial considerations. To achieve the goals of radiobiology experiments or medical procedures, it directs radiation safety practices to reduce radiation risks. Programmed education and training are essential for advancing radiation safety. These programmes equip people who work with radiation sources with the knowledge and abilities they need to comprehend the possible risks, safe handling techniques, and radiation safety protocols. Professionals are kept up to date on best practises and developments in radiation safety thanks to ongoing training [29, 30].

Conclusion

Radiobiology is a multidisciplinary field that integrates physics, chemistry, cellular and molecular biology to understand the complex effects of ionizing radiation on living organisms. From the historical discovery of X-rays and radioactivity to the development of modern radiation therapy, the field has evolved through pioneering research and technological advances. The fundamental concepts of radiation physics, dosimetry, and radiation chemistry underpin our knowledge of how radiation interacts with matter and induces biological effects, such as DNA damage, mutations, and cell death. Understanding radiosensitivity, repair mechanisms, and survival curves has become essential for both therapeutic applications and radiation protection. The study of acute and delayed radiation effects, as well as strategies like hyperthermia to enhance treatment outcomes, further emphasizes the need for precise risk assessment and safety protocols. Overall, radiobiology continues to play a vital role in improving cancer treatment, safeguarding human health, and advancing scientific understanding of radiation's impact on biological systems.

References

[1] Mould RF. Röntgen and the discovery of X-rays. *The British journal of radiology*. 1995 Nov;68(815):1145-76.

[2] Davis TJ, Gao D, Gureyev TE, Stevenson AW, Wilkins SW. Phase-contrast imaging of weakly absorbing materials using hard X-rays. *Nature*. 1995 Feb 16;373(6515):595-8.

[3] Haas RL, Floot BG, Scholten AN, van der Graaf WT, van Houdt W, Schrage Y, van de Ven M, Bovée JV, van Coevorden F, Vens C. Cellular radiosensitivity of soft tissue sarcoma. *Radiation Research*. 2021 Jul 1;196(1):23-30.

[4] Domenech H. *Radiation safety. Managment and Programs*. Suiza: Springer. 2017.

[5] Olive PL. DNA damage and repair in individual cells: applications of the comet assay in radiobiology. *International journal of radiation biology*. 1999 Jan 1;75(4):395-405.

[6] Sievert RM. The International Commission on Radiological Protection (ICRP). International Associations. Brussels, Belgium: Union of International Associations, Palais d'Egmont. 1957:3-7.

[7] Pötter R, Haie-Meder C, Van Limbergen E, Barillot I, De Brabandere M, Dimopoulos J, Dumas I, Erickson B, Lang S, Nulens A, Petrow P. Recommendations from gynaecological (GYN) GEC ESTRO working group (II): concepts and terms in 3D image-based treatment planning in cervix cancer brachytherapy—3D dose volume parameters and aspects of 3D image-based anatomy, radiation physics, radiobiology. *Radiotherapy and oncology*. 2006 Jan 1;78(1):67-77.

[8] Attix FH. *Introduction to radiological physics and radiation dosimetry*. John Wiley & Sons; 2008 Sep 26.

[9] Khan FM, Gibbons JP. *Khan's the physics of radiation therapy*. Lippincott Williams & Wilkins; 2014.

[10] Svensson GK. Quality assurance in radiation therapy: physics efforts. *International Journal of Radiation Oncology* Biology* Physics*. 1984 Jun 1;10:23-9.

[11] Martin A, Harbison S, Beach K, Cole P. *An introduction to radiation protection*. Crc Press; 2018 Oct 25.

[12] Kirsch DG, Diehn M, Kesarwala AH, Maity A, Morgan MA, Schwarz JK, Bristow R, Demaria S, Eke I, Griffin RJ, Haas-Kogan D. The future of radiobiology. *JNCI: Journal of the National Cancer Institute*. 2018 Apr 1;110(4):329-40.

[13] Charlesby A. *Atomic radiation and polymers: international series of monographs on radiation effects in materials*. Elsevier; 2016 Jun 6.

[14] Mettler Jr FA, Thomadsen BR, Bhargavan M, Gilley DB, Gray JE, Lipoti JA, McCrohan J, Yoshizumi TT, Mahesh M. Medical radiation exposure in the US in 2006: preliminary results. *Health physics*. 2008 Nov 1;95(5):502-7.

[15] Day DH, Hughes AE, Leake JW, Marples JA, Marsh GP, Rae J, Wade BO. The management of radioactive wastes. *Reports on Progress in Physics*. 1985;48(1):101.

[16] Alper T. *Cellular radiobiology*. Cambridge University Press; 1979 Aug 16.

[17] Solomon E, Borrow J, Goddard AD. Chromosome aberrations and cancer. *Science*. 1991 Nov 22;254(5035):1153-60.

[18] Alper T. *Cellular radiobiology*. Cambridge University Press; 1979 Aug 16.

[19] Fuks Z, Persaud RS, Alfieri A, McLoughlin M, Ehleiter D, Schwartz JL, Seddon AP, Cordon-Cardo C, Haimovitz-Friedman A. Basic fibroblast growth factor protects endothelial cells against radiation-induced programmed cell death *in vitro* and *in vivo*. *Cancer Research*. 1994 May 15;54(10):2582-90.

[20] Webb S, Nahum AE. A model for calculating tumour control probability in radiotherapy including the effects of inhomogeneous distributions of dose and clonogenic cell density. *Physics in medicine & biology*. 1993 Jun 1;38(6):653.

[21] Daly MJ. Death by protein damage in irradiated cells. *DNA repair*. 2012 Jan 2;11(1):12-21.

[22] Withers HR, Elkind MM. Microcolony survival assay for cells of mouse intestinal mucosa exposed to radiation. *International Journal of Radiation Biology and Related Studies in Physics, Chemistry and Medicine*. 1970 Jan 1;17(3):261-7.

[23] Deacon J, Peckham MJ, Steel GG. The radioresponsiveness of human tumours and the initial slope ofthe cell survival curve. *Radiotherapy and Oncology*. 1984 Dec 1;2(4):317-23.

[24] Fertil B, Malaise EP. Inherent cellular radiosensitivity as a basic concept for human tumor radiotherapy. *International Journal of Radiation Oncology* Biology* Physics*. 1981 May 1;7(5):621-9.

[25] Stone HB, Coleman CN, Anscher MS, McBride WH. Effects of radiation on normal tissue: consequences and mechanisms. *The lancet oncology*. 2003 Sep 1;4(9):529-36.

[26] Trotti A, Byhardt R, Stetz J, Gwede C, Corn B, Fu K, Gunderson L, McCormick B, Morris M, Rich T, Shipley W. Common toxicity criteria: version 2.0. an improved reference for grading the acute effects of cancer treatment: impact on radiotherapy. *International Journal of Radiation Oncology* Biology* Physics*. 2000 Apr 1;47(1):13-47.

[27] Morgan WF. Non-targeted and delayed effects of exposure to ionizing radiation: II. Radiation-induced genomic instability and bystander effects *in vivo*, clastogenic factors and transgenerational effects. *Radiation research.* 2003 May 1;159(5):581-96.

[28] Antipas V, Dale RG, Coles IP. A theoretical investigation into the role of tumour radiosensitivity, clonogen repopulation, tumour shrinkage and radionuclide RBE in permanent brachytherapy implants of 125I and 103Pd. *Physics in Medicine & Biology*. 2001 Sep 12;46(10):2557.

[29] Preston RJ. Radiation biology: concepts for radiation protection. *Health physics*. 2005 Jun 1;88(6):545-56.

Chapter 2

Radiation Physics

Anurag Luharia[1,*], PhD
Sanjay Dhoble[2], PhD
Anchineyan Pichandi[3], PhD
and Shweta Dahake[1], MSc
[1]Department of Radio physics and Radio safety, Datta Meghe Institute of Higher Education and Research, Wardha, India
[2]Department of Physics, Nagpur University, Nagpur, India
[3]Department of Central Physics, Health Care Global Enterprise Ltd, Banglore, India

Abstract

This chapter delves into the fundamental building blocks of matter, exploring the structure and properties of atoms, including their composition, atomic forces, and electron shells. The discussion extends to the nucleus, highlighting its stability, radiation emission, and the various types of radiation, such as alpha, beta, neutrons, and electromagnetic waves. The application of X-rays in radiology and radiotherapy is also examined, including their characteristics, interaction types, and image quality. Furthermore, the concept of radioactivity is introduced, covering its definition, applications, and discussion on naturally occurring and artificially produced isotopes. The half-life of radioactive materials is explained, along with the calculation of physical and biological half-lives, and the effective half-life of a radionuclide inside the human body. This abstract provides a concise summary of the key concepts and principles governing the behaviour of atoms, radiation, and radioactivity.

Keywords: atomic structure, radiation physics, radioactivity, radiotherapy

2.1. Introduction

Atoms are the fundamental building blocks of matter. Each atom is made up of a nucleus and one or more electrons that circle the nucleus like satellites orbit the globe. There are protons

---

* Corresponding Author's Email: anuragluharia@gmail.com

In: Fundamentals of Radiation Biology
Editors: Anurag Luharia, Ashish Uke, Gaurav Mishra et al.
ISBN: 979-8-89530-806-6

in the nucleus, which are positively charged particles. An electron has a negative charge, which is technically the 'opposite', hence the combined charges of both particles is zero. A neutral atom is one in which the number of electrons in orbit is equal to the number of protons in the nucleus. With the exception of hydrogen, all atoms have at least one neutral neutron in their nucleus. For a given element all nuclei in given atoms are similar; the number of protons and neutrons in the nucleus is what distinguishes one element from another, such as iron, copper, oxygen, and so on.

2.2. The Atom

2.2.1. Atomic Structure

After reviewing the fundamentals of atoms and elements, we can move on to discussing the subatomic particles that comprise them. Subatomic particles are defined as those that are even smaller than an atom [1]. There is a range of subatomic particles and quarks according to the standard model, out of them the primary building blocks are protons, neutrons, and electrons. The combination of these three form atoms and different combinations are responsible for different atoms. The nucleus is the name given to the core of an atom.

2.2.2. Atomic Forces

The force of attraction between particles with opposite charges and the force of repulsion between particles with comparable charges is a fundamental principle that can be used to explain a wide variety of electrical events [2]. Two electrons, for instance, will feel a force that separates them if they are close together. There exists a force that attracts an electron to a proton, and a force that repels a proton from an electron. As a general rule, charges of the same polarity repel one another and those of opposite polarity attract one another. As the square of the distance between the charged particles decreases, so does the strength of the force. In a nutshell, bringing the particles closer together substantially amplifies the force. Electrons don't get sucked into the nucleus because the attraction of the nucleus is balanced by the dynamic forces originating from the orbital motion of the electrons [3]. One can visualize this concept in analogy with the force of gravity that maintains a satellite in orbit around Earth.

2.2.3. Atomic Nuclei

Atoms have nuclei composed of protons and neutrons. Every single proton and neutron is the same as every other one. Protons are typically denoted with a "+" sign because of their positive electrical charge [4]. Since protons are positively charged particles and should resist each other, it is thought that the neutrons' lack of electrical charge helps keep the protons together. The unique properties of each atom are determined by the total number of protons and neutrons in its nucleus.

Nuclei appear to be extremely distinct from atoms at first glance. While atoms are mostly empty space, the interior of a nucleus is highly dense, making nuclei over 100,000 times smaller and far more complicated. Despite these distinctions, atoms and nuclei share many similarities.

The atom's nucleus is so tiny that it can barely be seen. Its radius is roughly 1/100,000 that of a whole atom. The nucleus of an atom would be about the size of a pea if the whole thing were a football field. Protons and neutrons are relatively large for their size compared to electrons [5]. Therefore, an atom's nucleus contains nearly all of its mass. The nucleus is incredibly dense due to its large mass and comparatively small size.

- **Electrons**

The electrons in orbits are generally depicted as a cloud surrounding the nucleus. Subatomic particles with a negative charge, electrons are the antipode to positively charged protons [6]. In order to be electrically balanced, atoms prefer to have the same number of electrons as protons. Electrons are responsible for electrical properties of the element and many reactions involving ion exchange or bonding. They have a mass of 9.10×10^{-31} kilograms and due to their light weight are actively participating in reactions including radiation induced reactions in body tissues.

In the periodic table the number of electron shells are more and much further from the nucleus, in elements beyond hydrogen. There is a rule for maximum number of electrons that can be accommodate in several "shells", these shells are denoted by the letters K, L, M and N. The maximum number of electrons that the nth shell can contain is provided by the formula:

$$\therefore \text{Number of electrons in a shell} = 2n^2$$

This means that the maximum number of electrons that can fit into the innermost (K = 1) shell is a 2, the next shell (L = 2) is 8, the next shell (M = 3) a maximum of 18, and the fourth shell (N = 4) a maximum of 32. When applied to simple atoms without any extra shells, the equation can be used to count the number of electrons in any of the first four shells. Atoms are the smallest units of all matter, including solids, liquids, and gases. That's why scientists regard atoms to be matter's fundamental unit. Molecules are collections of atoms bound together through chemical bonds. Only a handful of gases, like helium, are made up of individual atoms. Learn how atoms, molecules, and compounds are all connected by exploring the interactive applet provided below.

2.2.4. Atomic Stability

As mentioned earlier, the protons inside the nucleus are all positively charged and are supposed to repel each other, but in practicality this does not happen. The binding energy is a factor which is stated to keep the atom intact. In some atoms the binding energy is sufficient to keep the nucleus in place. This type of atoms (and hence elements) are characterized by a stable nucleus. On the contrary some other atoms' nuclei are unstable because their binding energy is insufficient to keep the nucleus together [7]. Unstable atoms and their nuclei eventually fall apart due to this issue and the atoms or elements are termed to be radioactive atoms. They shed neutrons and protons in an effort to achieve atomic stability.

2.2.5. Definitions of Atomic Number and Atomic Mass Number

The atomic number is a number which describes the number of protons inside the nucleus of the atom, denoted by Z. In other words, the number of protons in an atom of a given element is assigned a value that is specific to that element [8]. Hydrogen atoms, for instance, are the only ones with one proton and an atomic number of 1. Whereas Carbon atom has 6 protons, Oxygen has 8 and the atomic number is 6 and 8 respectively. The number of protons in the nucleus decides or describes the atom and its behaviour. In other words, it is the fundamental measure which defines and atom. We can identify a hydrogen atom by its single proton. When there are two protons in an atom, it is always helium. We can identify a beryllium atom by its distinctive four-proton nucleus If Co-60 nucleus contains 27 protons and after decaying it now has 28 protons, then the element now becomes nickel.

Equally strong negative and positive charges are balanced out by one another. When an electron orbits a positively charged proton, the resulting net charge is zero. That is, there must be exactly one electron for every proton in a neutral atom. A single proton in a neutral atom can only be balanced by a single electron. Two protons indicate that there are also two electrons in a neutral atom. If there are ten protons in an atom, then there must also be ten electrons. That's the gist of it. Atoms with an equal number of electrons and protons are considered neutral.

The mass number of an atom is calculated as the total of protons and neutrons in the atomic nuclei. To put it another way, a normal carbon atom, which has 6 protons and 6 neutrons in its nucleus, has a mass number of 12. Atomic mass unit is the mass of an atom of an element with single nuclide [9]. The standard definition is 'one twelfth of total mass of carbon-12. Hydrogen has an atomic mass of 1.00797 amu, while carbon has an atomic mass of 12.011 amu.

2.2.6. Electron Shells

Electron shells or Energy levels are discrete regions around an atom's nucleus which is occupied by electrons. The electrons of an atom are very small negatively charged particles that orbit the atom's central nucleus, which is positively charged [10]. A person's energy level might be seen of as a series of stairwells. You can stand on either step, but not in the space in between. Electrons are the same way. The only place they can't be is in the void between energy levels.

The first four atomic energy levels are; Level I electrons, often known as K electrons, have the lowest possible energy. Higher-level electrons have greater energy, and this energy grows by a definite, quantifiable quantity as you move out from the nucleus. If electrons take in enough energy, they can "jump" from one energy level to the next. In contrast, electrons release energy in the form of light if they fall from a higher to a lower energy level. That's why there are fireworks in the background there. When the fireworks go off, the electrons in the air gain momentum and amplify their energy. They discharge the energy as light as they return to their initial states. Since the electrons in various atoms are arranged in different ways, the resulting light is of various hues.

2.2.7. Nuclear Stability and Radiation Emission

- The nucleus has an abundance of energy when it is at a different level. In order for the nucleus to return to its initial ground state, some of its excess energy must be released as a gamma photon. Similar to X rays, these gamma photons come from the nucleus of an atom, but their energy can be as high as a million electronvolts (MeV) [11].
- Because of a 'layer' structure comparable to that of the atom, the community of coexisting nucleons in any nucleus can have a wide range of energy states. The nucleons' binding energy can take on different values depending on the number of 'layers' around them.
- Particularly stable nuclei have been observed to have 2, 8, 20, 28, 50, 82, or 126 nucleons, drawing an intriguing parallel to the stability of the atoms of the noble gases, whose outermost electron layers are believed to be complete.
- The nucleons can be said to experience collective movements that lead to different nuclear energy levels, on top of their multilayer structure. In the event that the entire cluster begins to vibrate, for example, the vibrational energies can take on only a finite range of values as prescribed by quantum mechanics [12].
- Last but not least, keep in mind that these nuclei are not always spherical and can change shape or even begin to rotate. These rotations have energies that are 'quantified,' meaning they can only take on certain predetermined quantities.

2.2.8. Different Kinds of Radiation

Radiation can be broken down into four categories: alpha, beta, neutrons, and electromagnetic waves like gamma rays. They are distinct from one another in terms of size, power, and penetrativeness.

- The first type of particle is an alpha one. These are the heaviest form of radiation particles, each of which consists of two protons and two neutrons. Alpha particles are emitted by many naturally occurring radioactive elements on Earth, including uranium and thorium [13]. Most people have heard about radon, which is a common example. An alpha particle doesn't travel very far due to its extreme heaviness and high charge. Because of this, an alpha particle cannot penetrate paper. You can't even feel an outside alpha particle hitting your skin. However, vulnerable organs like the lungs can be damaged if alpha-emitting material is inhaled or ingested.
- The second type of radiation is the beta. An unbound electron is an electron that is not part of any atom. It's negatively charged and has a relatively low mass. Tritium, which is ubiquitous because it is created by cosmic radiation in the atmosphere, gives off beta rays. Fossil and other artifacts can be dated by carbon-14 dating, which

generates beta particles. Carbon dating basically just takes advantage of the fact that radioactive carbon-14 exists [14]. The amount of carbon-14 remaining in a fossil can be determined by measuring the beta particles, which in turn provides an estimate of the age of the fossil. When compared to alpha particles, beta ones have a slightly greater range. A tiny bit of shielding would be sufficient to stop them. They may enter your body, but they cannot completely permeate it. Beta particles can be used in medical imaging if they are released by an injected substance. When used in conjunction with radioactive material injected directly into a tumor, they can be highly effective in the treatment of cancer.

- Neutrons count as the third. This particle exists in the nucleus of an atom and is neutral in charge. Neutrons are emitted as a by-product when uranium atoms go into fission in a nuclear reactor. Neutrons travel far because they have no electric charge and hence no interaction with matter. Large volumes of water or other materials made of very light atoms are the only thing that can stop them.
- Electromagnetic radiation, which includes X-rays and gamma rays, is the final type of radiation. Because of their widespread application in medical settings, they are likely the most recognizable form of radiation to the general public. These rays are similar to sunlight, but much more powerful. Neither mass nor charge are present in this form of radiation. Energy levels can be extremely low, as in dental x-rays, or extremely high, as in medical equipment sterilization irradiators.
- Both gamma rays and x-rays have the ability to pass through human tissue [15]. This is why they are so helpful in the medical field; they can reveal the exact location of a fracture, the extent of tooth decay, or a tumor. To protect delicate internal organs and the persons who may be exposed to this radiation, shielding with solid materials like concrete and lead is utilized. When I have dental x-rays, for instance, the technician covers me with a lead apron before snapping the photo. This apron shields the rest of my body from the x-rays. The technician hides behind a wall, which is often made of lead, for safety.
- Background radiation is present in our environment, but it should not cause alarm. Radiation comes in many forms, and some of them are quite useful.

2.2.9. Non-Ionizing Radiation

Non-ionizing radiation sources are used and emitted by humans on a daily basis. This type of radiation lacks the necessary energy to ionize molecules and atoms [16]. Non-ionizing radiation is used in many common household appliances and technological advancements, such as microwave ovens, GPS systems, cell phones, TV broadcasts, FM and AM radio, baby monitors, cordless phones, garage door openers, and ham radios. The magnetic field of the earth is another source, as is being near power lines, electrical outlets, and other electrical devices. These are classified as ELF waves, which stands for "extremely low frequency."

2.3. Applications of X-Rays in Radiology and Radiotherapy

The rays that make up an x-ray beam are, at their core, the same as those that make up visible light, ultraviolet light, infrared light, and so on. Electromagnetic waves encompass any wavelike disturbances caused by moving electric charges. For every given material, a rise in frequency (v) will always be accompanied by a matching drop in wavelength (A), and a decrease in frequency will always be accompanied by an increase in wavelength (A). In other words, the relationship between frequency and wavelength is negative.

X-rays have extremely small wavelengths; for example, the wavelength range usable in conventional radiography is roughly to (1A = 10^{-8}, or 1 one-hundred millionth of a centimeter). X-rays have tremendous frequencies of between 3 x 10^{19} and 6 x 10^{18} hertz due to their incredibly short wavelengths [16]. Radio waves, with wavelengths measured in the thousands of meters, and gamma rays, with wavelengths measured in the tens of angstroms, are both examples of electromagnetic waves.

Each electromagnetic wave carries a very little quantity of energy that varies with its frequency, as we will try to describe in further depth below. A "photon" or "quantum" is a "fragment of energy" of this type. Human-made machines are responsible for producing the x radiation utilized in roentgenography and therapy [17]. These rays are produced if an electron stream slows down unexpectedly. Some radioactive elements' nuclei give off gamma rays, which are essentially equivalent to X rays in every other way.

2.3.1. X-Ray Characteristics

We will now go through some of the more relevant characteristics of x-rays.

1. They are extremely elusive electromagnetic waves that have a high penetrating power.
2. They don't conduct electricity; thus, magnetic or electrical fields have no effect on them.
3. Their wavelengths vary greatly, from roughly 0.04 A to more than 1000 A, indicating their heterogeneity. Their radiographic usability range is between 0.1 A to 0.5 A. Alternatively, we may say that their photon energies span a broad spectrum (polyenergetic).
4. As they move through stuff, they give off negligible amounts of heat.
5. They emerge from the cylinder in parallel lines that gradually spread outward.
6. In a vacuum, they can only move at the speed of light, which is 186,000 miles per second (3 x 10^{10} cm per second).
7. Because of their capacity to strip atoms of their orbital electrons, they can ionize gases indirectly.
8. They can be used for fluoroscopy because they induce particular crystals to glow, and they can also be used to intensify screens for radiography.
9. They aren't going to work with a lens.
10. By reacting with photographic film, they create a hidden image that may be revealed through chemical processing.

11. Mainly by ionization and excitation, they cause alterations in chemical and biological systems. Because of this, they can be used therapeutically.
12. They give off radiation that is dispersed and secondary.

- *X-Ray Image Quality*
  Definition: The ability of an x-ray beam to penetrate matter is one measure of its quality. The "penetrating power" of an x-ray beam is measured by its capacity to penetrate tissue. The quantification can be done by surveying its reaction on an x-ray film or deposition of enrgy upon entering the body [18].
- *Strength and Quality of X-Rays*
  Examining what x-ray energy actually is will help clarify how it relates to quality (or penetrating power). An individual x-ray can be thought of as a quantum of energy, or photons, represented by the formula.

$$\therefore E = h\nu$$

where,

E is the photon's energy measured in ergs,
h is a constant called Planck's constant, and
ν (Greek nu) is the x-ray's frequency measured in hertz.

According to this formula, the energy of a photon is in direct proportion to the frequency of the waves [19]. This really means that high-frequency x-rays are more powerful than low-frequency ones. However, a wave of high frequency must have a shorter wavelength, and a wave of considerably low frequency has to have a longer wavelength in order to travel at the same speed as light. Since the energy of an x-ray beam determines its penetrating power, we can restate the claims made in the previous paragraph as in Figure 2.1.

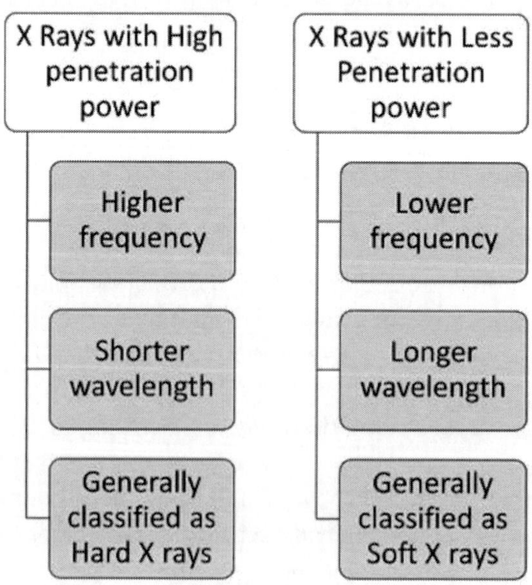

Figure 2.1. The relation of penetration Power of X ray with respect to its characteristics.

- *X-Ray Interaction Types*
  The energy entering a system is measured by the energy of the photons entering the system and the number of photons with the same energy [20]. Each photon in an x-ray or gamma ray beam has one of three probable ways of travel or interaction, a. It can simply pass through the medium b. It may interact with the medium to completely get absorbed into it or c. It may interact and get deflected by the particles of the medium.

In two distinct ways, photons deposit their energy, are by complete absorption or partially absorption and then scattering, depending on the nature of the encounter.

2.3.1.1. Coherent Scattering

Coherent scattering which is also known as Rayleigh or *elastic scattering* is yet another form of photon interaction which occurs when the energy of the x-ray or gamma photon is small in relation to the ionization energy of the atom [21]. Such radiations sometimes trigger other electrons in the atom to vibrate at a close or similar frequency relative to the incident photon. Thus, the whole atom acts as a unit and recoils when bombarded by a low-energy photon.

Upon interacting with the attenuating medium, the photon loses its energy to the atom but liberate the electron from its bound state (i.e. the photon energy is well below the binding energy of the electron) so no energy transfer occurs. There is no energy deposition and thus no dose resulting from coherent scattering. The only change is a change of direction (scatter) of the photon, hence 'unmodified' scatter. Coherent scattering is not a major interaction process encountered in radiography at the energies normally used.

2.3.1.2. Photoelectric Interaction

Photoelectric effect is the phenomenon when a light photon interacts with an element and results in ejection of electron from the atom/ matter [22,23]. The setup for this involves use of appropriate material/element and right biasing.

In a short amount of time, after the ejection, the electron's energy is depleted, and it travels back to its position. In this process the energy of the photon is stored in the material near the point of interaction with the photoelectric material.

A photoelectric interaction is impossible if the binding energy of the electron to the atom is more than the energy of the incident photon. For the photon to overcome the binding energy and eject the electron from the atom, the photon must have enough energy to do so. During the interaction incident photon's energy is split into two parts. One share goes to free the electron from the atom, here some of the energy is sacrificed to its binding energy. The remainder is deposited as kinetic energy on the electron in the vicinity of the contact location.

Because of the emptiness left in the electron shell due to the interaction, usually the K or L shell, an electron will descend to fill it. In many cases, an x-ray photon can be observed when the filled electron loses energy. The binding energy of the participating falling electrons determines how much energy is emitted in the form of characteristic radiation. Sometimes x-ray photons are turned into regular light photons by this method [24].

2.3.1.3. Compton Interaction

When a photon is created via an interaction where just a fraction of the incident energy is absorbed, we call this a Compton interaction [25]. After the interaction, this photon travels away from the origin in the opposite direction of the original photon. Since the interaction results in a change in the path taken by the photon, it is considered a scattering process. As a result, the material interacting with the with the primary x-ray beam becomes equivalent to a secondary radiation source. That is a reason why the patient's body is the most important object producing scattered radiation during an X-ray procedure.

2.3.1.4. Coherent Scattering

One type of interaction that produces scattered radiation is a scattering-based interaction that does not deposit any energy in the material; this interaction can occur at low photon energies but is usually not significant in most diagnostic procedures and goes by a variety of names [26].

2.3.1.5. Pair Production

Photon-matter interactions happen at energies greater than 1.02 MeV. In a pair-production interaction, the photon interacts with the nucleus to convert its energy into matter by creating a pair of particles, an electron and a positively charged positron.

2.4. Introduction to Radioactivity

The concept of unstable nuclei was explained earlier. The decay of radioactive nuclei can result in emission of photons, electrons, protons, neutrons, or alphas (two protons and two neutrons bound together), release of energy. To define in a sentence, we say the ability to emit energy and subatomic particles spontaneously by a nucleus is known as radioactivity, and it is essentially a feature of individual atomic nuclei.

We can use radioactivity for a variety of applications, including application as heat sources, medical imaging, targeted cancer treatments, as a radiometric dating tool, and for reprocessing nuclear fuel. However, the effect of radioactivity varies depending on the type and energy of the particles produced during nuclear decay.

Several naturally occurring elements and artificially produced isotopes of the elements exhibit radioactive decay, in which an unstable nucleus spontaneously decomposes, or decays, into a more stable configuration by emitting certain particles or forms of electromagnetic energy [27, 28].

2.5. Discussion of Radioactivity

In radioactive processes, particles or electromagnetic radiation are emitted from the nucleus. The most common forms of radiation emitted are classified as alpha (a), beta (b), and gamma (g) radiation. Nuclear radiation occurs in other forms, including the emission of protons or neutrons or spontaneous fission of a massive nucleus.

The naturally occurring radioactive atoms are Uranium-238, uranium-235, and thorium-232 [29]. The half-lives are comparable to the age of the elements, and this is the reason why they have not decayed away since their formation in stars. Potassium-40, a commonly found isotope of potassium on Earth and is the primary source of ionizing radiation in the human body due to its presence in potassium of tissue. Carbon-14 has a half-life of 5,720 years, tritium, which has a half-life of 12.3 years, beryllium-7, which has a half-life of 53 days, and Beryllium-10, which has a half-life of 2,700,000 years are all examples of natural radioactive species produced in the upper atmosphere by cosmic ray bombardment [30].

We can also generate radioactivity by manmade processes. By irradiating carefully chosen target materials with reactor neutrons or by using the charged particle beams or gamma ray beams of accelerators, it is possible to create radionuclides that are not found in nature or as fission products.

Originally proposed by Ernest Rutherford in 1907, the concept of a radioactive material's half-life is typically described as the amount of time it takes for half of the atoms in the substance to decay or transform into a different substance [31].

The idea of half-life is frequently used in nuclear physics, and it describes the rate at which atoms decay through radioactivity, as well as the length of time an atom may survive radioactive decay. The half-life of a radionuclide is the time taken by the radionuclide to decay to half of its original value or quantity.

Half-life is calculated using formula:

$$T_{1/2} = \frac{\ln(2)}{\lambda}$$

Here,

$T_{1/2}$ - Half Life

λ – decay constant

2.6. The Concept of Biological Half Life

After entering the body of a patient, a radionuclide or radiopharmaceutical decays in two ways. It will decay by radionuclide's physical half-life, and its biological half-life. Biological Half-life is the period of time, taken by the radiopharmaceutical to reduce the amount of a drug in an organ or the body tissue to half its original value. Important thing to be considered for T_{bio} is that we study biological half-life of a radiopharmaceutical to understand and predict the decay in target organ [32]. The total reduction of a drug in the body is dictated by a time period called effective half-life. It is denoted by T_{eff}.

The effective half-life of a radionuclide inside a human body is the time taken by the radionuclide to decay to half of its original value, after being administered [33]. It is calculated by formula:

$$\frac{1}{T_{\text{eff}}} = \frac{1}{T_{\text{phys}}} + \frac{1}{T_{\text{bio}}}$$

where,

T_{eff} - effective half -life
T_{phy} – physical half -life
T_{bio} – biological half -life

Conclusion

This chapter provided a detailed exploration of radiation physics, starting from the fundamental structure of atoms and nuclei to the diverse types of radiation, including alpha, beta, neutron, and electromagnetic waves. It explained the principles governing atomic stability, radioactivity, and the processes by which unstable nuclei emit radiation to achieve stability. The characteristics, interactions, and applications of X-rays in radiology and radiotherapy were thoroughly discussed, highlighting their critical role in medical diagnosis and treatment. Concepts such as electron shells, atomic forces, radiation interactions (photoelectric effect, Compton scattering, pair production), and the calculation of half-lives were examined to build a comprehensive understanding of how radiation behaves and interacts with matter. This foundational knowledge is essential for safe and effective use of radiation in healthcare, research, and industry.

References

[1] Weinberg S. The discovery of subatomic particles revised edition. Cambridge University Press; 2003.
[2] Binnig G, Quate CF, Gerber C. Atomic force microscope. *Physical review letters*. 1986 Mar 3;56(9):930.
[3] Meyer ER. Atomic force microscopy. *Progress in surface science*. 1992 Sep 1;41(1):3-49.
[4] Ebran JP, Khan E, Nikšić T, Vretenar D. How atomic nuclei cluster. *Nature*. 2012 Jul 19;487(7407):341-4.
[5] Hofstadter R, Bumiller F, Yearian MR. Electromagnetic structure of the proton and neutron. *Reviews of Modern Physics*. 1958 Apr 1;30(2):482.
[6] Bolonkin A. Femtotechnology: Nuclear matter with fantastic properties. *Am. J. Eng. Applied Sci.* 2009;2(2):501-14.
[7] Bohr N, Wheeler JA. The mechanism of nuclear fission. *Physical Review*. 1939 Sep 1;56(5):426.
[8] Loveland WD, Morrissey DJ, Seaborg GT. *Modern nuclear chemistry*. John Wiley & Sons; 2017 Apr 10.
[9] Audi G, Wapstra AH. The 1993 atomic mass evaluation:(I) Atomic mass table. *Nuclear Physics A*. 1993 Dec 6;565(1):1-65.
[10] Bohr N. I. On the constitution of atoms and molecules. *The London, Edinburgh, and Dublin Philosophical Magazine and Journal of Science*. 1913 Jul 1;26(151):1-25.
[11] Dirac PA. The quantum theory of dispersion. *Proceedings of the Royal Society of London. Series A, Containing Papers of a Mathematical and Physical Character*. 1927 May 2;114(769):710-28.
[12] May TC, Woods MH. Alpha-particle-induced soft errors in dynamic memories. *IEEE transactions on Electron devices*. 1979 Jan;26(1):2-9.
[13] Christie M. Radiocarbon dating. *WikiJournal of Science*. 2018 Jan;1(1):1-7.
[14] Filburn T, Bullard S, Filburn T, Bullard S. How Do Nuclear Reactors Work?. Three Mile Island, Chernobyl and Fukushima: *Curse of the Nuclear Genie*. 2016:1-3.
[15] Failla G, Henshaw PS. The relative biological effectiveness of X-rays and gamma rays. *Radiology*. 1931 Jul;17(1):1-43.

[16] Maqbool M, editor. *An introduction to medical physics*. Springer; 2017 Nov 11.
[17] Belfield WT, Rolnick HC. Roentgenography and therapy with iodized oils. *Journal of the American Medical Association.* 1926 Jun 12;86(24):1831-3.
[18] Withers PJ, Bouman C, Carmignato S, Cnudde V, Grimaldi D, Hagen CK, Maire E, Manley M, Du Plessis A, Stock SR. X-ray computed tomography. *Nature Reviews Methods Primers*. 2021 Feb 25;1(1):18.
[19] Singh V. Einstein and the quantum. In *The legacy of Albert Einstein: A collection of essays in celebration of the year of physics* 2007 (pp. 165-191).
[20] Hubbell JH. Review of photon interaction cross section data in the medical and biological context. *Physics in Medicine & Biology*. 1999;44(1):R1.
[21] Roy SC, Kissel L, Pratt RH. Elastic scattering of photons. *Radiation Physics and Chemistry*. 1999 Aug 1;56(1-2):3-26.
[22] Pratt RH, Ron A, Tseng HK. Atomic photoelectric effect above 10 keV. *Reviews of Modern physics*. 1973 Apr 1;45(2):273.
[23] Balabanoff ME, Al Fulaiti H, Bhusal S, Harrold A, Moon AC. An exploration of chemistry students' conceptions of light and light-matter interactions in the context of the photoelectric effect. *International Journal of Science Education.* 2020 Apr 12;42(6):861-81.
[24] Chastain J, King Jr RC. *Handbook of X-ray photoelectron spectroscopy*. Perkin-Elmer Corporation. 1992;40:221.
[25] George IM, Fabian AC. X-ray reflection from cold matter in active galactic nuclei and X-ray binaries. *Monthly Notices of the Royal Astronomical Society*. 1991 Mar 15;249(2):352-67.
[26] Johns PC, Yaffe MJ. Coherent scatter in diagnostic radiology. *Medical Physics*. 1983 Jan;10(1):40-50.
[27] Pfützner M, Karny M, Grigorenko LV, Riisager K. Radioactive decays at limits of nuclear stability. *Reviews of modern physics*. 2012 Apr 30;84(2):567.
[28] Malainey ME, Malainey ME. Radioactive Isotopes and Their Decay. *A Consumer's Guide to Archaeological Science: Analytical Techniques*. 2011:27-34.
[29] Alasadi LA, Abojassim AA. Mapping of natural radioactivity in soils of Kufa districts, Iraq using GIS technique. *Environmental Earth Sciences*. 2022 May;81(10):279.
[30] Wiens RC. Radiometric Dating. A Christian perspective. *Science in Christian Perspective: The American Scientific Affiliation*. Available online at: http://www. asa3. org/ASA/resources/WIENS. html. 2002.
[31] Lawson RS. *An introduction to radioactivity*. UK: Manchester royal infirmary. 1999.
[32] Damon DH, Lobb RR, D'Amore PA, Wagner JA. Heparin potentiates the action of acidic fibroblast growth factor by prolonging its biological half-life. *Journal of cellular physiology*. 1989 Feb;138(2):221-6.
[33] Pommé S. *The uncertainty of the half-life. Metrologia*. 2015 May 22;52(3):S51.

Chapter 3

Radiation Units and Measurements

Shweta Dahake[1,*], MSc
N. Gajendran[2], MSc
Shreya Naik[3], MSc
and Anurag Luharia[1], PhD
[1]Department of Radio physics and Radio safety, Datta Meghe Institute of Higher Education and Research, Wardha, India
[2]Department of Radiation Oncology, Regency Hospital Ltd, Kanpur, India
[3]School of Allied Health Science, Datta Meghe Institute of Higher Education and Research, Wardha, India

Abstract

This chapter explores the fundamental concepts and quantities used to measure radiation and its effects on materials and living organisms. The discussion covers various dosimetric quantities, including exposure, Kerma, absorbed dose, equivalent dose, and effective dose. The definitions and relationships between these quantities are explained, along with their units of measurement. The concept of radiation weighting factors and tissue weighting factors is also introduced, highlighting their importance in assessing the biological effects of radiation. The International Commission on Radiological Units (ICRU) and its role in establishing global standards for radiation measurement are also discussed. The abstract provides a concise summary of the key concepts and principles governing radiation-related measurement quantities, including radioactivity, radiation safety, and dosimetry. The text is intended to provide a comprehensive framework for understanding the complex relationships between radiation and its effects on materials and living organisms, and to facilitate a deeper understanding of the principles and applications of radiation measurement.

Keywords: absorbed dose, equivalent dose, effective dose, kerma, radiation weighting factor

---

* Corresponding Author's Email: shwetadahake001@gmail.com

In: Fundamentals of Radiation Biology
Editors: Anurag Luharia, Ashish Uke, Gaurav Mishra et al.
ISBN: 979-8-89530-806-6

3.1. Introduction

Exposure and excess Dose of Radiation can harm both living organisms and non-living bodies in a variety of ways. It makes sense to assume that the amount of radiation absorbed by the substance would determine the severity of the damage. For short-term radiation effects, this holds true. However, the intensity of the radiation has little bearing on the severity of the stochastic effects. One such result is cell mutation, which can occur even at modest radiation doses and has long-lasting consequences. In this situation, the dose of radiation just affects the likelihood that harm, like cancer, will be initiated, but not its severity. Many businesses calculate the integrated dose their employees have gotten during a given time period to keep track of the deadly cancer risk factor. Exposure to high radiation levels can cause serious skin burns and tissue damage in addition to cancer. Radiation dosage estimations are commonly used in medicine to reduce radiation's potentially negative consequences.

3.2. Radiation-Related Measurement Quantities

Radiation exposure and radiation dose were coined to help assess the potential harm to materials based on the amount of radiation. It has been discovered that low sustained doses have an effect on both living and non-living entities, as well as high instantaneous doses. The issue of radiation damage to cells and detectors is gaining more and more attention as high radiation conditions become more widely available and used, such as in particle accelerators [1].

The following topics provide a comprehensive framework for investigating dosimetric quantities:

- *Measure of Radioactivity*
  - Particle number
  - Radiant energy
  - Flux and Flux energy
  - Fluence and fluence energy
  - Fluence rate and energy fluence rate
  - Particle radiance and energy radiance
- *Quantities of Interactions*
  - Cross section
  - Attenuation
  - Mass energy transfer
  - Stopping power
  - Radiation chemical yield
  - W value
- *The Dosimetric Parameters*
  - Energy imparted
  - Exposure
  - KERMA

- Air KERMA rate constant
- Absorbed dose

Following are some of the dosimetric quantities that are discussed:

1. Exposure

The third fundamental Non-stochastic quantity of interest in radiological physics is exposure. The oldest of the three, it was formerly known as “exposure dose” prior to 1962 and simply as the quantity measured in roentgen (R) units, as specified by the International Commission on Radiation Units and Measurements (ICRU) in 1928 [2]. The terms “exposure” and “radiation” are typically reserved for x-ray and γ-ray photons.

The quantity of air ionization caused by a single exposure to photons (x-rays or gamma rays) is the basis for the Roentgen scale [3]. To ionize and generate $2.58 * 10^{-4}$ coulombs of positive and negative charges in 1 kg of air, the required dosage is 1 R. Since it solely depicts dosage due to photons and is therefore not applicable to all tissues (such as bones), it is no longer utilized in dosimetry.

Definition

The International Commission on Radiological Protection (1980) defined exposure as “the quotient of dQ by dm, where the value of dQ is the absolute value of the total charge of the ions of one sign produced in air when all the electrons (negatrons and positrons) liberated by photons in air of mass dm are completely stopped in air, X as the symbol for this quantity.” Thus,

$$\therefore X = dQ/ dm$$

The ICRU clarifies that “the ionization arising from the absorption of bremsstrahlung emitted by the electrons is not to be included in dQ.” (This probably also holds true for the small radiative losses of kinetic energy that occur through the in-flight annihilation of positrons.)

It is evident that the exposure X is the ionization equivalent of the collision kerma K, in air, for x- and y-rays, if one has worked through the preceding statements to arrive at a fundamental grasp of their meaning [4].

The Meaning of W

The term “ionization equivalent” was used to describe the level of radiation exposure, but it must be defined more specifically [5].

2. Exposure Rate

The exposure rate at a point P and time t is given as:

Formula:

$$\dot{X}(t) = \frac{dX}{dt}$$

This equation is used to define X for all times within some extended period of irradiation. The exposure rate is a function of time t. The exposure occurring between selected time limit is then found by integration.

3. KERMA

Kerma is an abbreviation for Kinetic Energy Released to matter and is used to quantify the amount of energy transferred from radiation to matter [6]. Not the same as the absorbed dose, but similar. The Gray (joules per kilogram) is the SI unit for kerma.

Kerma is a measurement of the photon-electron energy transfer rate per unit mass at a certain location [7]. In contrast, the quantity known as "absorbed dose" quantifies the amount of energy deposited in a unit of mass at a certain location.

Energy transmission and deposition are about similar at radioactive energies [8]. At higher energies, however, a photon may connect with tissue at a given site, generating an electron with sufficient energy to deposit energy to a region distant from the interaction point.

Kerma is described in terms of the radiant energy R and the associated stochastic quantity (ICRU, 1980). The flow of energy in a volume V is given as:

Formula:

$$K = \frac{dE_{tr}}{dm}$$

where:

K = kerma (Gy)
dEtr = sum of initial kinetic energies of charged particles liberated
dm = mass

By *"Radiative losses,"* we refer to the process by which the kinetic energy of charged particles is converted into photon energy, either through the creation of bremsstrahlung x-rays or the annihilation of positrons in flight [9]. In the latter situation, only the positron's kinetic energy at the instant of annihilation is considered radiative energy loss (it is transferred to the subsequent photons combined with the positron's rest-mass energy, totaling 1.022 MeV).

Emitted, transferred, or received particle energy (not including rest energy) is known as radiant energy R.

- **The Components of Kerma**

Energy transmitted to electrons and positrons per unit mass of medium makes up the kerma for x- or gamma rays [10]. There are two potential sinks for a fast electron's kinetic energy:

1. Energy is dissipated as ionization and excitation in or near the electron track due to Coulomb-force interactions with the atomic electrons of the absorbing substance [10]. These interactions are known as collision interactions.
2. X-ray photons (bremsstrahlung, or "braking radiation") are emitted as the electron decelerates as a result of radiative interactions with the Coulomb force field of atomic nuclei. When compared to electrons, x-ray photons have a greater depth of penetration and can transport their quantum energy further from the charged-particle's path [11].

4. Kerma Rate

The kerma rate at a point P and time t is given by

Formula:

$$\dot{K}(t) = \frac{dK}{dt}$$

where:

K˙(t)\ = kerma rate at time t

K = kerma (kinetic energy released per unit mass)

In units of J/kg (erg/g) is preferably used. Sometimes rad/s are also used.

5. Absorbed Dose

Absorption dose is defined as the amount of energy deposited in a medium by ionizing radiation per unit mass of the material [12]. J/kg is the unit of measure for this. The gray (Gy) has been selected as the unit of measure for absorbed dosage, with 1 Gy equalling 1 J/kg. The absorbed dose can also be measured in rad, in addition to the more common Gy.

Despite Gy's widespread adoption, rad is still occasionally encountered in contemporary writing. In 1953, the Rad replaced the Roentgen as the unit for measuring radiation exposure from x-rays and γ-rays [13]. It is the amount of energy absorbed by one kilogram of tissue at a rate of one microjoule per second.

The absorbed dose D is the theoretical value of the energy per mass delivered to matter at a place. The absorbed dosage is the primary measure of success in radiological physics [14].

3.3. Radiation Safety Quantities

3.3.1. Equivalent Dose

Radiation's biological impact cannot be described by its absorbed dose; it is a common understanding. Absorbed dosage cannot be used to characterize harm in any media [15]. This information just tells us how much energy the medium has absorbed, but not what effect this deposited energy has had on the medium. In this regard, absorbed dosage is universally applicable across all forms of radiation. In other words, if a photon and a beta-particle both deposit the same amount of energy, then there is no difference between them in terms of absorbed dose. Therefore, absorbed dosage is not the appropriate measure for assessing the consequences of radiation. Dosimetry's primary focus is on protecting workers, hence a measure of the radiation's harmful effect on tissues, known as the equivalent dose, has been established [16].

The concept is straightforward: the biological efficiency of a given type of radiation and its source location is multiplied by the absorbed dose. The formula can be written as:

$$\therefore H_{T,R} = w_R \bullet D_{T,R},$$

where $H_{T,R}$ represents the equivalent dosage caused by radiation type R, $D_{T,R}$ represents the mean absorbed dose provided by radiation R, and w_R represents the radiation weighting factor.

The weighting factor for radiation is calculated as:

$$\therefore w_R = Q_R \bullet N_R.$$

here Q and R denote the standard and modified quality of radiation, respectively. N_R is assumed to be 1 while dealing with radiation from outside sources. Some authoritative body sets an N_R value for internal sources. To determine the weighting factor, it is usually sufficient to know the quality factor and accept the default value of $N_R = 1$.

The equivalent dose is also expressed in terms of J/kg, as the weighting factor is a dimensionless number. However, the unit is now known by its more precise name sievert and its associated sign, Sv. The rad equivalent for man (rem) is an ancient unit that is still occasionally used [17]. One Sv is equal to one hundred rem, thus making the switch is easy.

3.3.2. Effective Dose

After taking into account differences in radiation type and organ sensitivity, the absorbed dose (described above) becomes the effective dose. Long-term health impacts (such as cancer and genetic changes) may be a measure of how dangerous an exposure [18].

Effective Dose is a measure of the dose to a particular organ due to a particular type of radiation [19]. It takes into account the tissue weighting factor and equivalent dose. It is used to determine appropriate regulatory limitations to protect a population from potential adverse long-term health impacts. It also facilitates comparisons between the predicted health impacts of various exposure scenarios between specialists. This value cannot be used to forecast the consequences on an individual's health, as it is only an estimate based on calculations and not a physical quantity [20]. Sievert (Sv; international unit) and rem (rem; U.S. unit) are the units for an effective dose.

3.3.3. Effective, Equivalent, and Absorbed Doses: A Comparison

- *Absorbed Dose*
  - Dose absorbed is the measure of how much energy was deposited in a given mass by radiation.
  - Mass may be anything from liquid to solid to gas to human beings.
  - Milligrays (mGy) is the unit of measure for absorbed dosage.
- *Equivalent Dose*
  - Each organ receives a calculated equivalent dosage.
  - It is based on the effective dose of radiation, which is calculated from the absorbed dosage to an organ.
  - The millisievert (mSv) is the unit of measurement for organ-equivalent dose.
- *Effective Dose*
  - The whole-body effective dosage is determined.
  - It's the accumulation of doses to all organs, with each dosage adjusted for the organ's radiation sensitivity.
  - Millisieverts (mSv) are the unit of measure for effective dosage.

3.4. Linear Energy Transfer

Linear energy transfer (LET) is the amount of energy which an ionizing particle deposits in the material traversed per unit distance. It is similar to retarding force on a charged particle through matter. It is closely related to stopping power, since both equal the retarding force. The unrestricted linear energy transfer is identical to linear electronic stopping power [21].

3.5. Radiation Weighting Factor

The Commission now believes that the detail and precision inherent in using a formal Q-L relationship to modify absorbed dose to reflect the higher probability of detriment resulting from exposure to radiation components with high LET is not justified because of the uncertainties in the radiobiological information [22]. In place of Q or more precisely 0, the Commission now selects radiation weighting factors, w, based on a review of the biological information, a variety of exposure circumstances and inspection of the results of traditional calculations of the ambient dose equivalent. (AlO) The Commission now specifies modifying factors which apply to the tissue or organ absorbed dose and are based on the type and quality of the external radiation field or on the type and quality of the radiation emitted by an internally deposited radionuclide.

3.6. Tissue Weighting Factors

The relationship between the probability of stochastic effects and equivalent dose is found also to vary with the organ or tissue irradiated. It is, therefore, appropriate to define a further quantity, derived from equivalent dose, to indicate the combination of different doses to several different tissues in a way which is likely to correlate well with the total of the stochastic effects [23]. The factor by which the equivalent dose in tissue or organ T is weighted is called the tissue weighting factor, IV. The values of w are chosen so that a uniform equivalent dose over the whole body gives an effective dose numerically equal to that uniform equivalent dose. The sum of the tissue weighting factors is then unity. This weighted equivalent dose (a doubly weighted absorbed dose) has previously been called the effective dose equivalent, but this name is unnecessarily complicated, especially in more complex combinations such as collective committed effective dose equivalent [24]. The Commission has now decided to use the simpler name effective dose, E. The unit of effective dose is J kg^{-1}', with the special name sievert (Sv).

3.7. Commonly Used Units

1. Radioactivity

The amount of ionizing radiation given off by a radioactive material is the unit of measurement for its radioactivity [25]. Ionizing radiation comes in many forms, each with the potential to cause harm to human tissue. The rate at which, radioactive material disintegrates (transforms) or decays. Becquerel (Bq) and Curie (Ci) standard units of radioactivity, respectively [26]. Since a curie is such a huge measurement, picocuries (pCi) are more commonly used to display radioactivity data. One picocurie is equal to one trillionth of a curie. If the number is larger, then the material emits more radiation.

The SI base activity unit is the curie (Ci). A disintegration rate of 1 Ci is equal to 3.7 x 10^{10} Bq per second.

2. Collective Dose

The sum of all doses absorbed by a population from a specific radiation source over a given time period is known as the collective dose.

- ***Committed dose equivalent ($H_{T,50}$)***
  Committed dose equivalent is the dose equivalent to reference organs or tissues (T) that a human will receive from ingesting radioactive material over the course of 50 years after the initial ingestion [27].

3. Committed effective dose equivalent ($H_{E,50}$)

The sum of the products of the applicable weighting factor and the committed dose equivalent to the organ or tissue (HE,50 = wTHT,50) for each organ or tissue that is irradiated.

4. Dose Equivalent

Tissue absorbed dose multiplied by the quality factor multiplied by any additional relevant modifiers equals the absorbed dose equivalent (HT) at the target site. The rem and sievert (Sv) are the units of dosage equivalence [28].

5. Effective Dose(E)

Total dosage to all tissues and organs multiplied by their weighted equivalent is the effective dose (E). The formula for the equivalent dose (E) is HT times the tissue weighting factor (wT).

6. Effective Dose Equivalent (H_E)

To calculate the effective dose equivalent (HE), multiply the dose equivalent to the organ or tissue by the relevant weighting factor and add the results.

- ***Rad***
  One rad is equal to one hundred ergs per gram, or one thousandth of a joule per kilogram, or 0.01 Gy.
- ***Reference man***
  An idealized standard of human anatomy and physiology agreed upon on a global scale [29]. Researchers and public health professionals can utilize these qualities to standardize experimental results and establish a framework for relating biologic insult to a common basis.

7. Relative Biological Effectiveness (RBE)

RBE measures how much less radiation is needed from a test radiation source to get the same level of biologic effect as the reference radiation source (often 200 keV x rays) [30]. The RBE of the test radiation will change based on the specific biologic effect in a selected species subjected to a certain exposure.

- **rem**
  The unique measurement for dose-equivalent quantities. One rem is equal to one sievert, thus multiply the absorbed dose in rads by the quality factor to get the dosage equivalent.

- **Sievert**
  The international system of units (SI) for dose equivalent quantities is the sievert (Sv). The dose in sieverts is calculated by multiplying the absorbed dose in gray by the quality factor (1 sievert = 100 rem).

8. Total Effective Dose Equivalent (TEDE)

The sum of the deep-dose equivalent (for exterior exposures) and the committed effective dose equivalent (for internal exposures) is the total effective dose equivalent (TEDE) [31]. Some groups use this term to specify that they are referring to all funding, not only that which comes from within the company. The ICRP and NCRP do not endorse this expression in their guidelines. Without adding the word "total," the term "effective dose equivalent" implies both external and internal contributions.

3.8. International Committee for Radiological Units

The International Committee for Radiological Units (ICRU), formerly known as the International X-Ray Unit Committee, was established at the Second International Congress of Radiology (ICR-2) in Stockholm, Sweden, in 1928[32]. The primary goal was to suggest a radiation measurement device for use in medical settings. Starting in 1950, the ICRU took on a much broader responsibility. One physicist and one radiologist from each participating country had the right to attend the initial meetings every three years at ICR congresses (except the thirteen-year period surrounding World War II), with the Chair being nominated by the ICR host country. In 1953, a Commission with a lifetime of service was chosen. From 1928 to 1934, L S Taylor (USA) was a member of ICRU; from 1934 to 1953, he was the organization's Secretary; from 1953 to 1969, he was its first permanent Chair; and from 1969 until his death in 2004, he was the organization's Honorary Chair.

The primary goal of the ICRU is to create standards that are recognised globally in areas such as:

1. measures of radiation and radioactivity's intensity; diagnostic radiology, radiation treatment, radiation biology, nuclear medicine, radiation protection, and industrial and environmental operations;
2. measurement and application methodologies suitable for these quantities;

Three, the physical information used to apply these methods and guarantee consistent reporting. In its publications, the ICRU recommends the most appropriate levels of radiation amounts and the most acceptable and safest methodologies for current usage based on its evaluation of the most up-to-date data and information relevant to the challenges of radiation measurement [33]. International organizations such as the International Atomic Energy Agency (IAEA), the World Health Organization (WHO), the International Commission on Radiological Protection (ICRP), the United Nations Scientific Committee on the Effects of Atomic Radiation (UNSCEAR), the International Organization for Standardization (ISO), and the International Bureau of Weights and Measures (BIPM) are kept in close contact with by the Commission. The ICRU's efforts are directly beneficial to a wide range of groups and institutions, as well as radiation workers, patients (especially those with cancer), and the general public [34].

Conclusion

This chapter has comprehensively described the units, measurements, and concepts essential to quantifying radiation and its interactions with matter. From fundamental quantities like exposure, kerma, and absorbed dose to more biologically relevant measures such as equivalent and effective dose, these parameters form the backbone of radiation dosimetry and protection. The inclusion of radiation and tissue weighting factors helps translate physical energy deposition into meaningful estimates of biological effect and health risk. The standardized units Gray, Sievert, Becquerel and their definitions ensure consistent measurement practices across applications in medicine, industry, and environmental monitoring. Understanding and correctly applying these concepts is vital for ensuring safety, optimizing treatment, and complying with regulatory standards in the use of ionizing radiation.

References

[1] Ahmed SN. *Physics and engineering of radiation detection.* Academic Press; 2007 Apr 12.

[2] Jennings WA. Evolution over the past century of quantities and units in radiation dosimetry. *Journal of Radiological Protection.* 2007 Mar 6;27(1):5.

[3] Exner FM, Packard C. A Biological Measurement of Radium Gamma Rays. *Radiology.* 1935 Oct;25(4):391-402.

[4] Attix FH. *Introduction to radiological physics and radiation dosimetry.* John Wiley & Sons; 2008 Sep 26.

[5] Jaeger RG, editor. *Engineering Compendium on Radiation Shielding: Volume I: Shielding Fundamentals and Methods.* Springer Science & Business Media; 2013 Jun 29.

[6] Huda W. Kerma-area product in diagnostic radiology. *American Journal of Roentgenology.* 2014 Dec;203(6):W565-9.

[7] Brede HJ, Greif KD, Hecker O, Heeg P, Heese J, Jones DT, Kluge H, Schardt D. Absorbed dose to water determination with ionization chamber dosimetry and calorimetry in restricted neutron, photon, proton and heavy-ion radiation fields. *Physics in Medicine & Biology.* 2006 Jul 12;51(15):3667.

[8] Talaat K, Xi J, Baldez P, Hecht A. Radiation dosimetry of inhaled radioactive aerosols: CFPD and MCNP transport simulations of radionuclides in the lung. *Scientific reports.* 2019 Nov 25;9(1):17450.

[9] Aharonian FA, Atoyan AM. Broad-band diffuse gamma ray emission of the galactic disk. *arXiv preprint* astro-ph/0009009. 2000 Sep 1.

[10] Nilsson B, Brahme A. Relation between kerma and absorbed dose in photon beams. *Acta Radiologica: Oncology.* 1983 Jan 1;22(1):77-85.

[11] Diehl R. Gamma-ray production and absorption processes. In *The Universe in Gamma Rays* 2001 (pp. 9-25). Berlin, Heidelberg: Springer Berlin Heidelberg.

[12] Rossi HH. Spatial distribution of energy deposition by ionizing radiation. *Radiation Research Supplement.* 1960 Jan 1;2:290-9.

[13] Piciu D, Piciu D. Specific Measurements, Units, and Terms. *Nuclear Endocrinology.* 2017:9-11.

[14] Pötter R, Haie-Meder C, Van Limbergen E, Barillot I, De Brabandere M, Dimopoulos J, Dumas I, Erickson B, Lang S, Nulens A, Petrow P. Recommendations from gynaecological (GYN) GEC

ESTRO working group (II): concepts and terms in 3D image-based treatment planning in cervix cancer brachytherapy—3D dose volume parameters and aspects of 3D image-based anatomy, radiation physics, radiobiology. *Radiotherapy and oncology*. 2006 Jan 1;78(1):67-77.

[15] Ritz C, Baty F, Streibig JC, Gerhard D. Dose-response analysis using R. *PloS one*. 2015 Dec 30;10(12):e0146021.

[16] Ainsbury EA, Bakhanova E, Barquinero JF, Brai M, Chumak V, Correcher V, Darroudi F, Fattibene P, Gruel G, Guclu I, Horn S. Review of retrospective dosimetry techniques for external ionizing radiation exposures. *Radiation protection dosimetry*. 2011 Nov 1;147(4):573-92.

[17] Cameron J. *Radiation dosimetry. Environmental health perspectives*. 1991 Feb;91:45-8.

[18] Kapaj S, Peterson H, Liber K, Bhattacharya P. Human health effects from chronic arsenic poisoning–a review. *Journal of Environmental Science and Health, Part A*. 2006 Oct 1;41(10):2399-428.'

[19] Martin CJ, Harrison JD, Rehani MM. Effective dose from radiation exposure in medicine: past, present, and future. *Physica Medica*. 2020 Nov 1;79:87-92.

[20] International Commission on Non-Ionizing Radiation Protection. Guidelines for limiting exposure to time-varying electric and magnetic fields (1 Hz to 100 kHz). *Health physics*. 2010 Dec 1;99(6):818-36.

[21] Rørvik E. A Comparison of Biological Dose Estimates in Proton and Carbon Ion Therapy Based on Averaged and Full Linear Energy Transfer Spectra (Master's thesis, NTNU).

[22] Valentin J. Relative biological effectiveness (RBE), quality factor (Q), and radiation weighting factor (wR): ICRP Publication 92. *Annals of the ICRP*. 2003 Dec 1;33(4):1-21.

[23] Wrixon AD. New ICRP recommendations. *Journal of radiological protection*. 2008 May 22;28(2):161.

[24] Drexler G. The dosimetric quantities in the new ICRP recommendations. *Radiation Protection Dosimetry*. 1992 Oct 1;43(1-4):93-8.

[25] Tykva R, Sabol J. *Low-level environmental radioactivity: sources and evaluation*. CRC Press; 1995 Apr 13.

[26] Ashbaugh CE. Gemstone irradiation and radioactivity. *Gems & Gemology*. 1988;24(4):196-213.

[27] Eckerman KF, Wolbarst AB, Richardson AC. Limiting values of radionuclide intake and air concentration and dose conversion factors for inhalation, submersion, and ingestion: Federal guidance report No. 11. Environmental Protection Agency, Washington, DC (USA). Office of Radiation Programs; *Oak Ridge National Lab*.(ORNL), *Oak Ridge,* TN (United States); 1988 Sep 1.

[28] Brateman L. The AAPM/RSNA physics tutorial for residents: radiation safety considerations for diagnostic radiology personnel. *Radiographics*. 1999 Jul;19(4):1037-55.

[29] Brownell KD. Dieting and the search for the perfect body: Where physiology and culture collide. *Behavior therapy*. 1991 Dec 1;22(1):1-2.

[30] Stewart RD, Streitmatter SW, Argento DC, Kirkby C, Goorley JT, Moffitt G, Jevremovic T, Sandison GA. Rapid MCNP simulation of DNA double strand break (DSB) relative biological effectiveness (RBE) for photons, neutrons, and light ions. *Physics in Medicine & Biology*. 2015 Oct 9;60(21):8249.

[31] Elkhatib H, Awad MA, El-Samanoudy MA. Modeling of atmospheric dispersion and radiation dose for a hypothetical accident in radioisotope production facility. *Progress in Nuclear Energy*. 2021 Apr 1;134:103674.

[32] Zoetelief J, Pernička F, CARLSSON G, Dance DR, DREXLER G, JÄRVINEN H, KRAMER H, NG K. Dosimetry in diagnostic and interventional radiology: international commission on radiation units and measurements and IAEA activities. *Standards and Codes of Practice in Medical Radiation Dosimetry*. 2002:387.

[33] Keall PJ, Glide-Hurst CK, Cao M, Lee P, Murray B, Raaymakers BW, Tree A, van der Heide UA. ICRU REPORT 97: MRI-Guided Radiation Therapy Using MRI-Linear Accelerators. *Journal of the ICRU*. 2022 Dec;22(1):1-00.

[34] Fisher DR, Fahey FH. Appropriate use of effective dose in radiation protection and risk assessment. *Health physics*. 2017 Aug;113(2):102.

Chapter 4

Radiation Detection Methods

Sanjay Dhoble[1,*], PhD
Albert Paul Varghese[2], MSc
Nandini[3], MSc
and Maruf Ahmad[4], MSc
[1]Department of Physics, Nagpur University, Nagpur, India
[2]School of Allied Health Science, Datta Meghe Institute of Higher Education and Research, Wardha, India
[3]Department of Radiology and Imaging Technology, Noida International University, Greater Noida (UP), India
[4]Department of Radiology, Centurion University of Technology and Management, Jatni, Bhubaneswar, Odisha, India

Abstract

This chapter explores the fundamental principles and applications of radiation detectors, including gas-filled, liquid, and solid-state detectors. The discussion covers the detection methodologies, operational regions, and characteristics of various detectors, such as ionization chambers, proportional counters, and scintillation detectors. The text also delves into the design and performance of gas-filled detectors, including their response to dose linearity, energy dependence, and directional dependence. The pros and cons of using ionization chambers are discussed, highlighting their benefits, such as high stability and linear response to dose, as well as their limitations, including limited sensitivity and susceptibility to environmental changes. The abstract provides a concise summary of the key concepts and principles governing radiation detection and measurement and is intended to provide a comprehensive framework for understanding the complex relationships between radiation and its effects on materials and living organisms, ultimately humans.

Keywords: ionization chamber, geiger-mueller detector, proportional counter, scintillation detector, semiconductor detector

---

* Corresponding Author's Email: sjDhoble@gmail.com

In: Fundamentals of Radiation Biology
Editors: Anurag Luharia, Ashish Uke, Gaurav Mishra et al.
ISBN: 979-8-89530-806-6

4.1. Introduction to Categories of Detectors

If the energy of the radiation is greater than the ionization potential of the gas, then the gas molecules will be ionized as the radiation passes through. When an external electric field is applied, the resulting charge pairs can be induced to move in opposite directions. As a result, an electric pulse is generated that can be detected by a separate sensor. The so-called gas-filled detectors have been built using this method. A detector with gas within would typically have an enclosure, positive and negative electrodes. Depending on the detector's configuration and mode of operation, a high potential difference is applied between the electrodes, often in the range of a few hundred to several thousand volts. The externally applied electric field is perturbed by the generation and movement of charge pairs caused by the passage of radiation in the gas, resulting in a pulse at the electrodes. With the right calibration, the ensuing change in charge, current, or voltage at one of the electrodes can be used to infer the particle beams energy and/or intensity.

It seems to reason that the system would function optimally if a large number of charge pairs could be generated and, before recombining to produce neutral molecules, easily collected at the electrodes. The creation of charge pairs and their kinetic behaviour in the gas are under our control due to the gas we use, the detector's geometry, and the applied voltage.

General design issues for gas filled detectors and their behaviour under various situations are discussed in this chapter. This chapter will also cover some of the most popular types of gaseous detectors.

Ionizing radiation can also be detected through the use of a liquid environment as the ionizing medium, in addition to the more common air-based detection methods. The pulse can be generated by passing radiation through a liquid, which creates charge couples that can be guided to electrodes. The height of the pulse is a suitable indicator of the energy deposited if the liquid guarantees a good proportionality between the energy deposited and the number of charge pairs formed. A surprising variety of liquids actually meet the criteria for usage as detection media due to their relatively good proportionality. It seems to reason, then, that a liquid would have a significantly larger probability of charge recombination than a conventional gas. This is correct, but it is also important to keep in mind that a greater density guarantees the creation of a greater number of charge pairs. Liquids, in principle, can be utilized as ionizing mediums to detect and measure radiation (we shall explore these two competing aspects later in the chapter).

The focus of this chapter is on electronic detectors that employ liquids as detection media, with the exception of a brief discussion of bubble chambers. As we shall see, the bubble chambers do not function like common electronic detectors, in which the voltage or current is detected at the readout electrode. Instead, bubbles are created by the particles and shot for later inspection. Liquid scintillation detectors are another type of detector that use the light produced by liquid molecules that have been stimulated by incident radiation. The scintillation detectors section will talk about equipment like this.

Although gas filled detectors and liquid detectors have proven to be quite beneficial in many applications, it is clear from the preceding explanation that their employment is rather restricted for a variety of reasons. In low radiation settings, the generation of a large number of electron-ion pairs in a gas detector can degrade the performance of high-resolution systems. This suggests that the likelihood of producing charge pairs would increase if we used a detector filled with liquids or solids rather than a gas. However, it turns out that density is merely one of several parameters that affect the mechanism of charge pair creation.

It was discovered that semiconductors possessed significantly better charge pair generation properties than gases. It has been found that diamond, another solid, can produce charge pairs at a high rate. Solid state detectors, a term that is frequently used only to refer to semiconductor detectors, encompass all detectors that employ solids as active sensing media. Using solids as active detection media, we will also cover the method of radiation detection and measurement in this chapter. Some of the most popular solid-state detectors will also be discussed.

Equipment to receive signals from radiation detectors, process them, and create a convenient output evolved in tandem with the development of radiation detectors and is therefore essential to both. Williams, in 1931, building on Greinacher's work from 1926, created the first linear amplifier to enhance the pulse created in a shallow ionization chamber by the passage of a single alpha particle. The first working photomultiplier was created in 1940. Amplifiers using vacuum-tube circuitry were plentiful in the early 1950s. Their effectiveness was gradually enhanced, for instance in 1956 when feedback circuits were introduced. Low power consumption, small size (integrated circuits), and dependability led to the widespread adoption of transistor circuits over vacuum tube circuits in the late 1950s and early 1960s. As a result, numerous highly effective portable radiation detectors emerged rapidly. To accommodate increased counting rates, instruments were lengthened. Radiation detectors benefited from the incorporation of computing technologies in the 1960s. It is difficult to foresee the future without the microprocessors (central processing units on integrated circuit chips) that will revolutionize radiation measuring devices.

Semiconductor detectors are solid-state detectors analogues of gas-filled ionization chambers with ionization, serving as their fundamental operating principle. The p-n junction between two semiconductors is the site of the ionization. The signal-to-noise (S/N) ratio of semiconductor detectors is low at ambient temperature but improves after being chilled, for example with liquid nitrogen. Energy resolution is excellent in the semiconductor detector.

On the other hand, the underlying principle behind scintillation detectors is the phenomenon of luminescence. Some materials have the unique property of emitting a flash of light whenever they absorb a quantum of radiation. Radiation energy is directly correlated to flash brightness. A photoelectron multiplier boosts the intensity of the flash. Although not as good as semiconductor detectors' energy resolution, it is good enough for many applications.

4.2. The Following Is An Overview of Various Detectors Based on Their Detection Methodology

1. *Sensor packed with gas*
   - Plasma Chamber
   - High-Pressure Xenon Ions
   - Ratio-based counters
   - Geiger-Muller Detector
2. *Sensors based on liquid scintillation*
   - Organic

  - Emulsions in water
3. *Solid- and Solid-State Detectors*
  - NaI (Tl)
  - BGO
  - Scintillator, Plastic
  - Sensor Based on Semiconductors

4.2.1. Gas Filled Detector

4.2.1.1. Electron-Ion Pair Generation in Gas Filled Detectors

Radiation can either excite and ionize particles in a gas, or have no effect at all [1]. These interactions could occur via a variety of processes. Cross section, stopping power, and the average energy required to produce an electron-ion pair in a gas all play a role in the methods by which interactions occur. For the vast majority of gases and radiation types, it has been determined that the W value is between 25 and 45 eV per charge pair and depends only weakly on other parameters. Where the W-value designates the quantity of power involved [2].

To differentiate them from secondary charges, which are produced indirectly in the active volume, the charges created by the incident radiation are referred to as primary charges. Similar to how main charges are generated, these secondary charge pairs are created through ionization triggered by primary charge pairs rather than incident radiation [3].

All ionizations within the detector's active volume are represented by the W-value. The yield of the primary charge pairs can be useful information in some cases. However, it is not always possible to estimate this number empirically due to the practically inevitable secondary ionizations that occur at nominal applied voltages.

4.2.1.2. The Path and Spread of Radiation in Gases

When radiation passes across an area, it creates electrons and ions, both of which quickly lose energy as they collide with molecules of the surrounding gas [4]. Their path in the gas volume is largely determined by the nature and magnitude of the force acting upon them. Therefore, charges' behaviors with and without an electric field are very different. Since electrons have such a low mass, they disperse at an incredibly high rate. As a result, electrons have a very different diffusion coefficient than ions do in the same gas. Due to its mass and charge dependency, the diffusion coefficient can take on very different values for various ions [5]. It gets more complicated because it is dependent on the gas through which the ion is travelling. Since the ions generated by the incident radiation are the focus of attention in radiation detectors, we can only consider the ions' diffusion in their own gas. Diffusion properties can be altered by including a little amount of an admixture gas in the filling gas; thus, it is important to determine the right value for the diffusion coefficient based on the specific gases and their concentrations [6].

4.2.1.3. Electric Field-Induced Diffusion

Because the diffusion is no longer isotropic in the presence of an electric field, the scalar diffusion coefficient can no longer be used to describe it. The electric field inside the active volume is generated by the bias voltage that is applied [7]. Because of their low mass, electrons are subject to a powerful electric force. However, if the applied electric field is not strong enough to generate discharge in the gas, it has no effect on the distribution of ions. Because electrons and ions react differently in an electric field, each form of charge has its own area of study.

The output is nothing but the change in electric field inside the active volume, hence the drift of ions and electrons is crucial for measuring output.

- **Operational Regions of Gas-Filled Detector**

The diagram below shows the various functional zones of a detector filled with gas. A detector can be operated in a variety of modes that vary in charge production and movement inside the detector chamber based on the bias voltage applied [8]. Detectors are typically tailored to function solely in the range of the applied voltage that is typical of the mode for which they were designed. Ionizing radiation can be detected through six primary operational modalities, three of which (ionization, proportional, and Geiger-Mueller region) are considered viable and practical for this purpose. These areas of activity are briefly addressed.

1. Recombination Region

The recombination region in a radiation detector is where charge carriers generated by incident radiation may recombine, which can detrimentally impact the detector's performance by diminishing the number of charge carriers available for signal generation and amplification. Charges generated by the passage of radiation quickly cancel out to make neutral molecules when an electric field is not present. Minimizing recombination is crucial for achieving high energy resolution and efficiency in detecting and measuring radiation. Some of the charges start to move toward the opposing electrodes as soon as the bias voltage is applied. By increasing this voltage, we can reduce the recombination rate and boost the detector current. The range of applied voltage corresponds to the point where recombination is quite minor. The energy deposited by incoming radiation is not accurately reflected by the current recorded at the detector's output due to significant recombination in this region [9]. As a result, using the detector in this area is pointless from a radiation characteristics measurement standpoint.

2. Ion Chamber Region

As the applied voltage rises, more and more of the electron-ion pairs formed in the recombination area are collected. The so-called ion chamber region officially begins at this point [10]. Since all the generated charges are efficiently collected by the electrodes, increasing the high voltage further has no effect on the measured current in this region. Saturation current, which is measured by the corresponding electronics in this region, is directly proportional to the energy deposited by the incident radiation. Ionization chambers are the name given to detectors that are optimized for this frequency range.

Charge pair recombination in the ion chamber region is extremely unlikely to be entirely ruled out [11]. With careful planning, though, ionization chambers can be constructed with vanishingly small slopes on their plateaus.

3. Proportional Region

Secondary ionization occurs when the charges created during initial ionization have enough energy to create additional electron-ion pairs. With enough energy, these charges could cause further ionization [12]. This process can only take place if the electric potential between the electrodes is strong enough to allow the charges to accelerate to extremely high speeds. Due to their extremely low mass, electrons are primarily responsible for the following ionizations that occur as the bias voltage is increased. The proportional detectors take advantage of the multiplication of charges at high fields to boost the strength of the output signal [13]. In this type of detector, the output pulse is kept proportionate to the deposited energy despite the multiplication of charges. For this Particular reason, we refer to these devices as proportional detectors.

4. Limited Proportionality Region

The detector's active volume fills up with charges as the bias voltage is raised. Since positive charges are heavier and hence move more slowly than electrons, they tend to congregate in a cloud between the electrodes.

As a shield, this cloud weakens the electric field the charges experience. Therefore, the final number of charges produced is not always proportional to the original number of charges. The term "region of limited proportionality" describes this area. Due to the lack of linearity that results from a loss of proportionality, radiation detectors are not used in this area.

5. Geiger-Mueller Region

If the voltage is raised any higher, the local electric field could become so strong that a massive avalanche of charge pairs is created in the gas. As a result, the readout electronics experience a massive pulse of many volts, i.e. being able to produce a significant output pulse from a single original ionizing event. The so-called Geiger-Mueller zone officially begins at this point. Since each incident particle triggers a breakdown and a sizable pulse in this location, it is possible to precisely count individual particles [14]. Detectors used in this region are unsuitable for spectroscopy due to the fact that the output pulse does not vary with the type of radiation being detected or the amount of energy deposited.

Furthermore, such detectors typically feature a lengthy lag time. Dead time is the period of inactivity of the detector [15]. The detector or its supporting circuitry may be at blame for this. A high positive charge accumulation can weaken the internal electric field to the point where avalanche multiplication is no longer favored. During this interval, if radiation creates charge pairs, the charges do not multiply and no pulse is produced. Once the majority of the positive charges have been gathered by the relevant electrode, the detector can resume its operations. The concept of dead time will be further touched upon later in the chapter.

Breakdown: It takes longer for the cathode to be reached, because the many ions produced during the avalanche drift considerably more slowly than the electrons. These powerful positive charges can cause further ionization of the surrounding gas by striking the cathode wall [16]. This procedure typically has an efficiency of less than 10% and is too low to significantly boost the charge population at low to medium voltages. However, the output pulse's linearity degrades with increasing voltage because the chance of secondary ion emission rises at higher voltages. If the voltage is raised any further, the gas may begin to discharge. The height of the pulse is no longer reliant on the initial number of electron ion pairs, and the current reaches extremely high levels at this stage. The area makes use of Geiger Muller tubes.

6. Continuous Discharge Region

The region experiencing continuous ion discharges into the electrodes, regardless of the presence of radiation, and is not suitable for effective radiation detection. When the breakdown process, we examined in the previous part is subjected to extremely high voltage, it can progress to the process of continuous discharge [17]. As soon as a single ionization occurs, a continuous discharge begins and will continue unabated until the voltage is reduced. There is a risk of the detector being harmed by electric arcs if they form between the electrodes in this area. Radiation detectors obviously cannot function at such high voltages, thus taking care to keep it below the necessary level is essential.

7. Ionization Chambers

One of the first types of radiation detectors built is the ionization chamber. They continue to be one of the most popular detectors because of its straightforward design and well understood physical processes [18].

4.2.1.4. Electric Current and Voltage Characteristics

To prevent the chambers from being damaged by excessive current fluctuations caused by even slight differences in the power supply voltage, they are typically operated in the middle of the plateau region [19]. This guarantees steadiness and reduces the need for extremely stable power supplies, which can be prohibitively expensive. As we mentioned before, the plateau of any given chamber will have a slight slope, but this will typically be too minor to have any appreciable effect on the signal-to-noise ratio.

In an ion chamber, the intensity of the incident radiation has no effect on the shape of the current-voltage characteristic curve. Two quantitative distinctions emerge: the time at which the plateau zone begins, and the amplitude of the current at the output. Both of these dissimilarities can be traced back to the greater abundance of electron-ion couples at higher intensities. A stronger electric field will be required to prevent (or, more realistically, to reduce) charge recombination if the rate at which charge pairs are produced increases. Therefore, the plateau will rise to a greater voltage in this scenario. In addition, as we will see in the following section, the plateau current is proportional to the number of charge pairs in the plateau zone, and hence increases with increasing intensity.

4.2.1.5. Design of Gas filled Ion Chamber

The design of an ionization chamber can exhibit variations in its response to factors such as dose linearity, energy dependence, and directional dependence, which are important considerations in radiation dosimetry. An ion chamber's mechanical architecture revolves around four main parts: the anode (collecting electrode), the cathode (conductive outer wall), the gas enclosure and with a guard electrode to further reduce the chamber charge leakage.

The specific geometry of these components varies from one use to the next. Ion chambers often take on either a parallel plate or a cylindrical shape.

4.3. Geometry of Parallel Plate Ion Chamber

Parallel-plate ionization chambers are compact, disc-shaped devices with circular collecting electrodes separated by a narrow gap, typically 2 millimetres or less in width. The extremely thin upper polarizing electrode/entry window enables highly precise measurements of near-surface radiation dose. Two parallel plates are held at different electrical potentials in this straightforward setup. However, as we have seen, nonlinearity in the response can be avoided with careful design despite the fact that the curvature in the electric lines of force at the margins of such a detector is a possible source of nonlinearity [20]. In reality, ionization chambers with extremely fine parallel plates have been created. These types of ionization chambers are recommended for the Dosimetric measurement of electron beams with energies below 10 MeV and are commonly utilized for the assessment of surface radiation doses.

4.4. Geometry of a Cylindrical Ion Chamber

Cylindrical ionization chambers are chambers with active volumes ranging from 0.1 to 1 cm^3, where chamber walls are usually constructed using low-atomic-number materials to improve tissue and air equivalence. Compared to their parallel plate counterparts, cylindrical ionization chambers provide a number of benefits. Most significantly, the presence of a non-uniform electric field strength within their active volumes increases the efficiency with which they gather charge. An anode wire is typically stretched along the cylindrical axis of the metal chamber. With its wide ion collecting area and great ion collection efficiency, the cylinder's dual role as gas container and cathode is clear. Because of the anode's remarkable slenderness, the electric fields surrounding it are highly concentrated. Therefore, the electrons move toward the anode, whereas the ions speed toward the cathode. This enhances the efficiency of electron collection and speeds up the electron drift compared to the parallel plate geometry.

4.4.1. Pros and Cons of Using Ion Chambers

- It is important to keep in mind that there is no such thing as a multipurpose detector. While some detectors, like ionization chambers, can serve multiple purposes, the vast majority are custom-made for a given set of circumstances. As a result, weighing the benefits and drawbacks of detectors is subjective. Nonetheless, we will have a broad look at the benefits and drawbacks of ionization chambers because of their adaptability.
- Since the ionization current in the ion chamber region is rather insensitive to the applied voltage, the system's resolution is not degraded by the inevitable minor fluctuations and drifts in high voltage power sources. As a corollary, this allows the

use of cheaper power supply to bias the detector without risk. The amount of energy deposited by incident radiation is proportional to the saturation current [21].

- Ionization chambers can be used for measuring high radiation dose rates because they do not exhibit the "dead time" phenomenon most commonly shows in Geiger-Mueller tube detectors under such conditions. This is due to the lack of inherent signal amplification within the operating medium of ionization chambers, allowing them to recover more quickly from large current pulses compared to other detector types. In nuclear reactors, ionization chambers in Neutron Instrumentation System can be often used in current mode to detect neutrons.
- Since there is no gas multiplication in ionization chambers, their performance is not drastically impacted by even minor alterations to the gas quality, such as an increase in the concentration of electronegative pollutants. At least, this holds true for low resolution systems operating in strong to extremely strong radiation fields [22]. Furthermore, ionization chambers which have lacking amplification, can be used to be operated in either current or pulse mode. While ionization chambers are among the most popular types of detectors due to features like high stability, linear response to dose, and accurate ion collection efficiency, ensuring precise and reliable dosimetry measurements, they do have several notable drawbacks that should be considered.
- In most radiation conditions, detectors in the ionization region operate at a low electric field strength, so no gas multiplication occurs, therefore the amount of current passing through the ionization chamber is negligible. It is possible that the current would not be detectable at all in very weak radiation fields. Because of this, the system has limited sensitivity and cannot be used in low-radiation conditions.
- Moreover, for ionization chambers to detect alpha and beta particles, they require a thin end-window that allows these particles to penetrate. However, even a window of almost any thickness will prevent alpha particles from entering the chamber.
- Due to the low ionization current, low-noise electronic circuitry is required for an adequate signal-to-noise ratio [23].
- Ionization chamber responses may vary depending on factors like ambient temperature and pressure, making them susceptible to environmental changes. However, the effect is typically negligible and only a problem for systems with a high degree of resolution.

Some commonly used gas filled detectors in routine dosimetry are listed below:

- Free air Ion Chamber
- Thimble Chamber
- Farmer Chamber
- Well Chamber
- Spherical ion Chamber

4.5. Proportional Counters

The key feature is the detector's capacity to measure the energy of incident radiation. It accomplishes this by generating a detector output pulse that is proportional to the radiation energy absorbed by the detector due to an ionizing event, which gives rise to the detector's name. Pulse amplitude in proportional counters is proportional to the number of charge pairs generated by the incident radiation in a parallel plate ionization chamber [24]. In cases when the incident particle energy is low or the flux is low, this could mean that the pulse amplitude is insufficient to produce a good signal-to-noise ratio.

Therefore, the number of electron-ion pairs is directly proportional to the pulse amplitude. The incident radiation's principal charges can easily generate further charges, making this the simplest method for producing a large number of charge pairs [25]. This behavior was previously seen in the Avalanche Multiplication section.

We described how, with enough separation between impacts, primary charges can generate secondary ionizations in the gas. A huge pulse is produced at the output as a result of avalanche multiplication.

Therefore, application of very high electric potential between the two electrodes is essential for the avalanche to occur. Due to the same density of electric lines of force at the anode and cathode, parallel plate shape is not optimal for this application [26]. The applied voltage cannot be made proportionate to the output pulse amplitude, even if we manage to operate a parallel plate chamber at the breakdown voltage. The magnitude of the pulse varies with the location at which the radiation is interacting, of course.

Both of these issues are addressed by cylindrical geometry. Similar to a cylindrical ionization chamber, a proportional counter is cylinder-shaped, but its mechanics are designed to tolerate higher electric potentials.

In proportional counters, increasing the high voltage causes space charge to accumulate around the anode wire because heavy positive ions move more slowly. Ions are created at greater voltages and move much more slowly than electrons. The effective electric field intensity within the active volume is reduced as a result of the screening of the electrodes. When this occurs, it is no longer possible to ensure that the deposited energy is proportional to the height of the pulse. As a result, the beginning of the region of limited proportionality is always used to operate the proportional counters.

4.5.1. Choice of Filling Gas

Proportional counters, like ionization chambers, are compatible with a wide variety of gases. Since gas multiplication is fundamental to the detector's ability to function as a proportional counter, this holds true for all gases and gas mixtures. Typically, an inert gas such as helium or argon is used due to its reasonably high atomic number. Some of the additional considerations that should be examined while selecting a filling gas are outlined below.

4.5.2. Avalanche Multiplication Threshold

For each given gas at a given pressure, there exists a critical electric potential below which the Avalanche does not occur. This limit varies with the nature of the gas and the pressure at which it is being held.

It is common practice to employ a noble gas as the primary filling gas component since the threshold for gas multiplication in noble gases is substantially lower than in polyatomic gases [27]. Because of its relatively inexpensive price compared to other inert gases, argon is arguably the noble gas most frequently employed in proportional counters.

4.5.3. Quenching

The purpose of the quench gas is to mitigate the occurrence of multiple pulses induced by secondary electrons emitted from the cathode / reduce the effect of secondary pulses. In a proportional counter, the avalanche multiplication happens only in a small, contained area. But it produces a by-product that can set off more small-scale avalanches in the area. During the avalanche process, a photon is created with a wavelength somewhere in the ultraviolet part of the spectrum.

This de-excitation is the precise mechanism responsible for the emission of ultraviolet photons. by the molecules of the gas. Take argon as an illustration.

$\gamma + Ar \rightarrow e + AR^{+*}$ [Ionization]

$Ar^{+*} \rightarrow Ar^{+} + \gamma$ UV [De-excitation]

In the process of de-excitation, UV stands for the UV photon given off by argon.

In argon, these ultraviolet rays have a minimum energy of 11.6 eV. Unfortunately, the metals often used in proportional counters have an ionization potential lower than this energy [28]. As a result, a cathode wall may lose an electron if a UV photon hits it. The high electric field inside the chamber accelerates this electron between collisions with gas molecules if it enters the gas. As it gets closer to the anodec, it could potentially trigger another avalanche.

The addition of a gas component with a high absorption coefficient for UV photons is a simple solution to this issue. This is the case for polyatomic gases (like CH4) due to their many closely spaced vibrational and rotational energy levels. Polyatomic molecules typically dissolve following photon absorption, which can also be thought of as a non-radiative process. Secondary discharges can be reduced through a process known as quenching, and the agent employed for this purpose is known as a quencher. Quenching effect is represented in Figure 4.1.

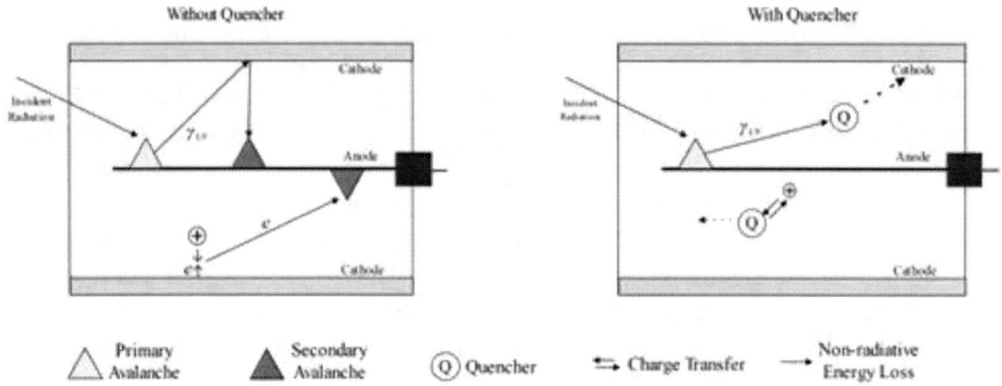

Figure 4.1. Positive effects of adding a quenching agent in a proportional counter.

4.5.4. Gas Gain

For choosing the Gas in a proportional chamber an important thing to consider is maximum attainable gain or multiplication factor. Most proportional counters have multiplication factor of the order of 10^4. If the voltage is raised to high values free electrons can cause multiple avalanches. Thus, we have to ensure that depletion happens time to time within a gas detector before these avalanches start to occur. A very good method of achieving this is addition of an electronegative impurity in the main filling gas. Freon is a good polyatomic gas [29]. The good thing about polyatomic gases is that they act both as electronegative impurities as well as quenchers.

Special Proportional Counters have been developed through these basic methods. Mostly they are named after the gas used in filling or the mechanism. A list of few of these counters is as follows:

- BF3 Proportional Counter
- Helium Proportional Counter
- Multi wire Proportional Counter

4.6. Geiger Muller Counters

When the voltage is increased to very high values, the process of avalanche multiplication starts and spreads throughout the detector. This produces breakdown in the gas, which is primarily attributed to ultraviolet photons emitted during the localized avalanches [30]. These photons posse's energies high enough to produce secondary electrons in the gas as well as in the electrodes and windows of the detector.

The electrons thus produced drift towards the anode under the influence of the effective field inside the chamber. The electric field is high enough for the electrons to attain high enough energy between the collisions to produce secondary avalanches. The secondary avalanche may produce more ultraviolet photons, which may produce more avalanches and so on.

This spread of avalanches throughout the detector volume is generally known as Geiger breakdown and the detector that behaves in this way is called a Geiger-Mueller or simply GM counter. The current flowing through the detector in this situation is extremely high and is limited only by the external circuitry. The voltage pulse is also quite high, generally of the order of several volts.

This is very adventitious as it eliminates the need for amplification. It is evident that the GM tubes cannot provide any information about the particle energy since every particle causing ionization in the gas produces the same pulse amplitude irrespective of its energy. Hence the GM detectors can be used for counting particles purposes only.

4.6.1. Pros and Cons of GM Counters

- Simple design: GM counters are perhaps the easiest to build and operate in terms of readout electronics.
- Resistance to environmental changes: Since the magnitude of the output pulse in GM detectors is very high, therefore they work almost independent of changes in temperature and pressure [31].
- The sensitive region of the GM counter operation is the plateau region where the count rate remains constant over a range of applied voltages.
- Following is some of the disadvantages of GM counters.
- Discrimination of Energy/Particle: The pulse height of the GM counters is not proportional to the energy deposited by the radiation and therefore they can not be used to measure dose or discriminate between types of radiations or their energies.
- Low dynamic range: The dead time losses in GM counters increase with radiation strength. The effect can be reduced by decreasing the size of the chamber, though at the expense of reduced sensitivity. Due to this the dynamic range of GM counters is very limited and the inability to measure high radiation rates due to the dead time of the tube.
- Quenching agents used in GM counters often decompose, which leads to the reduction in a lifetime.
- Dead Time: The process of dead time has been discussed earlier. This dead time plays an important role during the operation of GM counter. The dead time transform to the time between two consecutive pulses [32]. The dead time if very long, becomes a drawback for GM counters.

4.7. Liquid Filled Detectors

4.7.1. Charge Pair Generation and Recombination

The principal mechanism of liquid detector is the same as a gas filled detector. In liquids the energy needed to create a charge pair depends on the type of liquid used in the detector.

The creation of a charge pair in liquid is the same as in a gas. The energy states in liquid and gases are obviously different [33]. Liquids are having closely spaced and so the valence and conduction bands, which relates the energy required for electrons to move freely. When electrons become free, it simultaneously creates vacancies i.e., positive charge equivalent. Now as the incident radiation passes through the liquid it creates conducting electron-hole pairs.

Sometimes the electrons will occupy empty holes and diffuse by neutralizing. Thus, the atom will eventually de-excite by emitting in this process. This process is called recombination.

4.7.1.1. Drift of Charges

The drift velocity of electrons, is almost proportional to the applied electric field of the detector. Variety of drift velocities are observed for different noble gases and their mixtures. Drift velocity is affected by low electric field, it is slower. But at higher fields the relation between the field strength and drift velocity becomes less proportional and eventually independent.

In this non-linear behavior drift velocity is achieved by nonlinearity in the energy gained by electrons which is happening because of multiple collisions.

4.7.1.2. Liquid Ionization Chamber

Ionisation chamber is widely used in the liquid filled detectors category. These detectors are filled with liquid noble gases such as liquid argon. The favourable characteristics of liquid filled ionization chambers are enlisted below:

- *Stability:* These chambers are stable as less vulnerability is seen towards small degradation of the liquid with time, compared to other liquid detectors [34].
- *Proportionality:* Liquid ion chambers show excellent proportionality to the deposited energy.
- *Dynamic Range*: Liquid filled ionization chambers are best suited for moderate to high radiation fluxes.

Moreover, this chamber exhibits a favourable signal-to-noise ratio and effective water equivalence across a broad energy spectrum, rendering them a suitable choice for small active volume dosimeters. The basic principle of operation and construction of a liquid filled ionization chamber is the same as a gas filled ionization chamber. The entrant of radiation produces electron ion pairs. The resulting signal is measured at the anode.

4.7.1.3. Liquid Proportional Counters

Charge multiplication is a prerequisite for a detector to operate in the proportional region. Achieving charge multiplication in liquids is bit difficult as compared to gases. Nevertheless, several researchers have been successful in developing such detectors [35].

4.7.1.4. Cherenkov Detectors

Everyone is familiar with Cherenkov radiation in transparent media. The radiation detectors constructed on the basis of this phenomenon are called Cherenkov detectors. Let us see the emission process of Cherenkov radiation in brief.

When a charged particle in a medium moves faster than speed of light in that medium, it emits some radiation. These radiations are named as Cherenkov radiation.

Cherenkov radiation is composed of photons with wavelengths mostly in the visible region of the electromagnetic spectrum. The radiation is emitted in the shape of a cone with the path of the particle as its axis. The angle θ_c of the cone is related to the velocity v of the particle and the refractive index n of the medium. The angle of the cone is proportional to the energy of the particle producing the radiation [36].

A Cherenkov detector (basically a liquid filled detector) uses a liquid to produce Cherenkov light. This is again achieved by either interaction of particle to be detected and medium or by the generation of secondary particle and its further interaction. The light thus produced is detected by detectors surrounding the liquid. Though any type of detector can be used to detect light photons but the general practice is to use photomultiplier tubes due to their high photon detection efficiency.

4.7.1.5. Bubble Chamber

One of the earliest and extremely successful imaging detectors were Bubble chamber. The bubble chamber is a scientific instrument designed to detect and observe the paths of charged particles by capturing the tracks of bubbles that form in a liquefied gas, such as liquid hydrogen, contained within the chamber. This device was pioneered and developed by the physicist Donald Glaser in 1952. It was built such that it would track the particle in high energy collisions. The construction of a conventional bubble chamber consists of a sealed container filled with a liquefied gas, with an option to change the inside pressure quickly. Hydrogen and helium in their liquid states are the most prevalent liquids employed in bubble chambers. Additionally, a range of organic compounds can be utilized for applications demanding exceptionally dense liquids. While in operation one would momentarily superheat the fluid. When particles pass through this superheated fluid it would produce dense tracks of localized electron ion pairs. For the analysis of this the whole chamber would be illuminated and photographed with a high-definition camera. The photograph is then analyzed offline for particle identification and measurements. Particle identification is also possible through these chambers by simply applying an external magnetic field [37]. A disadvantage of bubble chambers is the difficulty in online analysis and triggering.

4.7.1.6. Liquid Scintillator Detectors

Liquid scintillation detectors offer a highly versatile solution for addressing a wide range of challenges in the field of nuclear radiation detection. Liquid scintillators operate on the principle of light emission by scintillation media when exposed to radiation. Later in the chapter scintillator detectors are discussed in detail [38].

4.8. Semiconductor Detectors

Semiconductors are solids with a crystalline structure and having electrical properties between conductors and insulators. Examples of pure semiconductors are Germanium (Ge) and Silicon (Si). GaAs is one of the materials that have shown to be very promising as an alternative to silicon, although at a much higher cost [39].

4.8.1. Structure of Semiconductors

Electrons in an atom occupy only discrete energy levels but when it comes to tightly bound solids, the discreteness is very much limited. These energy levels are grouped together in the broad energy levels called energy bands. The two bands involved in electrical properties are valence band and conduction band.

Valence band is a representation of a large number of very closely spaced energy levels at lower energies and conduction band is a representative of closely spaced energy levels at higher energies [40].

These bands have a considerable energy gap between them called as forbidden gap.

The valence band electrons are tightly bound to the atoms and need at least an energy equal to the band gap to move to the conduction band. The conduction band electrons are very loosely bound and are almost free to move around. The conduction band electrons take place in electrical conduction process.

When an electron from the valence band jumps to the conduction band, it leaves a net positive charge behind. This effective positive charge, called a hole, behaves like a real particle, and takes part in electrical conduction process. However, it should be noted that by movement of a hole we mean the shift of a net positive charge from one site to another due to the movement of an electron. A hole should not be considered a localized positive charge having defined mass.

4.8.2. Mechanism and Statistics of Electron-Hole Pair Production

When Radiation passes through a semiconductor material it causes the following phenomenon: Lattice Excitation takes place when the incident radiation deposits energy to the lattice increasing the lattice vibrations.

- Ionization in semiconductors happens when an electron hole pair.
- Atomic Displacement is a non-ionizing phenomenon occurring in the bulk and causing damage.
- In semiconductor detectors we are interested in the ionization process.

From the above explanation of the lattice structure we can conclude that in semiconductors (just like gases) the average energy needed to create an electron hole pair is independent of the type of radiation and totally depends on the semiconductor material and environmental conditions like temperature.

The process of ionisation is similar to the ionization process of gases but the number of charge carriers produced by radiation in a semiconductor is much higher than in gases [41]. Also, the energy required is approximately 4 to 8 times less than in gases. This property of the semiconductor detectors makes them far superior than gaseous detectors in terms of sensitivity.

4.8.2.1. Recombination

This recombination process is not very unique, a conduction band electron can immediately recombine with a valence band hole. In this example, the positive charge is a hole rather than an ion, but otherwise the process is similar to the electron-ion recombination we examined in the chapter on gas-filled detectors. In the end, one electron leaves the conduction band and a hole enters the valence band as a result of the process. It is important to keep in mind that, contrary to popular belief, the electron retains its specified mass throughout this process. Recombination does not destroy anything. The free electron is not changed in any way by being temporarily housed in the valence band. Electron-hole recombination is a complex process due to the fact that it occurs through multiple routes.

4.8.2.2. Conductivity of Charges

An external field can cause the free charges in a semiconductor to move around. Conductivity, which measures a material's capacity to conduct electric current, can also be used to characterize their motion, just as it can with metallic conductors. In contrast to metallic conductors, semiconductors can either have their conductivity enhanced or dampened by a variety of ways. The following are examples of some of these elements.

An electron in the conduction band can recombine with a hole in the valence band if it drops into the intermediate energy state. The net result of this operation is a reduction in the current and the elimination of one electron-hole pair from the free charge density [42].

Through a process called "hole emission," an electron in the valence band might go up to the next energy level. Since this result in a hole being left behind in the valence band instead of an electron, it can also be thought of as the emission of a hole from an intermediate energy level into the valence band.

In the process of electron emission, one electron from the valence band moves into the conduction band, where it contributes to the free charge density and, in turn, the current.

An electron can be imprisoned for a certain length of time if it drops to an energy level just below the conduction band. The time lag between when an electron is trapped and when it is released has the potential to introduce nonlinearity into the response.

4.8.2.3. Drift of Holes and Electrons

So-called photoconductive mode operation is the norm for semiconductor detectors. Creating an electric field across the material is a necessary step in this process. Electric fields cause charges to move in opposite directions when incident radiation creates electron hole pairs along the path of the detector. The speed at which the charges move is determined by the strength of the electric field. It has been discovered that for weak fields, the speed grows approximately linearly with the field strength.

The carriers' velocities begin to deviate from the aforementioned relation when the field is raised, and they eventually reach a maximum value. The charges in most detectors can reach saturation velocity in a negligible amount of time (picoseconds) [43].

4.9. Radiation-Detection: Optimal Materials

Radiation detectors cannot be made from just any semiconductor. Factors including resistivity, charge mobility, drift velocity, purity, operating temperature, and cost must all be considered. Although silicon has long been the go-to for particle detectors, other materials are beginning to gain ground. The elements germanium (Ge), gallium arsenide (GaAs), and cadmium, zinc, and tellurium (CdZnTe) are also frequently employed. Researchers are being pushed to design more complicated semiconductor structures as they work to create the next generation of radiation resistant silicon detectors. In this article, we will examine some semiconductor materials that are now in wide usage and learn about their features that make them suitable for use as radiation detectors. The goal of this exercise is to provide the reader with sufficient background knowledge to make an informed decision when choosing between these materials as detection medium.

The intrinsic carrier concentration of semiconductor materials is crucial because it can be used to approximate the signal-to-noise ratio at standard laboratory conditions. In contrast to silicon and germanium, the intrinsic carrier concentrations in GaAs and CdZnTe are much lower. This feature allows them to be used in environments where the temperature is always above freezing, which is both convenient and cost-effective. Therefore, detectors based on GaAs and CdZnTe have seen significant growth in popularity in recent years.

4.9.1. PN Junction

The pn-junction is formed when n- and p-type semiconductors are linked together. Radiation detector technology has also discovered these junctions to be incredibly beneficial in the construction of semiconductor circuits [44]. Because of the disparity in charge concentration across the junction, a current begins to flow when a p- and n-type semiconductor are brought together. In n-type semiconductors, electrons, which make up the vast majority of charge carriers, go in the direction of p-type material. The holes also tend to migrate towards the n-type part of the material.

An area devoid of electrical charges is formed as electrons and holes flow in opposite directions and cooperate to neutralize one another. Since electron hole pairs are created by incident radiation in this region—commonly referred to as the depletion region—it plays a crucial function in semiconductor radiation detectors. This current, made up of charges moving in opposite directions, can be measured. Unfortunately, the junction in this setup is not optimal for radiation detection for two reasons: (1) it is very thin, and (2) the potential difference across it is quite little. The challenge then is to increase the size of this chasm and set up an electric field strong enough to carry the charges generated by the radiation. To achieve this, a negative bias is applied across the junction. In the following paragraphs, I will elaborate on the features and qualities that define this type of junction.

There is something worth mentioning before we go any farther. It is not totally accurate to say that the depletion region is charge-free. There are always crystal defects and impurities, regardless of how high quality the semiconductor material is, and these introduce energy levels within the band gap. When electrons find such energy levels, they can use them to escape the valence band and enter the conduction band above. An electron-hole pair is produced as a result [45]. Some electrons can gain enough energy from thermal agitation to jump to the conduction band even if we believe the material is free of crystal defects and impurities. In conclusion, there are still some free charges present in the depletion region. However, there are only a tiny fraction of these charges, and the resulting current is negligible. To avoid current flow, there must be no free charges in the depletion region when a reverse bias is applied. However, a negligible current is always detected since free charge pairs exist. Dark or reverse current is the common name for this type of current.

4.9.2. Features of a PN-Diode with a Forward Bias

Generally, a PN diode works like a closed circuit in forward biased mode when operated beyond the barrier potential. For radiation detection the barrier is overcome by electron hole pairs produced by radiation. The incoming radiation creates electron-hole pairs in the depletion zone, which acts as the active medium. In the absence of radiation, this region almost completely lacks free charge carriers, resulting in negligible leakage current. A measurable electric current is produced when the charge pairs generated by the radiation move in opposing directions in response to the effective junction electric field. This current is proportional to the amount of energy deposited by the radiation under optimal working circumstances such as temperature.

The effective electric field intensity, capacitance, and the depth of the depletion region all have a role in the output signal and dynamic range of a semiconductor detector [46].

4.9.3. Modes of Operation of PN-Diode

PN-diodes have two main modes of operation, photovoltaic and photoconductive. Although semiconductor detectors are typically run in the photoconductive mode, a detector that runs in the photovoltaic mode is both theoretically and practically feasible to construct. The next two paragraphs will elaborate on these two modes. However, we will not devote much effort to discussing the photovoltaic mode because it is not particularly relevant to radiation detectors.

4.10. Thermoluminescent Detectors

Thermoluminescent dosimeters are passive radiation detection devices most commonly used to monitor individual occupational radiation exposure or measure patient radiation dose. The term thermoluminescence refers to the emission of light that is induced by temperature changes [47]. Radiation dose information can be stored in a thermoluminescent (TL) material for a lengthy period of time, or until the material is heated above a particular threshold. In the early 1950s, scientists discovered that TL materials may be used as radiation detectors. Since then, such detectors have seen widespread use in dosimetry for individuals.

4.10.1. Thermoluminescence: Principle

We observed how crystal defects and impurities in semiconductors and diamond can lead to energy levels outside the forbidden gap in the previous sections. These concentrations are undesirable in radiation detectors because they can behave as electron traps, distorting the signal. Even if TL materials also include similar layers, in this case the storage of information is an advantage [48].

4.10.2. TLD Badge or Thermoluminescent Dosimeter

Since 1975, the CaSO4: Dy Teflon disc-based TLD badge has been in widespread use for Personnel Monitoring. When used to track beta and gamma radiation exposure, the TLD badge has proven reliable. TLD monitoring service currently protects around 40,000 nuclear, medical, industrial, and research institution employees from radiation exposure.

A TLD card and a plastic cassette are both necessary components of a Personnel Monitoring TLD badge. The badge has a crocodile clip on the back that allows it to be connected to a person's clothing.

The most popular type of dosimeter is a film badge. They detect gamma, x-ray, and high-energy beta radiation and are worn externally. A badge is an inconspicuous piece of photographic film with an opaque cover that is encased in a metal badge holder. It can be attached to garments or worn as a ring. The film is exposed by the interaction of radiation with its atomic structure. The radiation exposure is measured by removing the film at regular intervals and developing it. Radiation exposure can be tracked indefinitely with a film badge.

Radiation levels of gamma, x-ray, and beta can all be measured with TLDs. They come in handy as rings or as tattoos. Small chips of lithium fluoride inside them can deflect electrons from their ground state when exposed to ionizing radiation. As a result, the electrons enter a metastable condition, from which they can be released back to their ground state by applying heat. When warmed, the electrons fall back to the ground state, releasing photons [49]. The light emitted from the chips is measured using a TLD readout equipment. Radiation dose absorbed by the TLD and the individual's dose of radiation exposure are both factors in the amount of light emitted. TLDs are slowly replacing film credits.

A pocket dosimeter is a small, portable device that looks like a fountain pen and may be clipped to a pocket for easy viewing. X-ray and gamma radiation detectors are often worn on the upper back. It is intended to be used in addition to a TLD, not in instead of one. The dosimeter for your pocket includes an ionization chamber, a scale, a lens for viewing the quartz fiber as it moves across the scale, and a scale. The quartz fiber receives an electrostatic charge until the meter reads zero. Some of the air molecules inside the dosimeter's chamber get ionized when it is subjected to radiation. This results in a proportional release of static electricity from the quartz fiber in response to the intensity of the radiation. As the charge is discharged, the fiber will shift to a new location on the radiation exposure scale.

The fundamental benefit of the pocket dosimeter over the film badge or TLD is that the user can examine the readings instantly, even while in a radiation-contaminated area. However, pocket dosimeters may provide an inaccurate reading of radiation exposure due to their electrical charge depletion. Two dosimeters should be used whenever possible to rule out the possibility of an inaccurate reading. The lower reading is more likely to reflect the true level of exposure [50].

Applications:

- Radiographic installations in healthcare (diagnostic and therapeutic) and industry: a geographic survey.
- Measuring the amount of radiation that escapes from the housing of X-ray generators.
- High beta source contamination must be watched for.
- Studies of population exposure to radiation from medical radiography and other sources.
- Calculating predicted brachytherapy and nuclear medicine radioactive isotope activity.
- Cobalt on Cesium implants are used to treat cancer of the uterine cervix, and patients having this treatment will have their rectum and bladder monitored for radiation exposure.
- Personnel monitoring

4.11. Scintillation Detectors

Scintillation materials work on a very basic principle: incoming radiation transfers some of its energy to the material's atoms when they collide. Therefore, these atoms enter transient excited states. Photons are emitted in the visible and ultraviolet ranges when they return to the ground state. This offers a replacement for ionization as a method of radiation detection and measurement [51].

4.11.1. Scintillation Detection of Radiation Entails the Following Fundamental Steps

- Radiation's effect on scintillating substances.
- Energy is transferred to the material's bound states.
- As the excited states return to the ground state, photons of light are released.
- The photodetector is accumulating photons.
- The signal from the photodetector is picked up by the circuitry.

Scintillation is not a highly efficient process because a typical scintillation material only has a 10% to 15% efficiency at emitting light after absorbing radiation. As we shall show, however, even with such a poor material, a highly effective radiation detector can be created. The key is to employ a very efficient photon detector for this purpose. The two main detectors for scintillation photons are photomultiplier tubes and photodiodes, both of which will be discussed in this chapter.

The scintillation photon is converted into an electron, and then this electron is multiplied into a very large number of electrons, according to the basic working principle of a photomultiplier tube (PMT). The photoelectric effect takes place in a thin material called a photocathode, where photons are converted into electrons. A huge number of electrons are released when photocathode-generated electrons are propelled toward a metallic structure known as a dynode. After being driven toward another dynode, these secondary electrons further increase in number. By recirculating the electrons via the dynodes, the process can be repeated multiple times. The completed process yields an output pulse with a sizable enough amplitude to be readily detected by the connected electronics. A PMT's gain can be greater than 105, making it a desirable tool for highly precise measurements. The negative is the conventional photoelectrode's low quantum efficiency of roughly 20% in the photon-electron conversion process. This means that almost 80% of the photons produced by scintillation are lost.

The photodiode detector is another option for picking up the photons given off by scintillation sources [52]. As we learned in the section on semiconductor detectors, a photodiode consists of a semiconductor that has been suitably doped. The scintillation photon creates electron-hole pairs in this detector, as opposed to single electrons in a PMT photocathode. Photodiodes are highly desirable due to their high quantum efficiency, which can reach up to 80% in low-radiation settings. Avalanche photodiodes are a specialized type of photodiode detector that can be used to take highly sensitive measurements in very weak radiation sources. The electron-hole pairs created by the incident radiation are amplified in such a device via an avalanche process. This mechanism is similar to electron multiplication in a PMT, but without the usage of dynode-like mechanical structures, the system is more robust against mechanical shocks. The electron hole multiplication ultimately raises a weak signal to a level where it may be detected by electronic equipment. Since photodetectors play such a crucial role in scintillation detectors, they warrant close study. Therefore, we will spend some time in the later parts of this chapter talking about the principles of operation, structures, benefits, and drawbacks of certain regularly used photodetectors.

4.11.2. Scintillation Mechanism and Scintillator Properties

Although there is a wide variety of scintillation materials available, they can be roughly classified as either organic or inorganic. The characteristics of these two types of materials will be discussed. We will examine why some scintillators are better suited for some uses than others. But first, let us take a high-level look at the salient features of scintillation materials that are pertinent to their application as radiation detectors.

- **Organic Scintillators**

Radiation detectors rely heavily on organic scintillators [53]. They can exist as a solid, a liquid, or a gas. Organic scintillators have the benefit of being able to be manufactured in almost any geometry, making them highly adaptable.

4.11.3. Scintillation Mechanism

Organic scintillators work through fluorescence or instantaneous emission of light after electronic transitions to the S state. Understanding the usual energy level diagram of organic scintillators is essential to grasping the nature of this activity. Electronic transitions from S0 ground levels to various vibrational levels in the S1 band (higher band transitions are of course also conceivable depending on the energy of the incident radiation) are triggered when the radiation imparts energy to the atoms.

Because of the generated instability, electrons in higher S1 vibrational states must descend to the S1 ground state via radiation-free transitions. Within a millisecond or two, these changes will have taken place. The electrons then decay into the S0 ground and vibrational levels, a process that takes many nanoseconds. Fluorescence photons, which are generated when electrons have more energy than they need, can be found, for the most part, in the ultraviolet or visible area of the electromagnetic spectrum. It is advantageous for scintillation detectors for electrons to decay from S1 vibrational states to S1 base level. This is because electrons lose energy whenever they undergo such decays. Since they absorb more energy during their radiation-induced transition from the S0 ground level to the S1 levels than they release during their S1 ground level to S0 level transitions, they emit less energy overall. This suggests that such materials have mismatched absorption and emission spectra, which works against the re-absorption of scintillation light. Sir George G. Stokes was the first to notice this phenomenon, and his subsequent formulation of a Stoke's law is named after him. Now that we have covered the fundamentals of how organic scintillators work, we can talk about the various forms these materials can take.

The three organic scintillators listed below are among the most common types used in radiation detectors used.

- Scintillators made of plastic
- Scintillating liquids
- Scintillating crystals

- **Plastic Scintillators**

Plastic scintillators have several uses and are widely available. They are manufactured artificially via a lengthy and laborious process.

However, the concept itself is straightforward: just combine the scintillator with a suitable base and proceed to polymerize the resulting mixture. However, things are not quite so easy in practice. Two major challenges are the need for extremely pure components and the need for substantial downtime between processes to allow the material to settle into the desired configuration [54]. Acrylic, polystyrene, or polyvinyltoluene monomer are commonly employed as the mixture's foundation. This base is then combined with a readily available scintillator. It just takes a small amount of this primary scintillator—about 1% by weight of the mixture—to generate a significant amount of usable light. Another scintillator is typically added to the mixture as well. In a moment, we will dive into the specific functions of each of these components. The plastic begins as a mixture that is polymerized. Many desirable features can be found in a plastic scintillator made using this process.

- As a chemical, it is very reliable,
- It is very optically consistent, and
- It is malleable enough to be sliced and milled into almost any form.

- **Liquid Scintillators**

Several different liquids can be employed as detectors since they emit scintillation light. The following three organic substances are typically found in liquid scintillators used in detecting systems [55].

- *The primary fluor*, also known as primary scintillator, is the most prominent scintillator in the compound. The light it emits, however, is in the ultraviolet portion of the electromagnetic spectrum, despite its high scintillation efficiency.
- *Wavelength Shifter*: UV photons emitted by the main fluor have low attenuation lengths in liquid, making a wavelength shifter an ideal solution. Most of them are trapped because the liquid is not totally transparent to them. The wavelength shifter brings these photons into the visible spectrum by modifying their wavelength. Since the wavelength shifters are scintillators that take up UV radiation and emit visible light, they are also frequently referred to as "secondary fluor." Blue light is the result of most practical wavelength changers.
- *Base Liquid*: A liquid with good light transmission qualities is used to create a homogeneous mixture of the aforementioned scintillators. The standards of purity for the ingredients of liquid scintillators are similarly rigorous to those of plastic scintillators because their basic building blocks are basically identical. All of the components, including the base, main fluor, and wavelength shifter, must be used in their purest forms. The scintillator's light-transmitting characteristics can be severely diminished by even trace levels of water.

Many different types of liquids, both pure and mixed, have been shown to be effective scintillators with features that make them useful for radiation detection. No generic names have been allocated to these fluids, however many of them are sold under brand names in commercial settings. The majority of liquid scintillators have their peak emission between 400 and 500 nm.

When it comes to temperature, most liquid scintillators are remarkably stable. Temperature fluctuations of less than 1 degree Celsius each decade is not unusual. There is a wide variation in the light yield of liquid scintillators, from around 50% to 80% of anthracene, however most producers create goods in the middle of that range. There is a close correlation between the dye content and the light output. As a result, optimizing dye concentrations according to system needs has become standard practice.

Large volume detectors have found great success with the use of organic liquid scintillators. The liquid's mass can be several hundred tons in neutrino detection investigations, for instance [56].

We have observed that contamination by outside elements is a serious issue with liquid scintillators. The scintillation properties of the liquid may degrade, and the transmission qualities of the scintillation light may be altered, by certain pollutants. When it comes to the second type of contamination, water is by far the most common. A liquid scintillator's light emission qualities can be severely diminished by even trace amounts of dissolved water. Thankfully, most liquid scintillators, especially those based on mineral oil, are not easily dissolved in water. However, because to the seriousness of water contamination's consequences, care must be taken to prevent the liquid from coming into contact with water under any circumstances. Moisture inside the container is a regular issue when working with a liquid scintillator. Water and other pollutants can be slowly dissolved in the liquid if the container is not properly cleaned and dried, reducing the liquid's efficiency over time.

Liquid scintillators are susceptible to contamination from atmospheric oxygen, which can dampen their luminescence. Air pollution, even at low concentrations, has been shown to reduce light production by 20-30%. Since it is nearly impossible to keep scintillators away from air or oxygen, it is standard practice to de-oxygenate the liquid at least once before putting it in a detector. The technique is fairly straightforward: just slowly circulate dry nitrogen through the liquid, and the oxygen will be bubbled out. After this is done, the liquid must not come into contact with air oxygen and must be stored in an atmosphere of highly purified nitrogen, argon, or another inert gas.

- **Inorganic Scintillators**

Crystalline structures are typical of inorganic scintillators. The atomic number and density of these materials are both higher than those of organic scintillators. Because of this, they are appealing for uses that call for a high capacity to deflect incident radiation. Their increased luminosity compared to organic scintillators is still another benefit [57].

4.11.4. Mechanism for Scintillation

4.11.4.1. Exciton Luminescence

Ionizing radiation creates electron hole pairs in an inorganic scintillator crystal. The pair can become completely free to travel about the molecule, or they can stay partially bound by the Coulomb attraction, depending on how much energy is lost to the molecule.

If the electron's energy is high enough, it can leave the valence band and enter the conduction band, where it is effectively unconstrained. As a result, the hole, which has an effective positive charge, gains the freedom to move about as well. However, if the departing energy is not particularly great, the electron remains only weakly connected to the hole. This can be thought of as the electron transitioning to a band below the conduction band.

However, the link between the electron and hole is weak because the electron can jump to the conduction band with only a minor increase in energy. Exciton is the name given to the system formed when an electron and a hole are bonded together. Interesting properties of excitons include their freedom of movement across a material and their susceptibility to confinement at impurity or defect sites.

When an electron drops to a lower energy level, scintillation photons may be released if the place in question comprises a bright center. Another mechanism for exciton trapping is charge transfer, in which case the resulting light is referred to as charge transfer luminescence.

4.11.4.2. Dopant Luminescence

Some scintillators have an impurity or dopant added to them in order to boost their scintillation capabilities. Scintillation light is produced when an electron is captured in a dopant level and then decays to a lower luminescence level.

4.11.4.3. Core Valence Band Luminescence

By depositing enough energy along its path into the lattice, incoming radiation can promote electrons from the deep core valence band to the conduction band. When an electron departs the central valence band, it creates a vacancy, also known as a hole [58].

A valence band electron swiftly moves into this vacant slot to restore system stability. This causes scintillation light to be released. Core valence band luminescence is the common name for this phenomenon.

Following is a list of commonly used inorganic scintillators:

- Thallium Doped Sodium Iodide (NaI: T l)
- Sodium Doped Cesium Iodide (CsI: Na)
- Thallium Doped Cesium Iodide (CsI: T l)
- Bismuth Germanate (BGO)
- Cadmium Tungstate (CWO)
- Lead Tungstate (PWO)
- Cerium Doped Gadolinium Silicate (GSO)
- Liquid Xenon

4.12. Exposure Measurement

Thimble chambers with an exposure calibration factor traceable to the NIST allow for accurate measurements of radiation exposure in roentgen. The chamber is positioned at the measurement site with its axis parallel to the beam axis, just as it was during the chamber calibration.

Care is necessary to ensure that no media besides air is present in the immediate proximity of the chamber, as this could cause radiation scattering. Exposure can be calculated from the chamber reading using the formula X = M * NX * PT, P * PST * Pion * where X is exposure in roentgens (R), M is the chamber reading (coulombs) measured under equilibrium conditions and corrected for any polarity effect, NX is the chamber exposure calibration factor (roentgen per coulomb) for the given quality beam. If the chamber were not present, the exposure measured at the point X would be the same as if it were measured in air. In other words, the chamber calibration factor NX already includes the correction for any disruption in the beam caused by the presence of the chamber. Thimble chambers are often utilized without a build-up cap and calibrated for low-energy beams such as superficial and orthovoltage x-rays. In order to calibrate the chamber and take exposure measurements in a specific beam, higher energy sources like cobalt-60 require the use of a Lucite (acrylic) accumulation cover [59]. Summary of the detectors and their specifications is given in Table 4.

Thus, exposure can be measured using a gas filled detector and absorbed dose can be calculated afterwards using other factors.

Table 4.1. Commonly used detectors weighted according to their performance

Class	Subclass	Comment (Technical)	Comment (Application)
Gas phase	Ionization chambers	Gas phase counters generally comprise a central anode and surrounding cathode.	Calibrates isotope yields in production processes and dose rate measurements in industrial plants, nuclear power plants, reprocessing plants, etc.
	Xe high-pressure ionization chambers	Detectors built with operating pressures up to 50 atm. Energy resolutions in the range of 2% to 3% at 662 keV achieved.	Detectors are rugged, thermally stable, and operate at room temperature.
	Proportional	Filled with a gas (e.g., Ar, 90% and CO_2, 10%) or P10 and operates at a higher voltage field than an ionization chamber.	Measures ionizing radiation and neutrons (when BF_3 is the counting gas).
	G-M counter	Operates at a still higher voltage field than a proportional counter.	Detects α and β^- particles and (with less efficiency) γ radiation.
Scintillation (solid)	NaI (Tl)	Sodium iodide crystals have a density of 3.67 and the highest light conversion efficiency of common scintillator materials.	Detectors are rugged, highly efficient, and are commonly used in field detection applications.
	BGO	Bismuth germinate (BGO) has a density of 7.13, but a light conversion efficiency only 15% to 20% that of NaI (Tl).	BGO detectors operate at room temperature, but have a higher energy resolution than sodium iodide.
	Plastic scintillators	Organic crystals, e.g., anthracene, dissolved in polystyrene or polyvinyl toluene. Typically, they have a light conversion efficiency 25% to 50% that of NaI (Tl).	Although the density of the materials is close to unity, they may be machined into large dimensions and complex shapes.
	$LaCl_3(Ce)$, $LaBr_3(Ce)$	Cerium-doped lanthanum halides have higher light output, higher density, comparable energy resolution to NaI (Tl), and good temperature stability (Pirard et al., 2005).	Modern detector material under ongoing development.
Scintillation (liquid)	Organic	Formerly, benzene was widely used for ^{14}C dating as it has good optical properties and C/CO_2 can be converted to benzene in high yield. Now largely replaced by accelerator mass spectrometry.	Very widely used in biochemical and related tracer studies, particularly of tritium or ^{14}C-labelled organic compounds.
	Aq. emulsions	A range of scintillant 'cocktails' comprising solutes, scintillation agents, and blending agents form emulsions with the aqueous test sample.	Routinely used for the measurement of tritiated water and the radioactivity levels of β^- and α emitting aqueous solutes.
Semi-conductor	HPGe	High-resolution γ spectrometry over an energy range of 40 keV to > 10 MeV.	Used to identify and measure complex mixtures of gamma emitting radionuclides.
	Silicon	Si (Li) X-ray detectors (a few hundred eV to 50 keV or so). Modern passivated implantation Si detectors are used for α particle detection.	Used, e.g., X-ray fluorescence, X-ray microanalysis, PIXE, and X-ray diffraction.

Conclusion

This chapter presented a comprehensive overview of radiation detection principles and the wide range of detectors used in radiation measurement. From gas-filled detectors like ionization chambers, proportional counters, and Geiger-Mueller tubes to liquid detectors, scintillation counters, semiconductor detectors, thermoluminescent dosimeters, and Cherenkov detectors, each method offers unique strengths and limitations depending on the application. The operating principles, advantages, drawbacks, and key design considerations were discussed in detail, highlighting how innovations in materials and electronics have continually advanced detector performance, sensitivity, and reliability. Understanding these detection technologies is fundamental to ensuring accurate radiation monitoring, effective dosimetry, and protection in medical, industrial, and research environments.

References

[1] Allen AO. Radiation chemistry of aqueous solutions. *The Journal of Physical Chemistry.* 1948 Mar;52(3):479-90.

[2] Saito N, Suzuki IH. Fine structure near the CK edge in the photon W-value of methane. *Chemical physics.* 1986 Oct 1;108(2):327-33.

[3] McLean FB, Oldham TR. Basic mechanisms of radiation effects in electronic materials and devices. Harry Diamond Laboratories *Technical Report.* 1987 Sep 1:2129.

[4] Toyoda N, Yamada I. Gas cluster ion beam equipment and applications for surface processing. *IEEE Transactions on plasma science.* 2008 Aug 12;36(4):1471-88.

[5] Scally S, Davison W, Zhang H. Diffusion coefficients of metals and metal complexes in hydrogels used in diffusive gradients in thin films. *Analytica Chimica Acta.* 2006 Feb 3;558(1-2):222-9.

[6] Acosta RH, Agulles-Pedrós L, Komin S, Sebastiani D, Spiess HW, Blümler P. Diffusion in binary gas mixtures studied by NMR of hyperpolarized gases and molecular dynamics simulations. *Physical Chemistry Chemical Physics.* 2006;8(36):4182-8.

[7] Caridi EA, Chang TY, Goossen KW, Eastman LF. Direct demonstration of a misfit strain-generated electric field in a [111] growth axis zinc-blende heterostructure. *Applied physics letters.* 1990 Feb 12;56(7):659-61.

[8] Kemmer J, Lutz G. New detector concepts. *Nuclear Instruments and Methods in Physics Research Section A: Accelerators, Spectrometers, Detectors and Associated Equipment.* 1987 Jan 15;253(3):365-77.

[9] Parsai EI, Shvydka D, Kang J. Design, and optimization of large area thin-film CdTe detector for radiation therapy imaging applications. *Medical physics.* 2010 Aug;37(8):3980-94.

[10] Steinhauser G, Buchtela K. Gas ionization detectors. In *Handbook of Radioactivity Analysis* 2020 Jan 1 (pp. 245-305). Academic Press.

[11] Fridman A, Chirokov A, Gutsol A. Non-thermal atmospheric pressure discharges. *Journal of Physics D: Applied Physics.* 2005 Jan 6;38(2): R1.

[12] Fleischer RL, Price PB, Walker RM. Ion explosion spike mechanism for formation of charged-particle tracks in solids. *Journal of applied Physics.* 1965 Nov 1;36(11):3645-52.

[13] Cartiglia N, Arcidiacono R, Baselga M, Bellan R, Boscardin M, Cenna F, Dalla Betta GF, Fernndez-Martnez P, Ferrero M, Flores D, Galloway Z. Design optimization of ultra-fast silicon detectors. *Nuclear Instruments and Methods in Physics Research Section A: Accelerators, Spectrometers, Detectors and Associated Equipment.* 2015 Oct 1; 796:141-8.

[14] Ahmed SN. *Physics and engineering of radiation detection.* Academic Press; 2007 Apr 12.

[15] Höbel M, Ricka J. Dead-time and afterpulsing correction in multiphoton timing with nonideal detectors. *Review of scientific instruments.* 1994 Jul 1;65(7):2326-36.

[16] Langmuir I. The pressure effect and other phenomena in gaseous discharges. *Journal of the Franklin Institute*. 1923 Dec 1;196(6):751-62.

[17] Stéphan C. Gas filled detectors. *Experimental techniques in nuclear physics*. 1997:57.

[18] Muir B, Nahum A. Ionisation Chambers. In *Handbook of Radiotherapy Physics* 2021 Dec 30 (pp. Vol1-321). CRC Press.

[19] Chuklyaev SV, Koshelev AS. Gas-Filled Ionization Chamber and Secondary-Emission Detector for Measuring γ-Ray Dose Rate. *Atomic Energy*. 2020 Jul;128(3):166-70.

[20] Peisert A, Charpak G, Sauli F, Viezzoli G. Development of a multistep parallel-plate chamber as time projection chamber end-cap or vertex detector. *IEEE Transactions on Nuclear Science*. 1984 Feb;31(1):125-8.

[21] Egerton RF, Li P, Malac M. *Radiation damage in the TEM and SEM. Micron*. 2004 Aug 1;35(6):399-409.

[22] Karalis A, Joannopoulos JD, Soljačić M. Efficient wireless non-radiative mid-range energy transfer. *Annals of physics*. 2008 Jan 1;323(1):34-48.

[23] Kubáň P, Hauser PC. Fundamental aspects of contactless conductivity detection for capillary electrophoresis. Part II: Signal-to-noise ratio and stray capacitance. *Electrophoresis*. 2004 Oct;25(20):3398-405.

[24] Curran SC, Cockroft AL, Angus J. LXXXVI. Investigation of soft radiation by proportional counters—V. Use as a detector of ultra-violet quanta and analysis of the gas multiplication process. *The London, Edinburgh, and Dublin Philosophical Magazine and Journal of Science*. 1949 Sep 1;40(308):929-37.

[25] Ziegler JF, Lanford WA. Effect of cosmic rays on computer memories. *Science*. 1979 Nov 16;206(4420):776-88.

[26] Yue GZ, Qiu Q, Gao B, Cheng Y, Zhang J, Shimoda H, Chang S, Lu JP, Zhou O. Generation of continuous and pulsed diagnostic imaging x-ray radiation using a carbon-nanotube-based field-emission cathode. *Applied Physics Letters*. 2002 Jul 8;81(2):355-7.

[27] Friedman H. Geiger counter tubes. *Proceedings of the IRE*. 1949 Jul;37(7):791-808.

[28] Sauli F. *Gaseous radiation detectors: fundamentals and applications*. Cambridge University Press; 2015.

[29] Vasilyev VA, Lévay B, Minkova A, Petrukhin VI, Horváth D. Atomic capture and transfer of negative pions stopped in binary mixtures of hydrogen with polyatomic gases. *Nuclear Physics A*. 1985 Dec 23;446(3-4):613-22.

[30] Charpak G, Sauli F. The multistep avalanche chamber: a new high-rate, high-accuracy gaseous detector. *Physics Letters B*. 1978 Oct 9;78(4):523-8.

[31] Foster B, Malos J, Saxon DH, Clark DE, Jamdani AK, Markou C, Miller DB, Miller DG, Roundup LW, Auty CG, Blair GA. The design and construction of the ZEUS central tracking detector. *Nuclear Instruments and Methods in Physics Research Section A: Accelerators, Spectrometers, Detectors and Associated Equipment*. 1994 Jan 15;338(2-3):254-83.

[32] Müller JW. Dead-time problems. *Nuclear Instruments and Methods*. 1973 Sep 1;112(1-2):47-57.

[33] Miyajima M, Takahashi T, Konno S, Hamada T, Kubota S, Shibamura H, Doke T. Average energy expended per ion pair in liquid argon. *Physical Review A*. 1974 Mar 1;9(3):1438.

[34] Asaadi J, Conrad JM, Gollapinni S, Jones BJ, Jostlein H, St John JM, Strauss T, Wolbers S, Zennamo J. Testing of high voltage surge protection devices for use in liquid argon TPC detectors. *Journal of Instrumentation*. 2014 Sep 2;9(09): P09002.

[35] Pinto SD. Gas electron multipliers. Development of large area GEMS and spherical GEMS.

[36] Gray LH. The absorption of penetrating radiation. *Proceedings of the Royal Society of London. Series A, Containing Papers of a Mathematical and Physical Character*. 1929 Feb 1;122(790):647-68.

[37] Williams MC. Particle identification using time of flight. *Journal of Physics G: Nuclear and Particle Physics*. 2012 Oct 19;39(12):123001.

[38] Beddar S, Tendler I, Therriault-Proulx F, Archambault L, Beaulieu L. Recent advances and clinical applications of plastic scintillators in the field of radiation therapy. *Plastic Scintillators: Chemistry and Applications*. 2021 Jul 11:425-60.

[39] Owens A, Peacock A. Compound semiconductor radiation detectors. *Nuclear Instruments and Methods in Physics Research Section A: Accelerators, Spectrometers, Detectors and Associated Equipment*. 2004 Sep 21;531(1-2):18-37.

[40] An JM, Franceschetti A, Dudiy SV, Zunger A. The peculiar electronic structure of PbSe quantum dots. *Nano Letters*. 2006 Dec 13;6(12):2728-35.

[41] Pearton SJ, Ren F, Patrick E, Law ME, Polyakov AY. Ionizing radiation damage effects on GaN devices. *ECS Journal of solid-state science and technology*. 2015 Nov 24;5(2): Q35.

[42] Lutz J, Schlangenotto H, Scheuermann U, De Doncker R. Semiconductor power devices. *Physics,* characteristics, reliability. 2011;2.

[43] Sadrozinski HW, Ely S, Fadeyev V, Galloway Z, Ngo J, Parker C, Petersen B, Seiden A, Zatserklyaniy A, Cartiglia N, Marchetto F. Ultra-fast silicon detectors. *Nuclear Instruments and Methods in Physics Research Section A: Accelerators, Spectrometers, Detectors and Associated Equipment*. 2013 Dec 1; 730:226-31.

[44] Monroy E, Munoz E, Sánchez FJ, Calle F, Calleja E, Beaumont B, Gibart P, Muñoz JA, Cussó F. High-performance GaN pn junction photodetectors for solar ultraviolet applications. *Semiconductor science and technology*. 1998 Sep 1;13(9):1042.

[45] Scholze F, Rabus H, Ulm G. Mean energy required to produce an electron-hole pair in silicon for photons of energies between 50 and 1500 eV. *Journal of Applied Physics*. 1998 Sep 1;84(5):2926-39.

[46] Spieler H. Fast timing methods for semiconductor detectors. *IEEE Transactions on Nuclear Science*. 1982 Jun;29(3):1142-58.

[47] Bos AJ. Theory of thermoluminescence. *Radiation measurements*. 2006 Dec 1;41: S45-56.

[48] McKeever SW. *Thermoluminescence of solids*. Cambridge University Press; 1985.

[49] Gadzuk JW, Richter LJ, Buntin SA, King DS, Cavanagh RR. Laser-excited hot-electron induced desorption: A theoretical model applied to NO/Pt (111). *Surface Science*. 1990 Sep 2;235(2-3):317-33.

[50] Durán A, Hian SK, Miller DL, Le Heron J, Padovani R, Vano E. Recommendations for occupational radiation protection in interventional cardiology. *Catheterization and cardiovascular interventions*. 2013 Jul 1;82(1):29-42.

[51] Derenzo SE, Choong WS, Moses WW. Fundamental limits of scintillation detector timing precision. *Physics in Medicine & Biology*. 2014 May 29;59(13):3261.

[52] Sysoeva E, Tarasov V, Zelenskaya O. Comparison of the methods for determination of scintillation light yield. *Nuclear Instruments and Methods in Physics Research Section A: Accelerators, Spectrometers, Detectors and Associated Equipment*. 2002 Jun 21;486(1-2):67-73.

[53] Brooks FD. Development of organic scintillators. *Nuclear Instruments and Methods*. 1979 Jun 1;162(1-3):477-505.

[54] Gu DD, Meiners W, Wissenbach K, Poprawe R. Laser additive manufacturing of metallic components: materials, processes, and mechanisms. *International materials reviews*. 2012 May 1;57(3):133-64.

[55] Marrone S, Cano-Ott D, Colonna N, Domingo C, Gramegna F, Gonzalez EM, Gunsing F, Heil M, Käppeler F, Mastinu PF, Milazzo PM. Pulse shape analysis of liquid scintillators for neutron studies. *Nuclear Instruments and Methods in Physics Research Section A: Accelerators, Spectrometers, Detectors and Associated Equipment*. 2002 Sep 1;490(1-2):299-307.

[56] Aglietta M, Alpat B, Alyea ED, Antonioli P, Anzivino G, Badino G, Ban Y, Bari G, Basile M, Benelli A, Berezinsky VS. *The most powerful scintillator supernovae detector*: LVD. Il Nuovo Cimento A (1965-1970). 1992 Dec; 105:1793-804.

[57] Weber MJ. Inorganic scintillators: today and tomorrow. *Journal of Luminescence*. 2002 Dec 1;100(1-4):35-45.

[58] Bott AW. Electrochemistry of semiconductors. *Current separations*. 1998 Dec; 17:87-92.

[59] Dosimeters C. A protocol for the determination of absorbed dose from high-energy photon. *Medical Physics*. 1983 Nov;10(6):741-71.

Chapter 5

Radiation Chemistry

Jayakrishnan Vaikkattil[1,*], MSc
Neha Rahul[2], MD, DrNB
Saraswathula Bharadwaj[3], MD
and Syed Asrar Ul Haq Andrabi[4], MSc

[1]Department of Nuclear Medicine, Manchester University NHS Trust, Manchester, UK
[2]Department of Radiation Oncology, Datta Meghe Institute of Higher Education and Research, Wardha, India
[3]Department of Radiodiagnosis, Datta Meghe Institute of Higher Education and Research, Wardha, India
[4]School of Allied Health Science, Datta Meghe Institute of Higher Education and Research, Wardha, India

Abstract

Radiation chemistry is a multidisciplinary field that investigates the chemical reactions and transformations that occur when materials are exposed to various types of radiation. Ionizing radiation, such as gamma rays and X-rays, can interact with matter at molecular and atomic levels, leading to significant changes in the chemical composition and behavior of substances. The primary focus of radiation chemistry is to understand how radiation-induced chemical reactions take place and how they can be controlled or harnessed for specific applications. Radiation chemistry has numerous practical applications and implications across various scientific and technological domains, including radiation processing, radiation biodosimetry, environmental radiation chemistry, and radiopharmaceuticals. The field involves the study of complex chemical processes that occur when materials are exposed to radiation, including the formation and reactivity of short-lived reactive species such as free radicals, excited states, and ion pairs. Understanding the physical events that occur in radiation chemistry is crucial for managing and predicting the chemical changes caused by radiation. The interactions of ionizing particles in biological media are essentially collisions with the electrons of the medium, leading to a series of physical events that ultimately result in chemical changes. The ability to forecast and manage these chemical changes is essential for improving applications like radiation processing and radiation treatment.

Keyword: free radicals, ionizing radiation, oxidative damage, radiolysis, radiosensitizers

---

[*] Corresponding Author's Email: jkvaikkattil@gmail.com

In: Fundamentals of Radiation Biology
Editors: Anurag Luharia, Ashish Uke, Gaurav Mishra et al.
ISBN: 979-8-89530-806-6

5.1. Introduction

Radiation chemistry is a fascinating field of study that focuses on the chemical reactions and transformations that occur when materials are exposed to various types of radiation. It investigates how radiation interacts with matter at the molecular and atomic levels, leading to significant changes in the chemical composition and behavior of substances. Radiation refers to the emission and transmission of energy in the form of particles or electromagnetic waves through space or a medium. It can be broadly classified into two categories: ionizing radiation and non-ionizing radiation. Ionizing radiation, such as gamma rays, X-rays, and high-energy particles, possesses enough energy to remove tightly bound electrons from atoms or molecules, resulting in the formation of charged particles known as ions. Non-ionizing radiation, such as ultraviolet (UV) rays, visible light, infrared radiation, microwaves, and radio waves, lacks the energy to cause ionization.

In radiation chemistry, researchers explore the complex chemical processes that occur when materials are exposed to radiation. These processes can involve direct interactions between radiation and molecules or indirect effects through the formation and reactivity of short-lived reactive species. Key reactive species in radiation chemistry include free radicals, excited states, and ion pairs. Free radicals, and in particular, it plays a crucial role as highly reactive species with unpaired electrons, which can initiate chain reactions and induce various chemical transformations. The primary focus of radiation chemistry is to understand how radiation-induced chemical reactions take place and how they can be controlled or harnessed for specific applications. Some of the key areas of study within radiation chemistry include such as radiolysis, radiation processing, radiation biodosimetry, environmental radiation chemistry, radiopharmaceuticals.

- *Radiolysis*: Radiolysis involves the study of the chemical changes that occur when a material is irradiated. It examines the formation and reactivity of free radicals and other reactive species, as well as the subsequent chemical reactions that take place.
- *Radiation processing:* Radiation processing involves the use of ionizing radiation to modify the properties of materials. For example, polymers can be crosslinked, leading to improved mechanical properties and heat resistance. Radiation processing is also used for sterilization, such as in the medical field for sterilizing medical equipment, and in food preservation to enhance the shelf life of food products.
- *Radiation biodosimetry*: Biodosimetry is the assessment of radiation exposure and its effects on biological systems. Radiation chemistry plays a crucial role in understanding the chemical changes that occur in biological molecules when exposed to radiation. This knowledge is essential for applications such as medical diagnostics and radiation therapy.
- *Environmental radiation chemistry*: Environmental radiation chemistry focuses on the study of chemical reactions occurring in natural systems influenced by radiation. It explores the degradation of pollutants in water or soil due to the presence of radiation, as well as the chemical effects of radiation on various environmental components.
- *Radiopharmaceuticals:* Radiopharmaceuticals are radioactive compounds used in medical imaging and targeted therapies. Radiation chemistry plays a key role in

developing and understanding the interactions between radiation and biological molecules, enabling the design of radiopharmaceuticals for diagnostic and therapeutic purposes.

Radiation chemistry has numerous practical applications and implications across various scientific and technological domains. It helps improve radiation safety measures, contributes to the development of new materials with tailored properties, and supports advancements in medical diagnostics and treatments. By studying the fundamental chemical processes induced by radiation, researchers can unlock new insights into the behavior of matter and utilize radiation's potential for beneficial applications.

5.1.1. Initial Physical Events

In initial physical events, ionizing radiation produces abundant secondary electrons that rapidly slow down (thermalize) to energies below 7.4 eV, the threshold to produce electronic transitions in liquid water. For both the primary charged particle and the secondary electrons, this slowing down process is accomplished by transfer of energy to the medium in a sequence of discrete events [1].

Stopping power (-dE/dx) treats the slowing down process as a continuous function, sometimes referred to as the continuous slowing down approximation. Depending on the amount of energy transferred to the electron, the molecule can undergo:

- Ionization (threshold in water ~ 13 eV)
- Excitation (threshold in water ~ 7.4 eV)
- Thermal transfer

The initial event is the transfer of ~ 7 - 100 eV, an amount of energy sufficient to cause (multiple) ionizations or excitations in water molecules. Transfer of energy to the medium in biological systems usually involves ionization of a water molecule, but can also involve the cellular macromolecules (e.g., DNA) directly. Through ionizations and excitations, the passage of a charged particle through biological medium creates three species in the local vicinity of the particle track: Direct ionization of water produces a radical ion and a free sub excitation electron (E < 7.4 eV) [2].

$$\mathbf{H_20} \xrightarrow{\text{rad}} \mathbf{H_2O^{+\cdot} + e^-}$$

Energy transfer can produce a wter molecule in an excited state.

$$\mathbf{H_20} \xrightarrow{\text{rad}} \mathbf{H_2O^{+\cdot} + e^-}$$

The time scale for the creation of these species is on the order of 10-16 seconds.

The interactions of ionizing particles in biological media are essentially collisions with the electrons of the medium and the interaction of radiation with matter initiates a series of physical events that ultimately lead to chemical changes physical events are categorized into three important stages [3]: primary processes, secondary processes, and subsequent chemical reactions are described below in details:

1. Primary Processes: The primary processes occur immediately after the absorption of radiation by the material. These processes involve the direct interaction of radiation with atoms or molecules and include:

a. *Ionization:* Ionization (threshold in water ~ 13 eV) Ionizing radiation, such as gamma rays and X-rays, possesses enough energy to remove tightly bound electrons from atoms or molecules, creating charged particles called ions. When the ionisation energy of the target material is higher than the energy of the radiation, this process takes place.
b. *Excitation*: Excitation (threshold in water ~ 7.4 eV) One or more electrons may be promoted to higher energy levels without being entirely removed during excitation, which occurs when radiation transfers energy to an atom or molecule. the excited species are in a metastable state and can undergo subsequent reactions [4].
c. *Electron capture*: In some circumstances, the absorbed radiation can lead to the capture of an electron from the surrounding medium by an atom or molecule, resulting in the production of negative ions.
d. *Energy deposition*: The absorbed radiation imparts energy to the material, resulting in the excitation or ionization of surrounding atoms or molecules through energy transfer processes.

2. Secondary Processes: Secondary processes occur, after the primary processes which involve the species formed as a result of ionization or excitation. These reactive species include:

a. *Free radicals*: With unpaired electrons, free radicals are extremely reactive organisms. They can be created directly by the radiation-induced bond-breaking processes or indirectly by ionisation. In later chemical processes, free radicals are essential [5].
b. *Excited states:* Excited states are atoms or molecules with electrons in higher energy levels due to radiation absorption. Excited states are capable of relaxing by mechanisms that either release energy through photon emission or transfer it to nearby molecules via collisions.
c. *Ion pairs:* Ion pairs are created when ionisation results in the production of an electron and a positive ion. These species with opposing charges may interact with other molecules in the solution or with one another.

3. Subsequent Chemical Reaction: Following the primary and secondary processes, the reactive species formed can participate in various chemical reactions, leading to chemical changes in the material. These reactions include:

a. *Reactions of free radicals*: Free radicals can undergo a range of reactions, such as hydrogen abstraction, electron transfer, addition or elimination reactions, and radical-

radical reactions. These reactions contribute to the overall transformation of the material [6].

b. *Recombination reactions*: Reactions between ion pairs and free radicals can result in the formation of neutral species, which ends their reactivity.
c. *Processes for transferring energy*: Excited states have the ability to ionise or excite nearby molecules by transferring any excess energy to those molecules.
d. *Crosslinking and polymerization*: In the case of polymers, the absorbed radiation can induce crosslinking or polymerization reactions, resulting in changes in the polymer structure and properties [7].

The order of primary processes, secondary processes, and subsequent chemical reactions is extremely complex and is influenced by a variety of elements, including the radiation's type and energy, the material's composition, and the presence of other molecules or substances in the system. The ability to forecast and manage the chemical changes caused by radiation is crucial for improving applications like radiation processing and radiation treatment. Understanding these physical events in radiation chemistry is also crucial for managing and predicting these chemical changes.

5.2. Radiolysis of Water

When ionizing radiation interacts with biological systems, the energy is absorbed. This initiate cascade of successive events the end result may be cell death.

Radiolysis of water results in the formation of highly reactive species-free radicals, which initiates the process of biological effect on cell; it is shown in Figure 5.1.

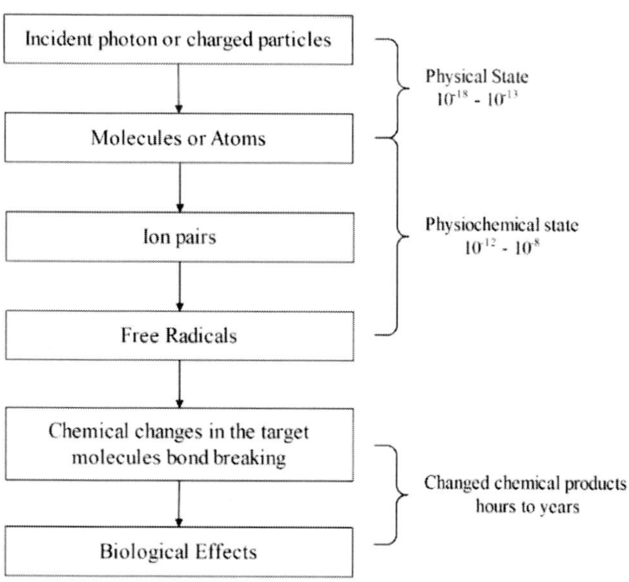

Figure 5.1. Radiobiologic effect on the body.

There are two primary types of effects observed in water radiolysis: *direct and indirect effects.*

- *Direct effect:* when radiation interacts with matter without involvement of water the effect is known as direct effect. Damage occurs as a result of ionization of atoms on key molecules in the biologic system. This cause inactivation or functional alteration of the molecule.

Direct ionization of atoms in molecules is a result of absorption of energy by photoelectric and Compton interactions. Ionization occurs at all radiation qualities and is the predominant cause of damage in reactions involving high LET radiations. Absorption of energy sufficient to remove an electron can result in bond breaks [8].

$$\text{Ionizing radiation} + RH \longrightarrow R^{o} + H^{+}$$

- *Indirect effect:* The living matter 70-90% H_2O. Therefore, when a living body is exposed to radiation most of the radiant energy will be absorbed by water. This will result in the interaction of radiation & H_2O molecule and a fast-moving electron [9].

$$H_2O \longrightarrow H_2O^{+} + e^{-} \text{ (fast moving electron)}$$

Having Kinetic energy, they travel significant distance, making recombination unlikely. Loss energy progressively and are captured by water molecule dipoles oriented towards the negative electrons. The equal is stable at RT and gives spectrum at 720 nm and the whole process takes 10^{-7} sec. electron is surrounded by four H_2O molecules hence it is known as hydrated electron or aqua [10].

The radiolysis of water can be broadly divided into four stages based on the physical, physiochemical, chemical, and biological effects that occur:

- **Physical stage:** $10^{-8} – 10^{-11}$ sec

The interaction of ionizing radiation in biological system is essentially collision or ionizing radiation with the electrons of the medium. Depending upon the energy of incident radiation the H_2O molecule is either ionized or excited, the physical event considerably increases the internal energy of the molecule. Ionization requires 32.5 eV energy to be dissipated in the system and is called average energy loss per ionization [11].

- *Absorption of Radiation*: Water molecules absorb ionizing radiation (e.g., gamma rays, X-rays, or high-energy particles).
- *Excitation and Ionization*: The absorbed energy leads to the excitation and ionization of water molecules, producing excited water molecules (H_2O^*) and ionized water molecules (H_2O^+).

- **Physicochemical stage**: $10^{-12} - 10^{-8}$ sec.

After absorption of the incident radiation, the ionized or excited molecule dissociates to give rise to free radicals by formation of primary and secondary species.

Primary Species

- *Excited Water Molecules (H_2O):* These can undergo dissociation to form hydroxyl radicals (•OH) and hydrogen atoms (•H).
- *Ionized Water Molecules (H_2O^+):* These can quickly react with other water molecules to produce hydroxyl radicals (•OH) and hydronium ions (H_3O^+).
- *Free Electrons (e^-):* Electrons ejected from water molecules can become solvated ($e^-_{a}q$) in water, leading to the formation of hydrated electrons.
- *Secondary Species:* The primary species further react with each other and with other water molecules to form secondary reactive species, such as hydrogen peroxide (H_2O_2), molecular hydrogen (H_2), and additional radicals.

- **Chemical stage**: 10^{-7} sec

The free radicals (•OH, •H, $e^-_{a}q$) thus formed and other reactive species formed in the previous stages undergo various chemical reactions with each other or with the cellular constituents

Hydroxyl Radicals (•OH) can react with each other to form hydrogen peroxide (H_2O_2), or with hydrogen atoms (•H) to form water. Hydrogen Atoms (•H) can react with each other to form molecular hydrogen (H_2). Hydrated Electrons ($e^-_{a}q$) can react with protons (H^+) to form hydrogen atoms (•H). Various other secondary reactions can occur, leading to the formation of complex molecules and further breakdown of water.

- **Biological stage:**

The possible biological effect due to exposure to radiation happens in a pattern starting from the initial exposure to final result observed on the organism. The sequence is shown in Figure 5.2.

This process takes hours to years. The biological stage refers to the biological effects and consequences of the radiolysis products formed in the chemical stage. The reactive oxygen species (ROS) generated during radiolysis, such as hydrogen peroxide and hydroxyl radicals, can cause oxidative damage to biological molecules, including DNA, proteins, and lipids. This stage involves interactions with cellular components, induction of DNA damage, cellular signaling pathways, and potentially leading to cell death or various biological responses. The biological effects can be influenced by factors such as radiation dose, dose rate, and the specific biological system under consideration.

Water is the major content in the cell. Bacterial spores - 20%, vegetative cells-40-50%, Therefore when cells are exposed to radiation the water molecules undergo dissociation (radiolysis) and produces free radicals.

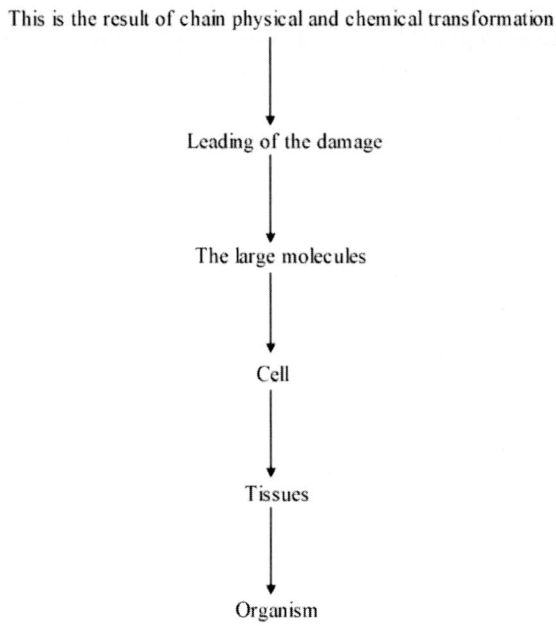

Figure 5.2. Biological damage due to radiation.

5.2.1. Excited Water Molecules

If the excited electron is not moving fast enough to escape the vicinity of H_2O^+ ion from which it is ejected. The electron may be recaptured by H_2O^+ ion to form highly energetic water molecule known as excited water molecule immediately dissociates to form free radicals and the energy required to break the bond is of the order of 5 eV.

$$H_2O^+ + e^- \longrightarrow H_2O^* \text{ (Excited water molecule)}$$

$$H_2O^* \longrightarrow H^* + O^oH$$

5.2.2. What Are Free Radicals?

Free radicals are electrical neutral atoms or molecules having an unpaired electron in their outer orbit. The presence of this unpaired electron imparts high chemical reactivity to the free radicals. They are formed within 10^{-7} s to hours.

Free radicals are electrophilic and therefore highly reactive, Free radicals can be electron acceptors (oxidizing) or electron donors (reducing) species.

For every 10^{-5} joules of low LET (Linear energy transfer) radiation:

- 2.6 hydrated electrons
- 2.6 hydroxy radical (OH^o)
- 0.4 hydrogen radical (H^o)

And a small amount of H_2 and H_2O_2 are produced if no scavengers and other reactant are present lifetime of e^-aq, OH^o and H^o is several hundred microseconds.

The free radicals are highly reactive, and the ^oOH (Hydroxy radical) is a powerful oxidizing agent and possesses great chemical reactivity. The life span of free radicals are very short 10^{-5} seconds.

H_2O^o and H_2O^- are unstable and dissociates

$H_2O^o \rightarrow H + {}^oOH$ (oxidizing radicals)

$H_2O^- \rightarrow H + OH^-$ (Reducing radicals)

^oOH and H^o are known as free radical.

5.2.3. Free Radicals May React in the Following Manner

1. Radical reaction or reaction among the free radicals.

$H^o + H^o \rightarrow H_2$ (Molecular hydrogen)

$^oOH + {}^oOH \rightarrow H_2O_2$ (Hydrogen peroxide)

$H^o + {}^oOH \rightarrow H_2O$ (water reconstitute)

2. Free radicals may react with water molecules

$H_2O + H^o \rightarrow H_3O^o \rightarrow H_2O + {}^oOH$

3. Free radicals may react with their own reaction products.

$H_2 + {}^oOH \rightarrow H_2O + H^o$

$H_2O_2 + {}^oOH \rightarrow HOO^o + H_2O$ ($HO_2{}^o$) Hydroperoxy radicals

$HO_2{}^o + {}^oOH \rightarrow H_2O + O_2$

$H_2O_2 + H \rightarrow HO_2{}^o + {}^oOH$

Free radicals may react with O_2, it is a strong oxidizing agent and its main radiosensitizing effect is connected with its high affinity to electrons. Free radicals formed may react with O_2 forming peroxide radicals, which are stable [12].

$H^o + O_2 \rightarrow HO_2{}^o$

$O_2 + e^-aq \rightarrow O_2^-$

$O_2^- + H^+ \rightarrow HO_2{}^o$

$O_2^- + H_2{}^o \rightarrow HO_2{}^o + OH^-$

$HO_2{}^o$ is less powerful oxidizing agent than ^oOH, but has a longer lifespan and can diffuse further from its site of formation to undergo further reaction.

$$HO_2^{o} + HO_2^{o} \longrightarrow H_2O_2 + O_2$$

4. H_2O_2 is an oxidizing agent and stable. It removes hydrogen from organic molecules. In biological system peroxide destroying enzymes such as catalase and peroxidases are present, which removes H_2O_2 and are of less consequences.

H_2O_2 may also be removed by free radicals.

$$H^{o} + H_2O_2{}^{o} \longrightarrow OH + H_2O$$
$$^{o}OH + H_2O_2 \longrightarrow HO_2^{o} + H_2O_2$$

5. Free radicals may react with organic molecules, forming organic free radicals, which may react with important biological molecule by removing H and causing damage to the molecule.

$$RH + {}^{o}OH \longrightarrow R^{o} + H_2O$$

Indirect

$$R'H + H^{o} \longrightarrow R'^{o} + H_2$$

Organic free radicals

$$RH \longrightarrow R^{o} + H^{o} \text{ ------- (Direct)}$$

If an organic biological molecule (RH) becomes a free radical either directly or indirectly it may react with O_2.

$$R^{o} + O_2 \longrightarrow ROO^{o}\ (RO_2^{0})\ \text{(Organic peroxyradical)}$$

RO_2^{0} may react with other R'H (organic molecules) and chain reaction may start

$$RO_2^{o} + R'H \longrightarrow ROOH + R'^{o}$$
$$R'^{o} + O_2 \longrightarrow R'O_2$$
$$RO_2^{o} + R'^{o} \longrightarrow ROOR'\ \text{(Organic peroxide)}$$

Hydroperoxides and peroxides are toxic substances. They get accumulated in the course of irradiation producing lesions/damages. These reactions are 30 times faster than the other competing reactions.

5.2.4. Action of Radiation on Aqueous Solutions

When radiation interacts with an aqueous solution, several effects can occur depending on the type of radiation and the concentration of the solution. When ionizing radiation, such as gamma rays, X-rays, or high-energy particles, interacts with an aqueous solution, several primary and secondary processes take place. Here are some key actions of radiation in aqueous solution:

- *Direct Ionization:*
  - High-energy radiation, such as gamma rays or X-rays, can directly interact with molecules in the solution.
  - The energy of the radiation can be sufficient to remove electrons from atoms or molecules, leading to ionization.
  - In the case of water (H_2O), radiation can ionize water molecules, resulting in the formation of hydrated electrons (e-) and various ions, including hydrogen ions (H^+) and hydroxide ions (OH^-).
  - The hydrated electrons are highly reactive and can participate in various chemical reactions [13].
- *Indirect Ionization:*
  - Radiation can indirectly ionize molecules in the aqueous solution through interactions with water molecules.
  - When high-energy radiation passes through the solution, it can ionize water molecules by transferring energy to them.
  - This ionization of water leads to the formation of ionized water species, such as H_2O (water cation), H_3O^+ (hydronium ion), and e^- (aq) (solvated electron).
  - These ionized water species can then react with other molecules present in the solution, causing further ionization and chemical reactions [14].
- *Water Radiolysis:*
  - Radiolysis of water refers to the decomposition of water molecules induced by radiation.
  - High-energy radiation, such as gamma rays, X-rays, or fast electrons, can break the chemical bonds within water molecules.
  - This breaking of bonds generates various reactive species, including hydrated electrons (e^-), hydrogen radicals (H^*), hydroxyl radicals ($^*OH$), and hydrogen peroxide (H_2O_2).
  - Hydrated electrons (e^-) are powerful reducing agents and can react with oxidizable molecules in the solution, leading to chemical transformations [15].
  - Hydrogen radicals (H^*) are highly reactive and can initiate hydrogen abstraction reactions with organic compounds.
  - Hydroxyl radicals ($^*OH$) are extremely reactive and can react with a wide range of molecules, causing oxidation, decomposition, or modification.
  - Hydrogen peroxide (H_2O_2) can undergo further reactions, including decomposition or redox reactions [16].
- *Redox Reactions:*
  - Radiation-induced redox reactions involve the transfer of electrons between species in the solution.

 - Hydrated electrons (e^-) generated during water radiolysis act as strong reducing agents and can reduce other species present in the solution, resulting in their oxidation [17].
 - Oxidizing species, such as hydroxyl radicals ($^*OH$), generated through radiolysis can oxidize other molecules in the solution.
 - These redox reactions play a significant role in radiation chemistry and can lead to the formation of new products or the degradation of existing compounds [18].

- *Chemical Reactions with Solutes:*
 - Radiation can induce chemical reactions with solutes dissolved in the aqueous solution.
 - Organic compounds, dissolved gases, or other solutes can react with the generated reactive species (e-, •OH, etc.), resulting in their modification, degradation, or cross-linking [19].
 - The specific reactions depend on the nature of the solute and the reactive species involved.
- *pH Changes:*
 - The ionization and radiolysis processes in an aqueous solution can alter the pH of the solution.
 - The formation of hydrogen ions (H+) and hydroxide ions (OH-) during water radiolysis affects the balance of acidic and basic species, leading to changes in pH [20].
 - The overall pH change depends on factors such as the radiation dose, solution composition, and the presence of the buffer systems.

5.3. The Oxygen Effect

The oxygen effect refers to the enhancement of radiation effects in the presence of molecular oxygen (O2) in an aqueous solution. It primarily occurs due to the interaction between radiation and molecular oxygen, leading to the production of reactive oxygen species (ROS). Here's a detailed explanation of the oxygen effect in an aqueous solution:

- *Radiolysis of Water in the Absence of Oxygen:*
 - In the absence of oxygen, the radiolysis of water primarily involves the direct and indirect ionization processes discussed earlier.
 - Direct ionization occurs when high-energy radiation directly interacts with water molecules, resulting in the formation of hydrated electrons (e^-) and various ions.
 - Indirect ionization involves the ionization of water molecules through interactions with ionized water species, such as H_2O^+ and H_3O^+.
 - The reactive species generated during water radiolysis (e^-, $^*OH$, H^*, etc.) participate in chemical reactions, leading to oxidative damage or chemical modifications [21].

- *Oxygen Effect:*
  - When molecular oxygen (O_2) is present in the aqueous solution, it can significantly enhance radiation-induced damage compared to the scenario without oxygen.
  - The enhanced damage is primarily attributed to the reaction between radiation-induced species and molecular oxygen, resulting in the production of reactive oxygen species (ROS).
  - The most notable ROS generated in the presence of oxygen are the superoxide radical ($^{*}O2^{-}$) and the hydroxyl radical ($^{*}OH$).
  - The superoxide radical ($^{*}O2^{-}$) is formed when radiation-induced electrons react with molecular oxygen. It is a potent oxidizing agent.
  - The hydroxyl radical (OH) is produced through reactions between radiation-induced species (such as e-) and $^{*}O2^{-}$ or other reactive oxygen species.
  - Both $^{*}O2^{-}$ and ^{-}OH can initiate and propagate oxidative reactions, causing increased damage to biomolecules and cellular components in the solution [22].
- *Oxidative Damage:*
  - The reactive oxygen species (ROS) generated in the presence of oxygen can induce oxidative damage to various molecules in the aqueous solution, including DNA, proteins, and lipids.
  - ROS can react with biomolecules, leading to the formation of DNA strand breaks, DNA base modifications, protein oxidation, lipid peroxidation, and other oxidative modifications.
  - These oxidative damages can disrupt cellular processes, impair cellular function, and potentially lead to cell death or genetic mutations [23].
- *Role in Radiation Therapy:*
  - The oxygen effect has important implications in radiation therapy, particularly in the treatment of tumors.
  - Tumor tissues often have higher oxygen levels compared to normal tissues. As a result, the presence of oxygen can enhance the effectiveness of radiation therapy in targeting and damaging tumor cells.
  - During radiation therapy, high-energy radiation is delivered to the tumor site, leading to the production of ROS in the presence of oxygen. This, in turn, increases the oxidative damage to the tumor cells and enhances the therapeutic effect [24].

5.4. Mechanism of Action of Chemical Modifiers of Radiosensitivity

Compounds that can change how cells or tissues react to radiation are known as chemical radiosensitivity modifiers. They might make cancer cells more sensitive to radiation or shield healthy tissues from its harmful effects. These chemical modifiers work through a variety of intricate, multi-cellular processes, and pathways that are different in their modes of action.

The regulation of DNA damage and repair mechanisms is a significant mechanism of action. Single strand breakage, double strand breaks, and base alterations are all results of radiation damage to DNA. The effectiveness and precision of DNA repair systems are both susceptible to chemical modifications. Some modifiers improve DNA repair procedures, fostering the prompt and precise repair of radiation-induced DNA damage. Cell survival may rise as a result, reducing genetic instability. Others may prevent DNA repair processes from working, increasing DNA damage and encouraging cancer cell death. Modulation of cellular redox state constitutes a further pathway. Reactive oxygen species (ROS), which can cause oxidative stress and harm to biological components, are produced because of radiation exposure [25]. A cell's ability to produce and scavenge ROS can be affected by chemical modifiers. By scavenging ROS and lowering oxidative stress, they might function as antioxidants. These modifiers can affect cellular viability and a cell's vulnerability to radiation damage by altering the redox status.

Modulation of cell cycle progression is another mechanism of action for chemical modifiers of radiosensitivity. Radiation has differential effects on cells in different phases of the cell cycle, with cells in the S and G2 phases being more sensitive. Chemical modifiers can alter cell cycle distribution, leading to synchronization of cells in radiation-sensitive phases or inducing cell cycle arrest. This can enhance the effectiveness of radiation by increasing the proportion of cells susceptible to radiation-induced damage. Some chemical modifiers can affect the expression and activity of proteins involved in signaling pathways related to DNA damage response, cell survival, and apoptosis. They can modulate these pathways to either sensitize cancer cells to radiation-induced apoptosis or promote cell survival and resistance to radiation. By influencing these signaling pathways, chemical modifiers can affect the cellular response to radiation and alter radiosensitivity. Certain modifiers can influence the tumor microenvironment, particularly the oxygenation status. Tumor hypoxia, characterized by low oxygen levels, is associated with radioresistance. Chemical modifiers can modify tumor oxygenation, improving oxygen delivery to hypoxic regions and making them more susceptible to radiation-induced damage. This can enhance the effectiveness of radiation therapy by overcoming the radioresistance associated with tumor hypoxia [26].

The mechanisms of action of chemical modifiers of radiosensitivity can be related to their influence on the radiation-induced chemical reactions and processes within the aqueous solution. Here are some mechanisms by which chemical modifiers can affect radiosensitivity in radiation chemistry:

- *Free Radical Scavenging:*
  - Radiation-induced ionizing events in the aqueous solution generate free radicals, such as hydroxyl radicals ($^{*}OH$) and hydrated electrons (e^{-}).
  - Chemical modifiers can act as free radical scavengers, neutralizing or quenching these reactive species.
  - By scavenging free radicals, the modifiers reduce the potential for oxidative damage to biomolecules and minimize the overall radiation-induced cellular damage [27].
- *Radioprotective Action:*
  - Chemical modifiers can have radioprotective properties by reducing the damaging effects of radiation on cellular components.
  - They may act by chelating metal ions that can participate in radiation-induced redox reactions or by interacting with radiation-induced reactive species to prevent their damaging effects.

  - Radioprotective compounds can also enhance cellular antioxidant defenses, reducing oxidative stress and minimizing radiation-induced damage [28].
- *DNA Damage Modulation:*
  - Chemical modifiers can influence the extent and nature of radiation-induced DNA damage within the aqueous solution.
  - Some compounds may bind to DNA, altering its structure and making it more or less susceptible to radiation-induced damage.
  - Other modifiers can interact with radiation-induced reactive species or participate in repair processes, affecting the efficiency or fidelity of DNA repair mechanisms [29].
- *Modification of Reactive Species Generation:*
  - Radiation-induced radiolysis of water produces various reactive species, including hydroxyl radicals ($^{*}OH$) and hydrated electrons (e^{-}).
  - Chemical modifiers can alter the yield or nature of these reactive species, affecting their reactivity and interactions within the solution.
  - For example, some compounds can act as electron donors, reducing the formation of hydrated electrons (e^{-}) and potentially modifying the radiation-induced redox reactions [30].
- *pH Regulation:*
  - Chemical modifiers can influence the pH of the aqueous solution, which, in turn, can affect the radiolysis processes and the reactivity of radiation-induced species.
  - By adjusting the pH, modifiers can modulate the balance between acidic and basic species, potentially altering the extent of ionization and the reactivity of the solution towards radiation-induced species.
- *Modulation of Redox Reactions:*
  - Radiation-induced redox reactions can contribute to cellular damage and oxidative stress.
  - Chemical modifiers can influence these redox reactions by interacting with radiation-induced species, altering their reactivity, or affecting the overall redox balance within the solution.
  - By modulating redox reactions, these compounds can potentially enhance or reduce the damaging effects of radiation [31].
- *Signal Transduction Pathways*:
  - Chemical modifiers can influence signaling pathways involved in radiation response.
  - They can modulate pathways related to DNA damage sensing and repair, cell cycle progression, apoptosis, inflammation, and angiogenesis.
  - By targeting these pathways, modifiers can enhance or suppress cellular responses to radiation, affecting the overall radiosensitivity of cells or tissues [32].
- *Hypoxia Modification:*
  - Hypoxic regions within tumors are often resistant to radiation therapy.
  - Chemical modifiers can modulate tumor hypoxia, increasing the oxygenation status of tumor cells and sensitizing them to radiation.

- They can enhance tumor oxygenation by improving blood flow or promoting the release of oxygen from hemoglobin.
- By increasing tumor oxygen levels, these modifiers improve the effectiveness of radiation therapy in hypoxic tumor regions [33].

Conclusion

This chapter has explored the fundamental principles and processes of radiation chemistry, emphasizing how ionizing radiation interacts with matter to produce chemical transformations. The radiolysis of water and formation of reactive species such as free radicals and hydrated electrons were discussed as central mechanisms driving radiation-induced chemical and biological effects. The distinction between direct and indirect actions of radiation was highlighted, along with the significant role of oxygen in enhancing oxidative damage. The chapter also reviewed applications in radiation processing, environmental remediation, and radiopharmaceutical development, as well as strategies for modulating radiosensitivity through chemical modifiers. By understanding the underlying chemical pathways and interactions, radiation chemistry provides crucial insights into both the risks and benefits of radiation in medicine, industry, and the environment.

References

[1] Goodhead DT. Initial events in the cellular effects of ionizing radiations: clustered damage in DNA. *International journal of radiation biology.* 1994 Jan 1; 65(1):7-17.

[2] Draganic I. *The radiation chemistry of water*. Elsevier; 2012 Dec 2.

[3] Kiefer J. *Biological radiation effects*. Springer Science & Business Media; 2012 Dec 6.

[4] Riley PA. Free radicals in biology: oxidative stress and the effects of ionizing radiation. *International journal of radiation biology*. 1994 Jan 1; 65(1):27-33.

[5] Halliwell B. Free radicals and antioxidants: a personal view. *Nutrition reviews.* 1994 Aug 1; 52(8):253-65.

[6] Nimse SB, Pal D. Free radicals, natural antioxidants, and their reaction mechanisms. *RSC advances.* 2015; 5(35):27986-8006.

[7] Singh B, Pal L. Radiation crosslinking polymerization of sterculia polysaccharide–PVA–PVP for making hydrogel wound dressings. *International Journal of Biological Macromolecules.* 2011 Apr 1; 48(3):501-10.

[8] Hutchinson F. Chemical changes induced in DNA by ionizing radiation. *Progress in nucleic acid research and molecular biology*. 1985 Jan 1; 32:115-54.

[9] Wurtman RJ. The effects of light on the human body. *Scientific american*. 1975 Jul 1; 233(1):68-79.

[10] Nimse SB, Pal D. Free radicals, natural antioxidants, and their reaction mechanisms. *RSC advances.* 2015; 5(35):27986-8006.

[11] Charlesby A. *Atomic radiation and polymers: international series of monographs on radiation effects in materials*. Elsevier; 2016 Jun 6.

[12] Chendil D, Ranga RS, Meigooni D, Sathishkumar S, Ahmed MM. Curcumin confers radiosensitizing effect in prostate cancer cell line PC-3. *Oncogene*. 2004 Feb; 23(8):1599-607.

[13] Hu B, Lai YH, So PK, Chen H, Yao ZP. Direct ionization of biological tissue for mass spectrometric analysis. *Analyst.* 2012; 137(16):3613-9.

[14] Alizadeh E, Orlando TM, Sanche L. Biomolecular damage induced by ionizing radiation: the direct and indirect effects of low-energy electrons on DNA. *Annual review of physical chemistry*. 2015 Apr 1; 66:379-98.

[15] Le Caër S. Water radiolysis: influence of oxide surfaces on H2 production under ionizing radiation. *Water*. 2011 Feb 28; 3(1):235-53.

[16] Burns WG, Sims HE. Effect of radiation type in water radiolysis. Journal of the Chemical Society, *Faraday Transactions 1: Physical Chemistry in Condensed Phases*. 1981; 77(11):2803-13.

[17] Gius D, Spitz DR. Redox signaling in cancer biology. *Antioxidants & redox signaling*. 2006 Jul 1; 8(7-8):1249-52.

[18] Greenstock CL. Redox processes in radiation biology and cancer. *Radiation Research*. 1981 May 1; 86(2):196-211.

[19] Hutchinson F. Chemical changes induced in DNA by ionizing radiation. *Progress in nucleic acid research and molecular biology*. 1985 Jan 1; 32:115-54.

[20] Von Sonntag C, Schuchmann HP. The elucidation of peroxyl radical reactions in aqueous solution with the help of radiation-chemical methods. *Angewandte Chemie International Edition in English*. 1991 Oct; 30(10):1229-53.

[21] Barr NF, Allen AO. Hydrogen atoms in the radiolysis of water. *The Journal of Physical Chemistry*. 1959 Jun; 63(6):928-31.

[22] Quintiliani M. The oxygen effect in radiation inactivation of DNA and enzymes. International Journal of Radiation Biology and Related Studies in Physics, *Chemistry and Medicine*. 1986 Jan 1; 50(4):573-94.

[23] Demple B, Harrison L. Repair of oxidative damage to DNA: enzymology and biology. *Annual review of biochemistry*. 1994 Jul; 63(1):915-48.

[24] Al-Waili NS, Butler GJ, Beale J, Hamilton RW, Lee BY, Lucas P. Hyperbaric oxygen and malignancies: a potential role in radiotherapy, chemotherapy, tumor surgery and phototherapy. *Medical science monitor*. 2005 Sep 1; 11(9):RA279.

[25] Coleman CN, Bump EA, Kramer RA. Chemical modifiers of cancer treatment. *Journal of Clinical Oncology*. 1988 Apr; 6(4):709-33.

[26] Hockel M, Vaupel P. Tumor hypoxia: definitions and current clinical, biologic, and molecular aspects. *Journal of the National Cancer Institute*. 2001 Feb 21; 93(4):266-76.

[27] Nair CK, Parida DK, Nomura T. Radioprotectors in radiotherapy. *Journal of radiation research*. 2001; 42(1):21-37.

[28] Nair CK, Parida DK, Nomura T. Radioprotectors in radiotherapy. *Journal of radiation research*. 2001; 42(1):21-37.

[29] Friedberg EC. A brief history of the DNA repair field. *Cell research*. 2008 Jan; 18(1):3-7.

[30] Shkrob IA, Marin TW, Chemerisov SD, Wishart JF. Radiation induced redox reactions and fragmentation of constituent ions in ionic liquids. 1. Anions. *The Journal of Physical Chemistry B*. 2011 Apr 14; 115(14):3872-88.

[31] Selenius M, Hedman M, Brodin D, Gandin V, Rigobello MP, Flygare J, Marzano C, Bindoli A, Brodin O, Björnstedt M, Fernandes AP. Effects of redox modulation by inhibition of thioredoxin reductase on radiosensitivity and gene expression. *Journal of Cellular and Molecular Medicine*. 2012 Jul;16(7):1593-605.

[32] Gillies McKenna W, Muschel RJ, Gupta AK, Hahn SM, Bernhard EJ. The RAS signal transduction pathway and its role in radiation sensitivity. *Oncogene*. 2003 Sep; 22(37):5866-75.

[33] Ashton TM, Fokas E, Kunz-Schughart LA, Folkes LK, Anbalagan S, Huether M, Kelly CJ, Pirovano G, Buffa FM, Hammond EM, Stratford M. The anti-malarial atovaquone increases radiosensitivity by alleviating tumour hypoxia. *Nature communications*. 2016 Jul 25; 7(1):12308.

Chapter 6

DNA Damage Caused by Ionizing Radiation

Vaibhav Sonwani[1,*], MD
Ashish Uke[2], MD
Suwarna Dangore[3], MDS
and Pratap Singh Parihar[4], MD, PhD
[1]Department of Radiation Oncology, HCG Cancer Centre, Nagpur, India
[2]Department of Radiation Oncology, Datta Meghe Institute of Higher Education and Research, Wardha, India
[3]Department of Oral Medicine and Radiology, Datta Meghe Institute of Higher Education and Research, Wardha, India
[4]Department of Radiodiagnosis, Datta Meghe Institute of Higher Education and Research, Wardha, India

Abstract

Ionizing radiation (IR) is the most common type of radiation used in radiotherapy, and it causes damage to cells by ejecting electrons from molecules, leading to ionization. The ejected electrons, in turn, ionize other molecules, causing a cascade of chemical changes that can disrupt the macromolecular structure of cells. DNA is the primary target of radiation-induced cell death, and its structure and function are critical in determining the fate of cells exposed to IR. The DNA damage response (DDR) is a complex system that coordinates the repair of radiation-induced DNA damage, and it involves the activation of various signaling pathways, including the ATM, DNA-PKcs, and ATR kinases. These kinases phosphorylate key proteins, including H2AX, which plays a crucial role in the recruitment of repair proteins to the site of DNA damage. The DDR also involves the activation of cell-cycle checkpoints, programmed cell death pathways, and DNA repair pathways. Understanding the mechanisms of the DDR is essential for developing effective strategies to enhance the therapeutic efficacy of radiation therapy and to mitigate the adverse effects of IR on normal tissues.

Keywords: cell-cycle checkpoints, DNA damage response (DDR), double-strand break repair, ionizing radiation, homologous recombination

* Corresponding Author's Email: vaibhavsonwani@gmail.com

In: Fundamentals of Radiation Biology
Editors: Anurag Luharia, Ashish Uke, Gaurav Mishra et al.
ISBN: 979-8-89530-806-6

6.1. Introduction

The most frequent type of radiation utilized in radiotherapy is ionizing radiation (IR), which comprises electromagnetic energy or photons. Less than 100 keV to several MeV (the maximum energy of the machine being utilized) are typical photon energies produced by 4-25 MV linear accelerators in radiation departments. The ability of this type of radiation to eject electrons from (ionize) molecules within cells is what causes the majority of its harmful effects. Nearly every photon linear accelerator creates has enough energy to result in these ionizations. However, the ejected electrons themselves, which continue to ionize molecules they collide with and increasingly slow down as they go, inflict most biological harm. Interactions increase in frequency and produce clusters of ionizations at the ends of electron tracks. The link between the ionizations' pattern and density and the DNA double helix's size.

The specifics of DNA's structure have previously been covered in previous chapters. Numerous ionization events can occur within a few DNA base pairs due to the sizes of radiation-induced ionization clusters. Contrary to other radiation types like ultraviolet (UV) or DNA-damaging medications like topoisomerase inhibitors, these clusters are a distinctive feature of infrared radiation (IR). Only a small portion of radiation damage occurs in clusters, but when this happens to DNA, the cell has a particularly tough time healing. Ionized molecules are extremely reactive and undergo a rapid cascade of chemical changes, which can cause chemical bonds to dissolve and disrupt the macromolecular structure. IR scatters its energy, harming every molecule in the cell.

However, most molecules (such as water, mRNA, proteins, and others) have several copies and undergo constant, rapid turnover, which limits the effects of destroying just a few molecules of one type. Contrarily, DNA is only found in two copies, has a very low turnover rate, is the largest molecule, thus providing the biggest target, and is essential for all cellular processes. Therefore, irreversible DNA damage can have catastrophic and frequently fatal consequences. According to overwhelming historical experimental evidence, DNA is the main target for radiation-induced cell death. Small polonium needles were used in elegant studies to irradiate individual cells, producing short-range alpha particles. Plasma membranes and cytoplasm could receive high amounts without experiencing cell death. Cell death occurred, though, as soon as the needle was positioned so that the nucleus got even one or two alpha particles. Other studies compared radioactively tagged compounds to homogenous cell irradiations with radioactively labelled chemicals that primarily irradiated the DNA (3H-labeled thymidine) or the plasma membrane (125I-concanavalin). Only the dose reaching the nucleus, not the plasma membrane or the cytoplasm, was tightly linked with cell death. Due to the significance of DNA, cells and organisms have evolved a complex set of mechanisms and pathways to protect them from damage from both inside and outside, including ingested chemicals, UV and IR, and oxidation and alkylation caused by metabolism. These include several methods of DNA repair to address the various types of DNA damage brought on by various sources. Base excision repair (BER), single-strand break repair (SSBR), double-strand break repair (DSBR), and interstrand crosslink repair (ICL) are examples of specialized repair methods that have been developed to identify and fix damage to bases, single-strand breaks, double-strand breaks, and crosslinks. There are additional DNA repair pathways, including those for repairing bulky lesions or DNA adducts like those caused by UV light and some medications like cisplatin (nucleotide excision repair [NER]) and those for repairing base pair mismatches in DNA that can occur during replication (mismatch repair [MMR]). However, since cells with mutations or deletions in the genes controlling these pathways are not more vulnerable to IR, it appears that neither MMR nor NER are crucial for survival after IR. These repair procedures are still crucial to stop mutations from developing due to DNA damage. On the other hand, BER, SSBR, and DSBR gene mutations or deletions can all result in enhanced radiosensitivity.

To give you an indication of the extent and type of the damage, 1 Gy of radiation will result in roughly 105 ionizations in each cell, more than 1000 DNA base damages, over 1000 single-strand DNA breaks (SSBs), and about 20–40 double-strand DNA breaks (DSBs). To further put this into perspective, 1 Gy only effectively destroys 30% of the cells in a common mammalian cell line. Even if there are many generated lesions per cell, there is only a small amount of cytotoxicity resulting from effective DNA repair. Since DSBs are breaks that interfere with chromosomal segregation in mitosis, they are regarded as fatal due to lesion types. DSBs can develop due to conversion from other forms of DNA damage or as a result of initial radiation lesions. For instance, DSBs might result from replication blockages that cannot be resolved because of DNA strand crosslinks, complicated base damage, or base loss. These radiation-induced replication-induced DSBs are chemically different from initial lesion-induced DSBs and can manifest hours after radiation. As a result of replication errors or stability problems, SSBs can potentially cause secondary DSBs. Nucleosomes, which resemble beads on a string, are formed when the DNA double helix is looped around a collection of proteins called histones at regular intervals. Numerous other proteins that regulate DNA metabolism, including as transcription, replication, and repair, are also linked to the DNA. Chromatin is made up of DNA and the proteins that go with it. After more folding and looping, the chromosomes ultimately take on their compact shape. This arrangement presents the cell with several difficulties while repairing DNA damage. Prior to damage detection, specialized proteins must be sufficiently numerous and mobile to do so within seconds or minutes of the damage occurring. Second, to provide access to repair proteins, the chromatin typically needs to be modified (the structure being opened up, for example). This may entail the removal of nucleosomes close to the break, among other changes.

The appropriate repair, accessory, and signalling proteins must subsequently be recruited, frequently through histone changes, and in a manner that is carefully coordinated. Activities like transcription and cell-cycle progression must be stopped to focus on repair. It's important to keep track of the repair process so that, after it's finished, the chromatin may be reset to its initial state, and normal cellular functions can continue. The DNA damage response (DDR) is an intricate and well-coordinated system that decides how radiation-induced DNA damage affects these coordinated activities.

6.2. The DNA Damage Response (DDR)

The DDR is an intricate and well-coordinated system that decides how radiation-induced DNA damage affects cells. The DDR is not just one pathway; it is a collection of closely linked signalling pathways, each regulating a different aspect of a cell's function [1]. As shown in Figure 6.1, the sensors of DNA damage and the transducers and effectors of the damage response are two different components of this system. A collection of proteins that actively search the genome for signs of damage make up the sensors [2]. These proteins subsequently communicate the damage via transducers to three major effector pathways, collectively determining the cell's destiny. Additional proteins acting as activators or adaptors can amplify and regulate the signal. The effector pathways include:

1. Programmed cell death pathways kill cells with damage
2. DNA damage checkpoints temporarily or permanently halt cells' progress through the cell cycle.
3. DNA repair pathways that physically repair DNA. Additionally, cellular reactions to radiation result in adaptive changes in gene transcription, mRNA translation, and protein modification and destruction.

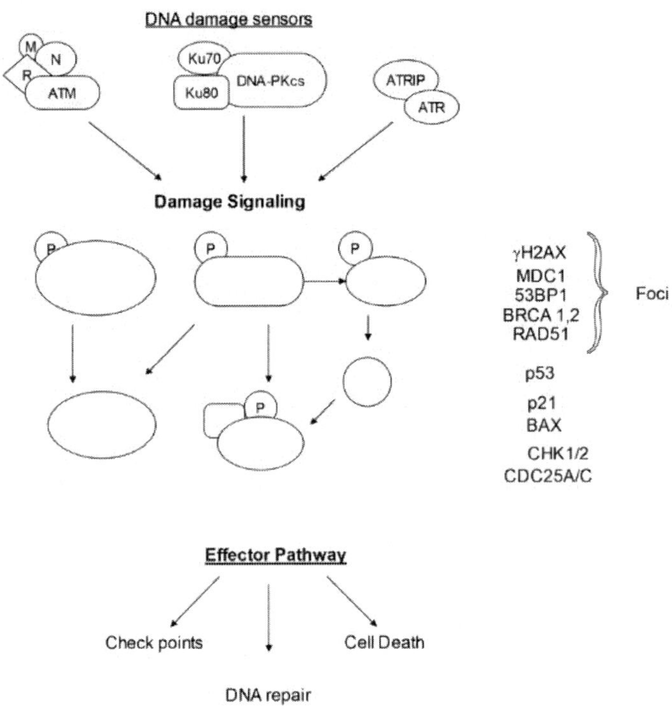

Figure 6.1. DNA damage sensors.

6.3. DNA Damage Sensors

Specific DNA lesions are identified by DNA damage sensor proteins, which then start the DDR. The DDR cascade and the recruitment of repair factors to the location of the lesions are both based on these initial processes. The initial damage-sensing protein must exist depending on the type of lesion [3]. For instance, certain glycosylases that are made to recognize and remove the damaged base from DNA can recognize base lesions, but poly (ADP-ribosylation)-polymerases (PARPs) are promptly activated when bases or phosphodiester links are lost from DNA. The MRN complex, made up of the proteins MRE11, RAD50, and NBS1, detects DSBs. Notably, the gene mutated in Nijmegen breakage syndrome (NBS) produces the NBS1 protein [4]. Patients with this disease are radiosensitive, as implied by its essential role in identifying and repairing DSBs. The Ku proteins can also identify and successfully bind the ends of DSBs (Ku70 and 80). The RPA complex coats single-stranded DNA segments produced during replication or DSBR [5]. The early DNA damage-detecting events control repair pathway selection and direct DDR signalling by activating several signal transduction proteins and processes.

6.4. DNA Damage Signalling Transducers

Signals are needed after DNA damage is detected to activate repair proteins, cell-death mechanisms, of cell-cycle checkpoints. The signal is transmitted from the sensors to the effectors through post-translational modification and/or relocalization of intermediary signalling proteins. A variety of enzymes can make these alterations and include phosphorylation (the addition of phosphate groups), ubiquitylation (the addition of ubiquitin peptides), sumoylation (the addition of sumo peptides), acetylation (the addition of acetyl groups), and poly (ADP-ribosylation). Post-translational modifications often alter the chromatin near the DNA damage to "mark" and prepare the region of the DNA damage and facilitate the recruitment of essential repair proteins [6]. In order to start downstream signalling to different effector pathways, modifications might change protein activity or complex formation.

6.4.1. Ataxia-Telangiectasia Mutated Protein

The activation of the ataxia-telangiectasia mutated (ATM) protein is among the earliest signalling processes identified in the DDR. oculocutaneous telangiectasia and progressive cerebellar ataxia arc the two clinical manifestations of the autosomal recessive condition ataxia-telangiectasia (AT) caused by a mutation in the ATM protein [7]. These people usually have high levels of radiosensitivity and are at higher risk of acquiring cancer. Through the assistance of MRN, the ATM protein is attracted to DSBs and is crucial for DSB signalling and repair. A kinase called ATM phosphorylates many proteins, including MRN and itself. Regarding cell-cycle checkpoints and programmed cell death, two key target proteins are CHK2 and p53. H2AX, a histone protein, is another significant target of ATM [8].

6.4.2. H2AX

H2AX is a subtype of histone H2A, a part of the central nucleosome structure that holds DNA in place. H2AX starts to get phosphorylated at the DSB location shortly after DSB formation. H2AX is the phosphorylated version of H2AX. A second enzyme named MDC1 controls the phosphorylation of H2AX proteins, which occurs over rather large chromatin areas (megabases) in both directions of the DSB [9]. By directly binding to both ATM and H2AX,

MDC1 functions as an adapter, amplifying H2AX mediated by ATM in both directions of the break. This amplification modifies the chromatin structure around the DSB considerably and is considered crucial for other DNA repair proteins to reach the break. The detection of H2AX foci using microscopy and certain antibodies is made easier by substantial regions of H2AX surrounding a single DSB [10]. In addition to ATM, two other kinases have been demonstrated to phosphorylate H2AX at the locations of DSBs: DNA-PKcs, an AT-related protein, and DNA-dependent protein kinase catalytic subunit.

6.4.3. DNA-Dependent Protein Kinase Catalytic Subunit

DNA-PKcs is a kinase that shares structural similarities with ATM and reacts only to DNA damage, especially to DSBs. DNA-PKcs, like ATMs, are unable to serve as a damaged sensor by themselves. The Ku70 above/Ku80 complex, which directly binds to the ends of DSBs and recruits DNA-PKcs to enable the phosphorylation of H2AX, performs this sensor function. Numerous target proteins involved in checkpoints and repair are also phosphorylated by DNA-PKcs [11].

6.4.4. ATR-ATRIP

The third kinase, ATR, which can phosphorylate H2AX in response to DNA damage, reacts swiftly to damage. ATR does not seem to have a major function in the signalling caused by radiation-induced DSBs, in contrast to ATM and DNA-PKcs. Alternatively, it phosphorylates H2AX in response to other kinds of DNA irregularities and damage, including single-stranded DNA and stagnant or damaged replication forks [12]. As a result, ATR plays a crucial role in the several kinds of damage that result from regular DNA replication. ATR and the mediator protein ATRIP (ATR interacting protein) are drawn to single-stranded DNA sequences coated with RPA. The DNA at DSB sites is processed due to the activation of the ATM-MRN complex. Intense DSB end resection during this phase can result in regions of single-stranded DNA activating ATR. As a result, ATR can be initiated "downstream" of ATM activation. As a result of replication issues that arise after irradiation, ATR is also activated. Radiation-induced DNA strand crosslinks and oxidized bases prevent DNA replication and trigger ATR. ATR phosphorylates a different collection of proteins involved in the DDR and some of the phosphorylation sites shared by ATM. As a result, following radiation therapy, ATR is also necessary for the DNA repair, checkpoint, and cell death components of the DDR effector pathways [13]. For instance, the ATR kinase phosphorylates important checkpoint proteins like CHK1, which establishes a direct connection to cell-cycle regulation.

6.4.5. Poly (ADP-ribosylation)-polymerase

Poly (ADP-ribose) (PAR) is created when the enzyme PARPs catalyzes the creation of a branching polymer from ADP ribose. As previously mentioned, those are the first things that happen to the chromatin and repair proteins when something goes wrong. In order to detect and signal radiation-induced DNA damage, such as abasic sites, SSBs, DNA nicks, and DSBs, at least two of the major PARP family members, PARP1 and PARP2, are required [14]. The functions of numerous proteins that are targets of PARP1 and PARP2 are changed due to PARylation. Ultimately, this leads to the regulation of signalling pathways, including those involved in inflammation or metabolic reactions known to happen after oxidative stress. Therefore, PAR-mediated responses may significantly impact inflammatory processes brought on by radiation, which are responsible for typical tissue toxicities. Many other cellular proteins are altered due to the activation of DNA-PKcs, PARPs, ATM, and ATR. The signals that activate the numerous downstream effectors of the DDR (most significantly apoptosis, cell-cycle checkpoints, and DNA repair) come from the phosphorylation and PARylation of these other proteins [15].

6.4.6. Effector Pathways: Programmed Cell Death – Apoptosis

P53 and MDM2 are two significant proteins that undergo phosphorylation due to ATM activation. The gene p53, which regulates genes that control both cell-cycle checkpoints and programmed cell death through the process known as apoptosis (see Chapter 3), is one of the most frequently altered tumour suppressors [16]. Therefore, activation of p53 following radiation can result in either a reduction in cell proliferation or a direct cause of cell death as shown in Figure 6.2.

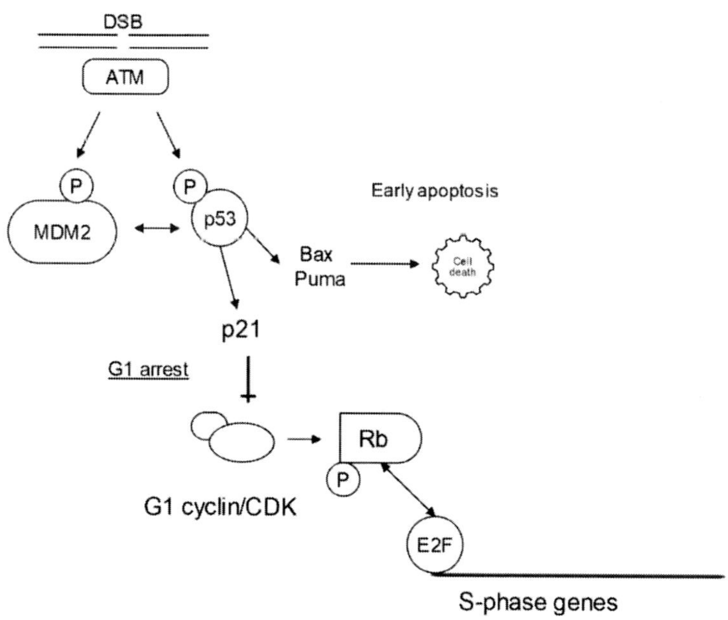

Figure 6.2. Effector Pathways.

The binding of the p53 protein to its partner MDM2 controls the p53 protein's abundance. Due to this connection, p53 is swiftly ubiquitinated and destroyed by the proteasome pathway. Thus, p53 is continuously produced in normal cells that are not under stress, but it is also destroyed and rendered inactive. ATM phosphorylates both p53 and MDM2 after DNA damage [17]. The p53 protein is no longer destroyed due to these processes, destabilizing the p53-MDM2 relationship and instead building up in the cell. Along with this stabilization, ATM's direct phosphorylation of p53 causes it to become activated as a transcription factor, which in turn causes the upregulation of many of its target genes. The pro-apoptotic genes BAX and PUMA are among these target genes; in some cells, these genes alone may be sufficient to cause cell death [18].

As a result, in some cells, DDR activation itself can trigger the quick induction of cell death through apoptosis. The ability of p53 to trigger apoptosis may aid in the protein's capacity to act as a tumour suppressor [19]. It may be more advantageous to the organism to kill the cell than to attempt to repair the damage because DNA damage can result in harmful mutations.

6.5. Effector Pathways: Cell-Cycle Checkpoints

Activating cell-cycle checkpoints is the second important effector route of the DDR. The progression of cells through the cell cycle's G1, S, and G2 stages is slowed down by IR treatment of the cells. This happens when DNA damage checkpoints are activated, which are particular locations in the cell cycle where the movement of the cell into the following phase can be stopped or retarded. In response to irradiation, the DDR activates four separate checkpoints at various times during the cell cycle [20]. These "checkpoints" can be viewed as delays that give cells extra time to repair DNA damage and stop the spread of mutations that result from it. Cell-cycle checkpoints decrease the likelihood that some lesions will undergo replication or mitotic processes, which could transform them into more harmful lesions by preventing proliferation.

Cyclin-dependent kinases (CDKs) are responsible for all cell cycle movement. CDKs phosphorylate other proteins to start the reactions necessary for cell cycle advancement. A CDK can only function when paired with a cyclin partner, thus their name. Various cyclin/CDK complexes are active at various stages of the cell cycle [21]. For instance, during G1, cyclinD/CDK4 is active; during G2 and mitosis, cyclinB/CDK1 is active; and during the S phase, cyclinA is active along with CDK1 and CDK2. After radiation, there are two primary methods by which the cyclin/CDK complexes are inhibited, which is necessary for checkpoint activation. The first is by activating other proteins that directly inhibit the cyclin/ CDK complex, the 'cyclin-dependent kinase inhibitors' (CDKIs) [22]. The second affects the phosphorylation and activity of the CDK enzyme.

6.5.1. G1/S Checkpoint

Cell-cycle checkpoints decrease the likelihood that some lesions will undergo replication or mitotic processes, which could transform them into more harmful lesions by preventing proliferation.

The decision of the cell to start DNA replication for continued cell division is made by a checkpoint found in cells at the junction between the G1 and S phases. As a result, this checkpoint is sensitive to nutrients, growth agents, and other circumstances that encourage proliferation. The activation of the E2F transcription factor [23], which is crucial for regulating many of the genes required to start DNA replication, controls the transition from G1 to the S phase. By interacting with the retinoblastoma (Rb) protein, E2F is inactive in G1. Normally, cyclinD/CDK4 and cyclinE/CDK2 phosphorylate the Rb protein as cells transition from G1 to S. As a result of this phosphorylation, Rb is liberated from E2F, enabling E2F to operate as a transcription factor and start the S phase. Irradiation causes p53 to stabilize and become activated, as previously mentioned. The CDKI p21 (CDKN1A) gene is one of the genes that p53 upregulates. The G1 cyclin/CDK complexes are inhibited by p21, which prevents Rb from being phosphorylated and keeps cells from entering the S phase [24]. Therefore, cells exposed to radiation in the G1 phase will experience a delay before transitioning into the S phase, which is reliant on both p53 and p21.

6.5.2. S-phase Checkpoint

The DNA synthesis rate is reduced dose-dependent in cells that are in the S phase at the time of irradiation. As a result, the time it takes for cells to duplicate their DNA significantly lengthens. Two closely similar proteins called CHK1 and CHK2 are in charge of regulating this S-phase checkpoint [25]. ATR and ATM have direct targets in CHK1 and CHK2, which are phosphorylated to activate them. They subsequently phosphorylate the CDC25A and CDC25C proteins, which results in their deactivation or destruction. The phosphatases CDC25A and CDC25C maintain CDK2 in its active, dephosphorylated state. As a result, CHK1 and CHK2 activation by ATR and ATM increases the amount of phosphorylated CDK2 and thus slows progression through the S phase. Although activation of ATM-CHK2 and ATR-CHK1 and inhibition of CDC25A/C is the primary mechanism for starting the S-phase checkpoint, several other proteins in the DDR can also affect this response. In the homologous recombination branch of DNA repair, the BRCA1 and BRCA2 proteins, which serve a key role, are included [26]. This implies a complicated interaction between DNA repair and checkpoint activation.

6.5.3. G2 Checkpoints

In the G2 phase, there are two checkpoints, both of which function similarly to those in the S phase. The 'early' G2 checkpoint, which is dependent on ATM-CHK2-CDC25A/C, applies to cells that are exposed to radiation when in G2. This checkpoint causes a stop in cell cycle progression at the end of G2 and is activated by relatively low radiation doses (1 Gy is sufficient) [27].

The mitotic cyclinB/CDK1 complex, which, like CDK2 in the S-phase, must be dephosphorylated on particular locations to become active, is the target of ATM-CHK2-CDC25A/C signalling in this instance. Because it affects cells that are exposed to radiation while they are in the G2 phase and quickly prevents their progression into mitosis, it is known as the early G2 checkpoint [28]. As a result, there is a drop in the number of cells within mitosis at short times after irradiation.

On the other hand, the 'late' G2 checkpoint applies to cells that have previously undergone radiation exposure when in the G1 or S phases, and it explains a G2 delay seen at longer durations following irradiation. These cells might go through short-lived G1 and S-phase checkpoints, but when they reach the G2 phase many hours later, they go through another delay before beginning mitosis. This delay, distinct from the early G2 checkpoint and can last for many hours following high radiation doses, is substantially dose dependent. Unlike all other damage checkpoints, this late G2 checkpoint is also ATM-independent. Instead, the principal signalling axis occurs from ATR to CHK1 to CDC25A/C [29]. The late G2 checkpoint is thus mechanistically similar to the S and early G2 checkpoints and likely arises from a fundamentally different and replication-associated type of DNA damage.

6.6. Checkpoints, Cancer and Radiosensitivity

The genetic alterations that occur during tumorigenesis cause one or more of the G1/S, S, and early G2 checkpoints to be impaired in many cancer cells. These checkpoint reactions have been connected to the disruption of the tumour suppressor function, which is necessary for oncogene-induced proliferation. This is believed to happen after growth-promoting oncogenes are activated, which causes "inappropriate replication" and DNA damage from replication stress. When in operation, the checkpoints prevent these cells from proliferating further, which can effectively restrict cancer growth. The observation that numerous early cancer lesions exhibit broad checkpoint activation lends credence to this theory. Mutations in the genes that control checkpoint activation will prevent the cell cycle from being delayed in response to irradiation. This might significantly impact the development of tumours and genetic instability following radiation, but it might not impact cellular radiosensitivity as a whole [30]. Even though checkpoints are frequently regarded as offering extra time for repair, this extra time appears to be more crucial for preserving genomic integrity than for promoting cell survival. For instance, while most cancer cells are not highly radiosensitive, they have abnormalities in the G1- and S-phase cell-cycle checkpoints due to mutations in the lack of tumour suppressor proteins like p53 or Rb. Loss of the protein p21 abolishes the radiation-induced G1/S checkpoint without appreciably affecting radiosensitivity, even in isogenic cell cultures. On the other hand, G2 checkpoints that stop cells from going through mitosis with DNA damage are crucial for cell survival following radiation.

Low-dose hyper-radiosensitivity is when cells fail to activate the 'early' ATM-dependent G2 checkpoint in response to very low radiation doses (1 Gy). Genetic disruption of the 'late' ATR-dependent G2 checkpoint also causes radiosensitivity, particularly when combined with defects in other checkpoints. Therefore, it has been suggested that blocking ATR signalling may preferentially radiosensitize cancer cells who, resulting from abnormalities in proteins like p53, lack other checkpoints. The G1 and S checkpoints may affect how responsive cells are to multiple (fractionated) doses of radiation, even though they don't always alter how radiosensitive cells are to single doses of radiation [31]. The relocation of cells in the cell cycle following irradiation will depend on whether checkpoints are present. Since DNA repair capacity varies over the cell cycle, this could indirectly impact cells' sensitivity to additional radiation doses. Cell-cycle checkpoints may become increasingly significant for radiation response *in vivo* and in some normal tissues due to the coordination of tissue architecture and growth kinetics.

6.7. Effector Pathways: DNA Repair

DNA lesions are detected by specialized sensing proteins that signal the cell that damage has occurred, initiating the DNA damage response. This response effectively focuses the cell's attention on the damage, stopping other processes like transcription and cell-cycle progression and, importantly, initiating DNA repair. Radiation induces a large burden of oxidized base lesions and SSBs, as well as more cytotoxic DSBs. The main repair pathways that tackle these lesions are BER, SSBR and DSBR pathways, of which DSBR is the most important for radio sensitivity [32]. Many of the involved repair proteins have been discovered through radiation response analysis, as evident from names such as 'XRCC' (X-ray repair cross-complementing) or 'RAD' (radiation).

6.7.1. Base Excision Repair and Single-Strand Break Repair

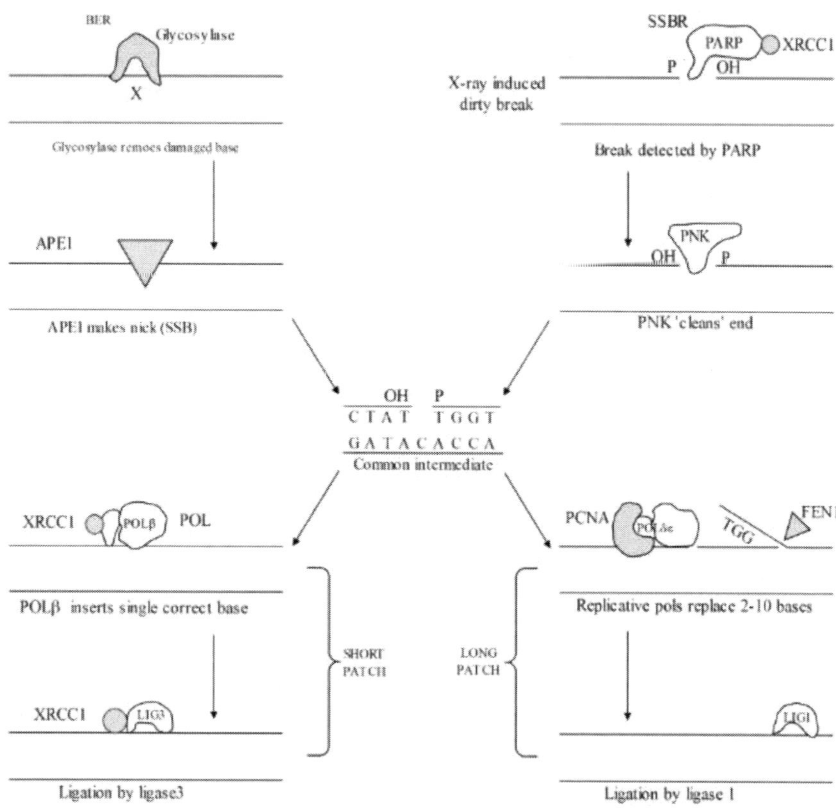

Figure 6.3. Base Excision Repair and Single-Strand Break Repair.

After radiation, base damages and SSBs are up to 50 times more common than DSBs in terms of quantity. Notably, comparable base damages and SSBs also happen without radiation since reactive oxygen species are produced by normal metabolism. Therefore, the BER and SSBR pathways have developed to repair such damage and maintain genome integrity efficiently, as shown in Figure 6.3.

As previously mentioned, PARP activation and PAR production on chromatin at the lesion sites are two of the early lesion-detecting activities. A rapid PAR response from SSBs and a basic site speeds up the recruitment of repair proteins. Then, poly (ADP-ribose)-glycohydrolase (PARG) eliminates PAR polymers [33].

Briefly, in BER, most of the DNA's damaged bases are found and removed by specialized glycosylase proteins, leaving a basic site in their place. When an AP endonuclease (APE) detects this, it will cut the DNA backbone, leaving a nickHR or NHEJ repairs a DSB or SSB. Short patch or extended patch are the two paths that subsequent repair takes. In a short patch, DNA polymerase (POL) is used to repair the broken base in the presence of XRCC1, and then ligase 3 (LIG3) is used to ligate the DNA ends. In a lengthy patch, DNA polymerase (or) in the presence of PCNA replaces up to 10 nucleotides surrounding the damaged site, while flap endonuclease 1 (FEN1) removes the overhanging nucleotides [34]. Next, ligase 1 (LIG1) ligates the remaining nucleotides. Many of the enzymes used in SSBR are also used in BER. Through its intimate interactions with ligase 3 and other proteins, XRCC1 recruitment, which is mediated by PAR and substantially supports BER and SSBR, is supported. The radiation-induced SSBs, which offer DNA ends with oxidized nucleotides and lack the phosphate group-linked ends required for ligation, are frequently more complicated than those produced endogenously. They need end processing since ligases and polymerases do not recognize them. Enzymes like PNK (polynucleotide kinase), PNKP (polynucleotide kinase 3′-phosphatase), or AP endonucleases can carry out this procedure. Repair can proceed after a clean end has been formed. Notably, decreased radiation damage repair and comparatively mild radio sensitization can result from mutation, deletion, or inhibition of any of the two primary BER/SSBR enzymes [35]. There are probably effective backup mechanisms, so a damaged SSBR pathway does not significantly affect radiosensitive cells. Unrepaired SSBs can eventually develop into DSBs, which can then be fixed by DSB repair equipment. However, targeting SSBR in cancers with DSBR abnormalities can be a desirable therapeutic approach.

6.7.2. Double-Strand Break Repair

Radiation can result in direct DSBs that, if repaired incorrectly or not at all, can damage chromosomes or chromatids. Homologous recombination (HR) and non-homologous end joining (NHEJ) are the two primary processes of DSBR. While NHEJ does not, HR uses the replicated homologous sister chromatid as a template for mending DSBs [36]. As a result, HR becomes a high-fidelity repair mechanism that preserves the original DNA sequence, as opposed to NHEJ, which is error-prone and frequently leads to DNA alterations that cannot be reversed. The chromatin structure and cell cycle phase determine whether HR or NHEJ repairs a DSB. 90% of the DNA typically resides in euchromatin, loosely packed and capable of transcriptional activity. NHEJ with quick kinetics is mostly used to repair DSBs within euchromatin. The choice of repair strategy for the 10% of DNA contained within the denser-packed superstructures of the transcriptionally inactive heterochromatin depends on the cell cycle stage. These DSBs must also be repaired by NHEJ when a duplicated sister chromatid is not present, such as during G1 and the early stages of S phase. HR will, however, repair these breaks if the damaged DNA has already undergone replication, as in the G2 phase. For DSBR to occur, heterochromatin must be remodelled, and this process depends on MRN activating A.T.M., which in turn phosphorylates KAP1 and the endonuclease ARTEMIS. Repair of DSBs within heterochromatin occurs with slower kinetics. The importance of proper DNA repair within heterochromatin is evidenced by the severe radio sensitivity of cells or patients lacking functional ATM [37].

When mending a DSB, several proteins assist in determining whether to use the NHEJ or HR pathway. Cells cannot try HR in G1 because CDK1 activity controls the DNA end resection necessary for HR. Additionally, H2AX phosphorylation encourages RNF8 and RNF168 to ubiquitylate H2A proteins in the nearby chromatin, which acts as a signalling hub for the recruitment of repair components specific to a certain pathway. The protein 53BP1, which drives repair towards NHEJ in G1 by promoting end resection at DNA breaks that directly oppose HR factors, is drawn to mono-ubiquitylated H2A [38]. In contrast, the chromatin's poly-ubiquitination chains draw the adaptor protein RAP80, which calls for the HR protein machinery.

6.7.2.1. Non-Homologous End Joining

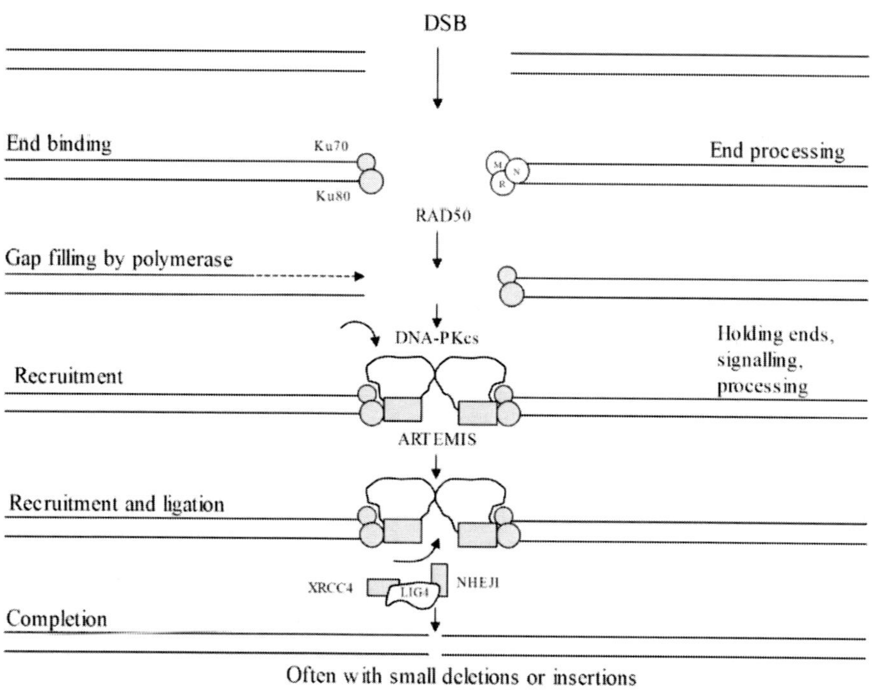

Figure 6.4. Non Homologus double strand break repair.

NHEJ merely connects two DNA DSB ends. The recruitment of the DNA-PKcs occurs first; then the Ku70/80 heterodimer binds to the ends of the DNA. Given its size, the protein can physically connect the two ends as a bridge, keeping them close together for future repair processes.

As shown in Figure 6.4., when coupled to the Ku complex at break sites, DNA-PKcs also turns on as a kinase. DSBs may have “overhangs” (non-blunt ends) or sugar group residues that prevent them from being ligated. To enable ligation by DNA ligase 4 with the assistance of XRRC4 and NHEJ1, the PNK, ARTEMIS endonuclease, and polymerases handle the broken DNA ends. However, this procedure can also lead to DNA loss or gain, resulting in irreversible mutations, insertions, and irreversible deletions. It is not surprising that the deletion of crucial NHEJ proteins like DNA-PKcs or ligase 4 leads in extreme radio sensitivity given that NHEJ is the only DSBR mechanism in G1 and is in charge of repairing 90% of DSBs in G2 [39]. The lack of sparing caused by dividing a single dose into many dose portions is another effect of inadequate repair capacity. As a result, the cellular dose-response curves have a high / value and are essentially straight. Patients with mutations in these genes frequently present with severe immunodeficiency because the NHEJ machinery also participates in the V(D)J recombination of antibodies and T-cell receptors. Similar to the ‘SCID’ mouse strain, which is frequently employed in laboratories, lacks DNA-PKcs activity, which underlies both its weakened immune system and radiosensitive phenotype [40].

6.7.2.2. Homologous Recombination

As a template for repair, HR uses replicated, intact homologous DNA as shown in Figure 6.5. By doing so, the cell cycle’s S and G2 phases are the only ones active. The repair procedure, which restores the DNA to its original state before the damage, can be error-free using DNA with the same sequence as a template.

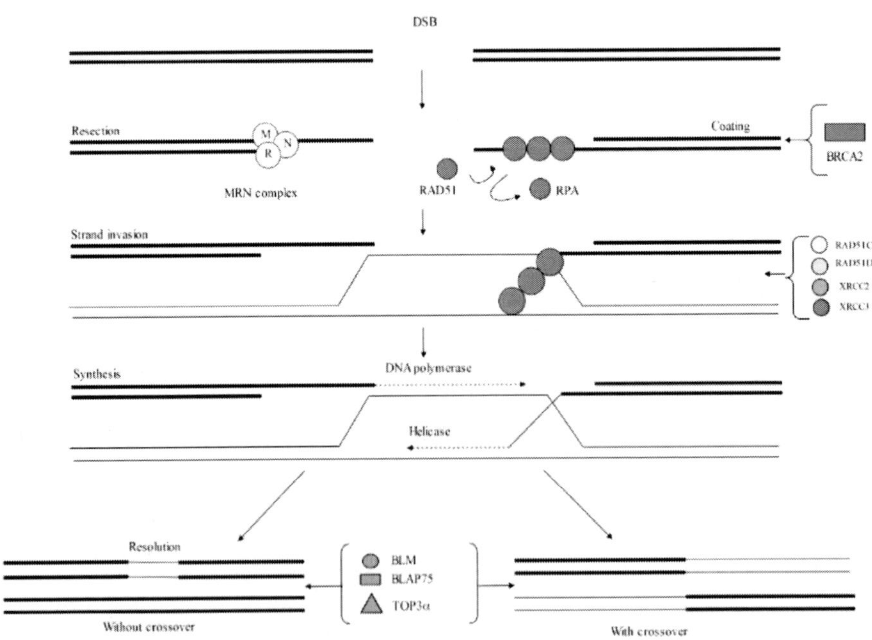

Figure 6.5. Homologous double strand break repair.

Each side of the split generates single-stranded areas. They are produced in large part by MRN and other exonucleases like Exo1. The coating of the exposed single-stranded regions with specialized proteins, such as RPA follows this. These single-stranded nucleoprotein filaments can now invade sister chromatid DNA that has not been damaged. This process is guided by the RAD51 protein placed onto these areas, with help from BRCA2 (the type 2 breast cancer susceptibility gene product). RAD51B, RAD51C, RAD51D, XRCC2 and XRCC3 are a few RAD51 paralogs that aid in the hunt for homologous DNA and sister chromatid invasion processes. Homologous recombination can be significantly hampered by the deletion or mutation of any one of these genes [41]. Helicases like BLM aid in releasing DNA from its tightly wound structure, enabling homology search, invasion, and annealing. DNA polymerases can precisely repair the break by synthesizing across the absent sections of the damaged spot when an intact DNA template is found and provided. The crossover structure that comes from this must be reversed to restore the chromatin to its initial state. This is accomplished using specialized nucleases, which first cut or resolve the junctions before ligating the neighbouring ends. Structure-specific endonucleases like the human MUS81 complex, SLX4 and SLX1, which are also involved in unravelling the DNA, assisting in the resolution of these complex structures created during strand invasion and template replication. In order to prevent DNA crossover, the RMI complex (BLM, BLAP75, TOP3) is crucial. As HR becomes a DSBR route, cells exhibit increased radiation resistance in the cell cycle's late S and G2 stages. The HR machinery also repairs the DNA interstrand crosslink (ICL) damage that results in the stalling of replication forks. ICL is particularly dependent on the Fanconi Anaemia (FA) family of proteins, and cells with FA gene mutations are more sensitive to DNA crosslinking agents. By ubiquitylating FANC-D2 and -I, the core FA complex (consisting of FANC-A, -B, -C, -E, -F, -G, -L, -M) activates downstream targets (FANC-D1, -J, -N), which in turn activates proteins to digest the crosslinked DNA, synthesize new DNA across the break, and assemble the repaired DNA sequence. BRCA2/FANC-D1 and RAD51/FANC-O are only a few of the names many HR proteins use to indicate their role in this process. Patients with FA mutations initially experience bone marrow failure, as the name suggests, but they are also more likely to develop acute myelogenous leukaemia (AML) [42]. Similar to this, people who carry germline mutations in the HR genes BRCA1 and BRCA2 are considerably more likely to acquire cancer throughout their lifespan, especially breast and ovarian cancer. Cells lacking in HR and FA proteins are somewhat radiosensitive due to the HR and FA pathways' functions in DSBR and replication-associated stress. Concerns have been raised about the possibility of second malignancies and normal tissue toxicity in breast cancer patients who also contain BRCA1/BRCA2 mutations as a result of this. The fact that the normal cells have a wild-type (non-mutated) allele that is functionally competent likely accounts for the lack of evidence for increased detrimental effects in this patient population after radiation. Exploiting HR flaws for therapeutic purposes is very popular. In cancers lacking BRCA1 or BRCA2, blocking SSBR with PARP inhibitors have been proven to be an effective therapy. Stalled replication forks become DSBs when PARP is inhibited and need repair of HR. Thus, a therapeutic ratio for this strategy is provided by the particular loss of BRCA in cancer cells [43].

6.7.2.3. Mismatch Repair

Mis-paired nucleotides, such as those other than A-T and C-G, are corrected through the MMR pathway. It includes a recognition phase, an excision and re-synthesis step, and a ligation step, just like all other repair pathways. Most research using MMR gene deletion cells did not discover a significant rise in radio sensitivity. However, given that MMR-deficient cells show altered susceptibility to specific chemotherapeutic drugs (such as cisplatin and temozolomide), this pathway is relevant to the treatment of cancer. Additionally, due to their inability to eliminate the changed base, MMR-deficient cells are more radiosensitive to thymidine analogues like IUdR. Therefore, the MMR status of cells may be significant for the outcome of radiation when combined with other treatments. Additionally, cancers with MMR deficiencies have an incredibly high mutational load, which results in antigens that make them vulnerable to immune checkpoint blockage. Based on this, the U.S. Food and Drug Administration approved an immune checkpoint inhibitor for tumours bearing MMR abnormalities in 2017 as the first pan-cancer treatment based on a genetic biomarker [44].

6.7.2.4. Nucleotide Excision Repair

NER can handle large lesions that disrupt the DNA helix at one strand, such as those brought on by UV light (thymine dimers) or DNA adducts brought on by cross-linkers like cisplatin. The NER proteins ERCC1 and XPF break the DNA surrounding the damaged spot [45]. This causes a sizable single-stranded gap that polymerases fill up to repair the DNA helix. NER gene dysfunction generally has little impact on IR sensitivity.

6.7.3. Radiation Quality, Cell Types and Cellular Context

The biggest problem for the cell could be the concentrated damage caused by IR. For instance, if base damage develops on the strand opposite a radiation-induced SSB, the transient nick created during BER may join with the radiation break on that strand to produce a DSB. These intricate lesion locations have greater mutagenicity and cytotoxicity because they need a lot of DDR coordination. Radiation treatments that result in more complicated lesions and clustered damage are comparatively more effective. DNA repair capacity varied between stem cells and differentiated cells, cancer cells and healthy cells, and between cell types of varied origins. These variances may differ in how radiation reacts with normal tissue and tumours. It has been demonstrated that stem cells, which are important for both, have a higher capacity for HR than differentiated cells, possibly indicating the significance of preventing mutations in these cells [46]. Most non-proliferative normal tissue cells (resting in G0) must rely on NHEJ for DSB repair because HR is only used by actively growing cells. Radiation therapy and other IR exposures can cause normal cells to multiply with DNA damage that has not been properly repaired, larger mutations, and chromosomal abnormalities. This can lead to the development of cancer. From vast cohorts of atomic bomb survivors and radiation-monitored personnel, it has been determined that radiation causes a dose-dependent increased relative risk of cancer. The DNA damage response is either absent or altered in cancer cells due to genetic abnormalities or transcriptional dysregulation. Genomic instability brought on by DDR flaws is regarded as an enabling factor in cancer growth. Because of these flaws, cancer cells are expected to perform DNA repair somewhat differently than healthy cells, which may present opportunities for targeted radiation therapy [47].

Conclusion

This chapter has provided an in-depth exploration of how ionizing radiation induces diverse types of DNA damage, emphasizing the pivotal role of double-strand breaks in determining cellular fate. The coordinated DNA damage response system—encompassing damage sensing, signaling transducers, cell-cycle checkpoints, DNA repair pathways, and programmed cell death—ensures that damaged cells can either repair lesions or be eliminated to preserve genomic integrity. The detailed discussion of homologous recombination, non-homologous end joining, and other repair mechanisms highlights how cells maintain stability despite constant threats to DNA. Understanding these processes not only informs radiobiology and cancer therapy but also reveals opportunities to selectively target tumors by exploiting their DNA repair vulnerabilities, ultimately enhancing the therapeutic efficacy and safety of radiation treatments.

References

[1] Zhou BB, Elledge SJ. The DNA damage response: putting checkpoints in perspective. *Nature.* 2000 Nov 23;408(6811):433-9.

[2] Jackson SP, Bartek J. The DNA-damage response in human biology and disease. *Nature*. 2009 Oct 22;461(7267):1071-8.

[3] McGowan CH, Russell P. The DNA damage response: sensing and signaling. *Current opinion in cell biology*. 2004 Dec 1;16(6):629-33

[4] Maser RS, Zinkel R, Petrini JH. An alternative mode of translation permits production of a variant NBS1 protein from the common Nijmegen breakage syndrome allele. *Nature genetics*. 2001 Apr;27(4):417-21.

[5] Wold MS. Replication protein A: a heterotrimeric, single-stranded DNA-binding protein required for eukaryotic DNA metabolism. *Annual review of biochemistry*. 1997 Jul;66(1):61-92.

[6] Kruman II, Wersto RP, Cardozo-Pelaez F, Smilenov L, Chan SL, Chrest FJ, Emokpae R, Gorospe M, Mattson MP. Cell cycle activation linked to neuronal cell death initiated by DNA damage. *Neuron.* 2004 Feb 19;41(4):549-61.

[7] Helt CE, Cliby WA, Keng PC, Bambara RA, O'Reilly MA. Ataxia telangiectasia mutated (ATM) and ATM and Rad3-related protein exhibit selective target specificities in response to different forms of DNA damage. *Journal of Biological Chemistry*. 2005 Jan 14;280(2):1186-92.

[8] Matsuoka S, Rotman G, Ogawa A, Shiloh Y, Tamai K, Elledge SJ. Ataxia telangiectasia-mutated phosphorylates Chk2 *in vivo* and *in vitro*. *Proceedings of the National Academy of Sciences*. 2000 Sep 12;97(19):10389-94.

[9] Dickey JS, Redon CE, Nakamura AJ, Baird BJ, Sedelnikova OA, Bonner WM. H2AX: functional roles and potential applications. *Chromosoma.* 2009 Dec;118:683-92.

[10] Monteiro FL, Baptista T, Amado F, Vitorino R, Jerónimo C, Helguero LA. Expression and functionality of histone H2A variants in cancer. *Oncotarget*. 2014 Jun;5(11):3428.

[11] Rivera-Calzada A, Maman JP, Spagnolo L, Pearl LH, Llorca O. Three-dimensional structure and regulation of the DNA-dependent protein kinase catalytic subunit (DNA-PKcs). *Structure.* 2005 Feb 1;13(2):243-55.

[12] Kumagai A, Lee J, Yoo HY, Dunphy WG. TopBP1 activates the ATR-ATRIP complex. *Cell.* 2006 Mar 10;124(5):943-55.

[13] Zhang J, Dai Q, Park D, Deng X. Targeting DNA replication stress for cancer therapy. *Genes*. 2016 Aug 19;7(8):51.

[14] Poly (ADP-ribose) polymerase. A molecular nick sensor. *Trends Biochem Sci.* 1994;19:172-6.

[15] Realini CA, Althaus FR. Histone shuttling by poly (ADP-ribosylation). *Journal of Biological Chemistry*. 1992 Sep 15;267(26):18858-65.

[16] Maya R, Balass M, Kim ST, Shkedy D, Leal JF, Shifman O, Moas M, Buschmann T, Ronai ZE, Shiloh Y, Kastan MB. ATM-dependent phosphorylation of Mdm2 on serine 395: role in p53 activation by DNA damage. *Genes & development*. 2001 May 1;15(9):1067-77.

[17] Khosravi R, Maya R, Gottlieb T, Oren M, Shiloh Y, Shkedy D. Rapid ATM-dependent phosphorylation of MDM2 precedes p53 accumulation in response to DNA damage. *Proceedings of the National Academy of Sciences*. 1999 Dec 21;96(26):14973-7.

[18] Moll UM, Wolff S, Speidel D, Deppert W. Transcription-independent pro-apoptotic functions of p53. *Current opinion in cell biology*. 2005 Dec 1;17(6):631-6.

[19] Fridman JS, Lowe SW. Control of apoptosis by p53. *Oncogene*. 2003 Dec;22(56):9030-40.

[20] Abraham RT. Cell cycle checkpoint signaling through the ATM and ATR kinases. *Genes & development*. 2001 Sep 1;15(17):2177-96.

[21] Malumbres M, Sotillo R, Santamaría D, Galán J, Cerezo A, Ortega S, Dubus P, Barbacid M. Mammalian cells cycle without the D-type cyclin-dependent kinases Cdk4 and Cdk6. *Cell*. 2004 Aug 20;118(4):493-504.

[22] Adams PD, Sellers WR, Sharma SK, Wu AD, Nalin CM, Kaelin Jr WG. Identification of a cyclin-cdk2 recognition motif present in substrates and p21-like cyclin-dependent kinase inhibitors. *Molecular and cellular biology*. 1996 Dec 1;16(12):6623-33.

[23] Iaquinta PJ, Lees JA. Life and death decisions by the E2F transcription factors. *Current opinion in cell biology*. 2007 Dec 1;19(6):649-57.

[24] Hung T, Wang Y, Lin MF, Koegel AK, Kotake Y, Grant GD, Horlings HM, Shah N, Umbricht C, Wang P, Wang Y. Extensive and coordinated transcription of noncoding RNAs within cell-cycle promoters. *Nature genetics*. 2011 Jul;43(7):621-9.

[25] Sørensen CS, Syljuåsen RG, Falck J, Schroeder T, Rönnstrand L, Khanna KK, Zhou BB, Bartek J, Lukas J. Chk1 regulates the S phase checkpoint by coupling the physiological turnover and ionizing radiation-induced accelerated proteolysis of Cdc25A. *Cancer cell*. 2003 Mar 1;3(3):247-58.

[26] Agarwal C, Tyagi A, Agarwal R. Gallic acid causes inactivating phosphorylation of cdc25A/cdc25C-cdc2 via ATM-Chk2 activation, leading to cell cycle arrest, and induces apoptosis in human prostate carcinoma DU145 cells. *Molecular cancer therapeutics*. 2006 Dec 1;5(12):3294-302.

[27] Vens C, Koritzinsky M, Wouters BG. Irradiation-induced damage and the DNA damage response. *Basic clinical radiobiology*. 2018 Aug 28:9.

[28] Lindqvist A, Rodríguez-Bravo V, Medema RH. The decision to enter mitosis: feedback and redundancy in the mitotic entry network. *Journal of Cell Biology*. 2009 Apr 20;185(2):193-202.

[29] Goldstone S, Pavey S, Forrest A, Sinnamon J, Gabrielli B. Cdc25-dependent activation of cyclin A/cdk2 is blocked in G2 phase arrested cells independently of ATM/ATR. *Oncogene*. 2001 Feb;20(8):921-32.

[30] Jeggo P, Lavin MF. Cellular radiosensitivity: how much better do we understand it?. *International journal of radiation biology*. 2009 Dec 1;85(12):1061-81.

[31] Woodward WA, Bristow RG. Radiosensitivity of cancer-initiating cells and normal stem cells (or what the Heisenberg uncertainly principle has to do with biology). In *Seminars in radiation oncology* 2009 Apr 1 (Vol. 19, No. 2, pp. 87-95). WB Saunders.

[32] Giaccia AJ, Schwartz J, Shieh J, Brown JM. The use of asymmetric-field inversion gel electrophoresis to predict tumor cell radiosensitivity. *Radiotherapy and Oncology*. 1992 Aug 1;24(4):231-8.

[33] Barkauskaite E, Brassington A, Tan ES, Warwicker J, Dunstan MS, Banos B, Lafite P, Ahel M, Mitchison TJ, Ahel I, Leys D. Visualization of poly (ADP-ribose) bound to PARG reveals inherent balance between exo-and endo-glycohydrolase activities. *Nature communications*. 2013 Aug 6;4(1):2164.

[34] Luke AM, Chastain PD, Pachkowski BF, Afonin V, Takeda S, Kaufman DG, Swenberg JA, Nakamura J. Accumulation of true single strand breaks and AP sites in base excision repair deficient cells. *Mutation Research/Fundamental and Molecular Mechanisms of Mutagenesis*. 2010 Dec 10;694(1-2):65-71.

[35] Ström CE, Johansson F, Uhlen M, Szigyarto CA, Erixon K, Helleday T. Poly (ADP-ribose) polymerase (PARP) is not involved in base excision repair but PARP inhibition traps a single-strand intermediate. *Nucleic acids research.* 2011 Apr 1;39(8):3166-75.

[36] Chakraborty A, Tapryal N, Venkova T, Horikoshi N, Pandita RK, Sarker AH, Sarkar PS, Pandita TK, Hazra TK. Classical non-homologous end-joining pathway utilizes nascent RNA for error-free double-strand break repair of transcribed genes. *Nature communications.* 2016 Oct 5;7(1):13049.

[37] Carone DM, Lawrence JB. Heterochromatin instability in cancer: from the Barr body to satellites and the nuclear periphery. In *Seminars in cancer biology* 2013 Apr 1 (Vol. 23, No. 2, pp. 99-108). Academic Press.

[38] Ward IM, Minn K, Van Deursen J, Chen J. p53 Binding protein 53BP1 is required for DNA damage responses and tumor suppression in mice. *Molecular and cellular biology.* 2003 Apr 1;23(7):2556-63.

[39] Ma Y, Schwarz K, Lieber MR. The Artemis: DNA-PKcs endonuclease cleaves DNA loops, flaps, and gaps. *DNA repair.* 2005 Jul 12;4(7):845-51.

[40] Taccioli GE, Amatucci AG, Beamish HJ, Gell D, Xiang XH, Arzayus MI, Priestley A, Jackson SP, Rothstein AM, Jeggo PA, Herrera VL. Targeted disruption of the catalytic subunit of the DNA-PK gene in mice confers severe combined immunodeficiency and radiosensitivity. *Immunity.* 1998 Sep 1;9(3):355-66.

[41] Baumann P, West SC. Role of the human RAD51 protein in homologous recombination and double-stranded-break repair. *Trends in biochemical sciences.* 1998 Jul 1;23(7):247-51.

[42] Estey E, Döhner H. Acute myeloid leukaemia. *The Lancet.* 2006 Nov 25;368(9550):1894-907.

[43] Lim J, Yang K, Taylor-Harding B, Wiedemeyer WR, Buckanovich RJ. VEGFR3 inhibition chemosensitizes ovarian cancer stemlike cells through down-regulation of BRCA1 and BRCA2. *Neoplasia.* 2014 Apr 1;16(4):343-53.

[44] Campbell BB, Light N, Fabrizio D, Zatzman M, Fuligni F, de Borja R, Davidson S, Edwards M, Elvin JA, Hodel KP, Zahurancik WJ. Comprehensive analysis of hypermutation in human cancer. *Cell.* 2017 Nov 16;171(5):1042-56.

[45] Budden T, Bowden NA. The role of altered nucleotide excision repair and UVB-induced DNA damage in melanomagenesis. *International Journal of Molecular Sciences.* 2013 Jan 9;14(1):1132-51.

[46] Van Bekkum DW. Radiation sensitivity of the hemopoietic stem cell. *Radiation research.* 1991 Oct 1;128(1s):S4-8.

[47] Morris ZS, Harari PM. Interaction of radiation therapy with molecular targeted agents. *Journal of Clinical Oncology.* 2014 Sep 9;32(26):2886.

Chapter 7

Chromosomal Aberrations and Gene Mutations

Ashish Uke[1,*], MD
Priyal Shrivastava[2], MD
Jaishriram Rathored[1], PhD
and Elangovan Doraisamy[3], MSc, DABR

[1]Department of Radiation Oncology, Datta Meghe Institute of Higher Education and Research, Wardha, India
[2]Department of Radio-diagnosis, Datta Meghe Institute of Higher Education and Research, Wardha, India
[3]Department of Radiation Oncology, UPMC Hillman Cancer Center, Pittsburgh, PA, USA

Abstract

Following chapter provides an in-depth exploration of genetics and chromosomal abnormalities, covering various topics such as the structure and function of cells, DNA, chromosomes, genetic disorders, and chromosomal abnormalities. It explains the basic units of life, cells, and the genetic material DNA, which carries information from one generation to the next. It also delves into the world of chromosomes, discussing their structure, function, and the genetic disorders that can occur due to mutations in DNA. The text categorizes genetic disorders into three main types: Mendelian disorders, multifactorial disorders, and chromosomal disorders. It provides examples of Mendelian disorders, such as sickle cell anemia and Huntington's disease, and explains their patterns of inheritance. Additionally, it discusses multifactorial disorders, such as heart disease and diabetes, which are influenced by multiple genetic and environmental factors. It also explores chromosomal abnormalities, including numerical and structural changes, and their effects on human health. It discusses various types of chromosomal abnormalities, such as aneuploidy, translocations, and deletions, and their associations with genetic disorders. Overall, this chapter provides a thorough understanding of genetics and chromosomal abnormalities, making it an essential resource for students, researchers, and healthcare professionals.

Keywords: chromosomal aberration, cytogenetic disorders, genetic diagnosis, gene mutation, mendelian disorders, multifactorial inheritance

* Corresponding Author's Email: ashishuke1@gmail.com

In: Fundamentals of Radiation Biology
Editors: Anurag Luharia, Ashish Uke, Gaurav Mishra et al.
ISBN: 979-8-89530-806-6

7.1. Introduction

Genetics is the study of heredity, genes, and variation. It is a fundamental aspect of biology that has revolutionized our understanding of life and its complexities. The discovery of the structure and function of DNA, the genetic material that carries information from one generation to the next, has been a major milestone in the field of genetics. The study of genetics has led to a deeper understanding of the mechanisms of inheritance, the causes of genetic disorders, and the development of new treatments and therapies.

Chromosomal abnormalities, which occur when there is a change in the number or structure of chromosomes, are a significant area of study in genetics. These abnormalities can have a profound impact on human health, leading to genetic disorders, birth defects, and infertility. Understanding the causes and consequences of chromosomal abnormalities is essential for the diagnosis, treatment, and prevention of genetic disorders.

The following chapter provides an in-depth exploration of genetics and chromosomal abnormalities, covering various topics such as the structure and function of cells, DNA, chromosomes, genetic disorders, and chromosomal abnormalities. It aims to provide a thorough understanding of the principles of genetics and the mechanisms of chromosomal abnormalities, as well as their effects on human health. Through this chapter, readers will gain a comprehensive understanding of the complex relationships between genes, chromosomes, and genetic disorders. They will also learn about the latest advances in genetic research and the development of new treatments and therapies for genetic disorders. By exploring the fascinating world of genetics and chromosomal abnormalities, readers will gain a deeper appreciation for the complexities of life and the importance of genetics in understanding human health and disease.

7.2. Chromosome, DNA, and Gene

Cells are the structural units of all life. The human body is made up of trillions of cells. They sustain the body's structure, absorb nutrients through food, and convert nutrients into energy while performing specialized tasks. Cells can replicate and transmit the body's genetic material [1]. The nucleus is the cell's command centre, receiving instructions on developing, maturing, dividing, and dying. It also contains DNA (deoxyribonucleic acid), known as nuclear DNA. The nucleus is surrounded by the nuclear envelope, which protects the DNA and isolates it from the rest of the components of the cell. DNA, or deoxyribonucleic acid, is the hereditary substance in humans and almost all other animals. Every cell in an individual's body possesses the same DNA. Most DNA can be discovered in the cell's nucleus, but a small amount is also present in the mitochondria (it is referred to as mitochondrial DNA or mtDNA).

DNA stores information in the form of a code composed of four chemical bases: adenine (A), guanine (G), cytosine (C), and thymine (T). Human DNA comprises around 3 billion bases, with over 95% being identical in all humans [2]. The order, or sequence, of each of these bases, establishes the information available for constructing and maintaining an organism, much as letters of the alphabet appear precisely to produce words and phrases. Once two DNA bases, A with T and C with G, bind, base pairs are created. Each base is also connected to a sugar molecule and a phosphate molecule. A nucleotide comprises three components: a base, a sugar, and a phosphate. Nucleotides are connected in two long strands to produce a spiral-shaped structure known as a double helix [3]. The structure of the double helix is comparable to that of a ladder, with the base pairs forming the steps and the phosphate and sugar molecules forming the vertical sidepieces.

The capacity of DNA to replicate or make copies of itself is a critical characteristic. Every single DNA strand in the double helix could be used as a template for replicating the base sequence. Cells must divide since each new cell must have an exact DNA duplicate in the old cells.

A gene is the most basic physical and functional component of heredity. The essential block of genes is DNA. Some genes act as blueprints for the creation of protein molecules. However, many genes lack protein coding. Human genes range from a few hundred DNA bases to more than 2 million bases. According to the Human Genome Project, a multinational scientific effort focused on discovering the sequence of the human genome and the genes it includes, humans have between 20,000 and 25,000 genes [4]. Every person has two genes, one from each of their parents. Although most genes are the same in all persons, a small number of genes (less than 1%) are unique.

7.2.1. Chromatid and Centromere

A chromatid consists of two identical replicas of a duplicated chromosome connected by a region known as the centromere. Each chromosome comprises two sister chromatids kept together at the centromere after DNA replication occurs during a cell cycle [5]. Each chromatid has the same DNA sequence as the original chromosome. Chromatins split and produce distinct chromosomes transferred to daughter cells during cell division.

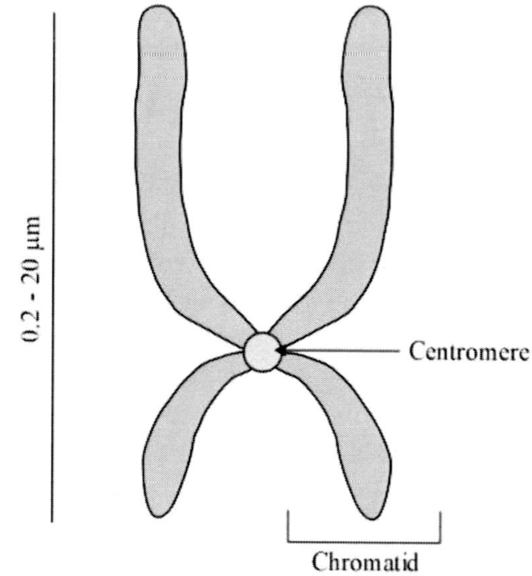

Figure 7.1. Illustration of a chromosome.

A centromere is a specialized region on a chromosome that acts as a site of attachment for spindle fibers during cell division. It plays a crucial role in ensuring the accurate segregation of chromosomes during Mitosis (cell division for growth and tissue repair) and Meiosis (cell division for sexual reproduction). The centromere acts as a binding site for proteins that form the kinetochore, which interacts with spindle fibres to facilitate chromosome movement and separation of sister chromatids during cell division.

7.3. Autosomal and Sex Chromosome

Autosomes are non-sex chromosomes that establish an organism's characteristics. They are known as somatic chromosomes since they determine an individual's physical traits. The majority of one's genome is made up of autosomes. For example, the human genome contains 46 chromosomes, 44 of which comprise autosomes [6]. Autosomes exist as homologous pairs, with 22 autosome pairings in the human genome. The same genes are found on both autosomal chromosomes and are ordered in the same order. An autosomal chromosome pair, on the contrary, differs from other autosomal chromosome pairs across the same genome. These pairs are marked from 1 to 22 based on each chromosome's number of base pairs. Allosomes are the names given to sex chromosomes. They determine a person's gender. Most animals and many plants also have sex determination. Humans have only two sex chromosomes within their genome, which are known as the X and Y chromosomes. XX determines a female individual, while XY determines a male human. A female has two copies of the same sex-determining genes in the same order on both X chromosomes (homomorphic).

Female gametes are generated from a single X chromosome and 22 autosomal chromosomes during Meiosis. Male gametes have an X or Y chromosome and 22 autosomal chromosomes. A female kid is born from combining two gametes containing both X chromosomes. The merger of a pair of gametes with an X or Y chromosome results in a male child. The fertilization of gametes, each carrying a haploid pair of chromosomes, leads to the development of a diploid human genome. Unfertilized ant and bee eggs develop into haploid males, whilst fertilized eggs evolve into females. A defective second copy of the same gene causes sex-linked genetic disorders such as hemophilia and muscular dystrophy [7]. Gene abnormalities on the X chromosomes cause red and green blindness. Because men only have one X chromosome, inheriting a defective version of the gene that causes red/green blindness might result in blindness. Unusual sex chromosomal combinations (for example, XXX, XXY) cause developmental issues in new-borns. Heteromorphic sex chromosomes are passed down to children at variable rates. As a result, they are less relevant in evolutionary processes like Mutation, selection, and genetic drift. Homomorphic chromosomes, on the other hand, go through processes of evolution that involve homologous recombination and mutation. Thus, sex chromosomes are disproportionate, according to Haldane's rule.

7.4. Genotype and Phenotype

The genotype of a person is their unique DNA sequence. This phrase refers to the collection of two alleles that a person inherited for a specific gene [8]. The phenotype of this genotype is its observable expression. The interaction of a person's genetics and environment determines his or her phenotype. The relationship between genetics and phenotype is only sometimes evident. This suggests that there may be discrepancies between your patient's genomic test results and clinical presentation [9].

Similarly, even within families, the phenotypic of patients with a specific genetic disease might vary substantially. The variety of phenotypes seen in patients having the same genetic disease. A patient with one variety may have modest symptoms, whereas another having the same variant may have severe disease. The reasons for varying expressivity, like diminished penetrance, still need to be fully understood. It could be more challenging to diagnose a hereditary illness if the symptoms are highly varied. In both dominant and recessive circumstances, variable expressivity is prevalent.

7.5. Cell Cycle and Cell Division

The cell cycle refers to the series of events in a cell as it grows, prepares for division, and divides into two daughter cells. It is a highly regulated and coordinated process that ensures the accurate duplication and distribution of genetic material (DNA) to maintain cell integrity and promote growth and tissue renewal. The cell cycle consists of four main phases: G1 (Gap 1), S (Synthesis), G2 (Gap 2), and M (Mitosis) [10].

a. *G_1 Phase:* G1 means the first gap phase needed before the DNA synthetic phase. It is present in the interval between the M and S phases; hence, it is called the post-mitotic and pre-synthetic phases. It is the most extended phase of the cell cycle, and hence, it contributes 25-50% of the total time of interphase. In this phase, RNA synthesis, Protein synthesis, ATP synthesis, Nucleotide synthesis and various enzyme androgynes synthesis occur. These enzymes, which are synthesized here, are used in DNA replication in the S phase. Due to this all-synthetic process, the cell volume increases, and hence, cells undergo division.
b. *The S Phase* is a synthetic DNA phase in which the DNA replication occurs, called the Synthetic Phase (S phase) [11]. This phase is the interval between the G1 phase and G2 phase, hence called the phase and pre-G2 phase. The enzymes, nucleotide, ATP, amino acids, and histone protein are synthesized and utilized in this phase. The total DNA content of the cell doubles after DNA replication. The amount of the DNA in the nucleus of the cell is denoted by "C." The number of chromosomes in a nucleus is denoted by "N." All cells except gametes in humans have two sets of chromosomes; hence, it is represented as 2N (Diploid). The gametes have only one set of chromosomes, denoted as N (haploid). Only DNA replication occurs during this S phase; hence, the amount of DNA gets doubled, which is the most crucial step during cell division. This means that if a Diploid cell has a 2C amount of DNA, it becomes 2C at the end of the S phase. All should note that there is no increase in the

number of chromosomes. The new chromatids of the chromosomes are not separated and are attached to the centromere; hence, we cannot consider an increase in chromosome number—only the DNA amount doubles. Therefore, if a human body cell has 2C DNA and 2N chromosome number, it has only 4C DNA but 2N chromosomes at the end of the S phase.

c. *G_2 Phase:* This is called the second gap phase, as it is required for the M phase. This phase is the interval between the S and M phases; therefore, it is called the post-phase and pre-M phases (Premitotic phase). No DNA replication occurs in this phase, but transcription and translation are the key features. In this phase, translation produces a special protein called Tubulin protein. There are two types of tubulin protein: alpha-tubulin and beta-tubulin [12]. These monomers come together and form a dimer of tubulin. Many Tubulin dimers form a polymer, i.e., a long chain of the tubulin protein called spindle fibers. These spindle fibers are useful in the M phase to separate chromosomes. In the G phase, all enzymes and proteins are produced, which is required to dissolve the nuclear membrane. The cell organelle is also duplicated, as two new cells are produced in the M phase.
d. *M phase:* It includes all dividing stages of the cell cycle [13]. This phase lasts for 1 hr in a human cell. In this phase, two cell division types occur: Mitosis and Meiosis. If the reproductive cell participates in cell division to produce gametes or spores, then it undergoes Meiosis. If the cell participates in body structure, then it undergoes Mitosis. No cell at a time undergoes both Mitosis and Meiosis or no cell undergoes half Mitosis and half Meiosis.
e. *G_0 Phase:* It is also called the Differential phase or quiescent phase of the cell cycle. After division, when a new daughter cell is produced, these cells again start the cell cycle from the beginning of the G phase. These cells undergo different growth and development processes, which are essential for the functioning of the cell's life cycle. Therefore, if a new cell wants to undergo cell division, it moves further from the G phase to the other phase sequentially. However, if a new cell undergoes complete development and does not enter into the further division phases, then such a cell undergoes a resting period. This resting period is called the G phase [14]. There are many cells that last for life in G, like neurons, RBC Heart cells, skeletal muscles, etc. The cells in the G phase are metabolically active but cannot divide. Differentiation is the process by which new cells gain their function in growth and development. If the checkpoints of the G phase reject any cell, then this cell undergoes into the G phase. The cell rejected from G is suspended in the G phase.

The process that occurs when the parent cell divides into two or more daughter cells is called cell division [15]. It is a fundamental biological mechanism that helps organisms to grow, develop, and repair damaged tissues. Cell division is classified into two types: Mitosis and Meiosis.

1. *Mitosis:* Mitosis is a kind of cell division that happens in somatic cells, the body's non-reproductive cells. In some organisms, it is in charge of growth, tissue healing, and asexual reproduction [16]. Mitosis is divided into various stages:
   - *Prophase*: Chromosomes condense and become visible. The nuclear envelope breaks down, and spindle fibres form.

- *Prometaphase:* The nuclear envelope completely disappears, and the spindle fibres connect to the centromeres that comprise chromosomes.
- *Metaphase*: Chromosomes align along the centre of the cell, known as the metaphase plate.
- *Anaphase:* Sister chromatids split and travel to opposing cell poles during anaphase.
- *Telophase*: The nuclear membrane reforms as the cytoplasm proceeds to divide when chromosomes reach the poles.
- *Cytokinesis*: The cytoplasm divides, producing two daughter cells, each with an identical set of chromosomes.

2. *Meiosis:* Meiosis is a form of cell division that happens in reproductive organ cells (such as the testes and ovaries) to create gametes (sperm and eggs). Meiosis consists of two rounds of division that result in the formation of four daughter cells with half the number of chromosomes as the parent cell. This reduction in chromosomal number is essential for sexual reproduction as it ensures that descendants receive genetic material from both parents. Meiosis is divided into two stages: Meiosis I and Meiosis II, each with prophase, metaphase, anaphase, and telophase [17]. Crossing over occurs during meiosis I, when homologous chromosomes couple up and transfer genetic material, boosting genetic diversity. Sister chromatids separate in Meiosis II, analogous to Mitosis, resulting in four haploid daughter cells. Cell division is tightly regulated to maintain the proper cell growth, proliferation, and differentiation balance in multicellular organisms. Defects in cell division regulation can lead to abnormal cell growth, genetic disorders, or cancer.

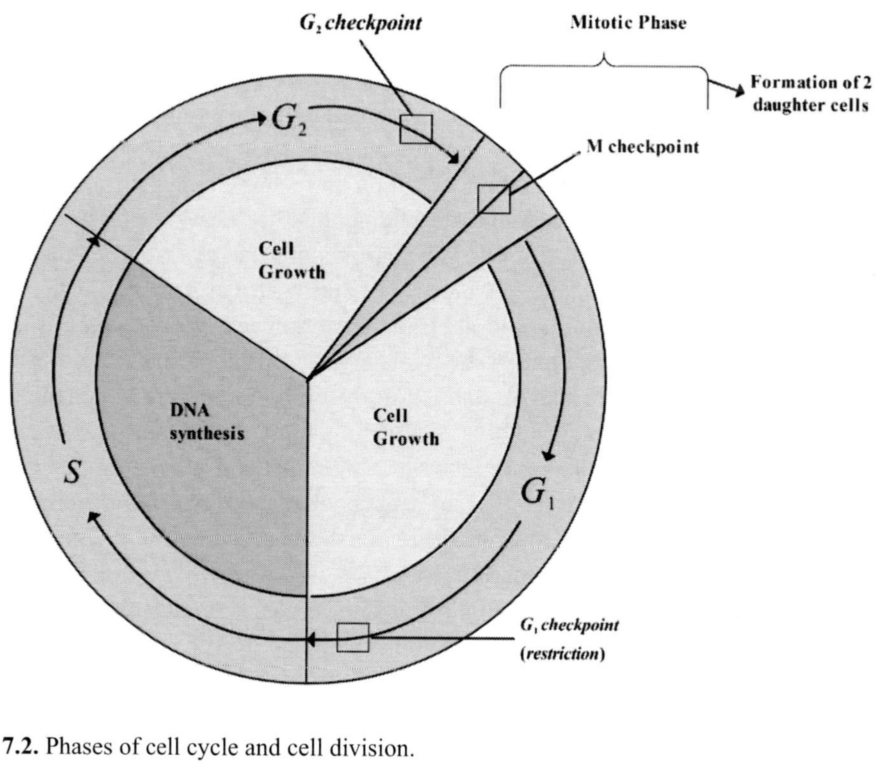

Figure 7.2. Phases of cell cycle and cell division.

7.6. Chromosomal Abnormalities

Chromosomal abnormalities, also known as chromosomal disorders or cytogenetic abnormalities, are structural or numerical alterations in an individual's chromosomes [18]. These abnormalities can significantly affect development, health, and overall functioning. They can be classified into two main types: numerical abnormalities and structural abnormalities. Chromosomal abnormalities can occur spontaneously or be inherited from parents. They can cause various side effects, such as physical, developmental, and intellectual problems and an increased risk of certain medical disorders. Genetic testing, such as karyotyping or chromosomal microarray analysis, can help diagnose chromosomal abnormalities and guide appropriate management and support for affected individuals.

7.6.1. Radiation-Induced Chromosomal Aberration

Radiation-induced chromosomal aberrations refer to structural changes or chromosome damage due to exposure to ionizing radiation [19]. Ionizing radiation includes high-energy particles such as X-rays, gamma rays, and certain types of radioactive materials. These radiation sources have enough energy to ionize atoms and molecules, potentially damaging DNA and chromosomes. When ionizing radiation interacts with cells, it can cause breaks in the DNA double helix, including breaks in the chromosomes. Repair mechanisms attempt to fix these breaks, but errors or incomplete repair can result in chromosomal aberrations. These radiation-induced chromosomal aberrations can significantly affect cell function, development, and health. Depending on the extent and location of the damage, radiation-induced chromosomal aberrations can lead to cell death, genetic mutations, chromosomal instability, or the development of cancers and other diseases [20]. It is important to note that the effects of radiation on chromosomal aberrations depend on various factors, including the dose and duration of radiation exposure, the type of radiation, and individual susceptibility. Studying radiation-induced chromosomal aberrations is crucial in understanding the risks associated with radiation exposure and setting radiation protection guidelines and standards.

Various types of Aberration are found depending on the location of the cells in the mitotic cycle at the moment of irradiation. When irradiation is given before the S phase, chromosome abnormalities occur. The daughter chromatids will get damaged if the lesion is not repaired before replication. Chromatid aberration is produced by irradiation after the S phase, i.e., during the G_2 phase, only one of the two chromatids is abnormal.

A portion of a chromosome breaks off and is lost, resulting in the loss of genetic material [21]. For example, if a radiation-induced break occurs in the middle of a chromosome and the broken segment is lost, it can lead to a chromosome deletion. Radiation can cause a chromosome segment to be duplicated. This can happen when a broken chromosome segment is reattached to its chromosome instead of its original location, resulting in the duplication of genetic material. Radiation-induced chromosome breaks can occur, followed by the reattachment of the broken segment being flipped or reversed compared to its original arrangement. When a broken section of one chromosome links to a separate chromosome, this is referred to as translocation. Radiation exposure can increase the likelihood of such translocation events. Radiation-induced breaks in chromosomes can lead to the formation of ring chromosomes [22]. In this Aberration, the broken ends of a chromosome fuse to form a ring-shaped chromosome. The loss of genetic material at the fusion points can occur, leading to altered gene expression.

Chromosomal Aberration plays a crucial role in biological dosimetry, which measures radiation dose received by individuals. Biological dosimetry assesses the biological effects of radiation exposure by analysing the damage caused to cells and chromosomes. Chromosomal Aberration is commonly used as a biomarker for estimating the absorbed radiation dose in cases of accidental or occupational radiation exposure [23]. Chromosomal Aberration exhibits a dose-dependent relationship with radiation exposure. As the radiation dose increases, the frequency of chromosomal Aberration also increases. By analyzing the type and frequency of chromosomal aberrations in a sample, it is possible to estimate the radiation dose to which an individual has been exposed. Biological dosimetry often involves the analysis of chromosomes from peripheral blood lymphocytes. The lymphocytes are stimulated to divide; then, their chromosomes are stained and examined under a microscope. Chromosomal aberrations, such as dicentrics, rings, or translocations, indicate exposure to ionizing radiation. Calibration curves are established to determine the relationship between chromosomal aberration frequency and radiation dose. These curves are created by exposing blood samples from individuals to know radiation doses in controlled laboratory settings. The frequency of chromosomal aberrations in these samples is then quantified, allowing for the construction of dose-response curves specific to the particular type of radiation and biological system. By comparing the frequency of chromosomal aberrations in an exposed individual's sample to the calibration curve, it is possible to estimate the absorbed radiation dose. Chromosomal Aberration can be detected and analyzed at different time points following radiation exposure [24]. The timing of sample collection is essential as the frequency and types of chromosomal Aberration may vary depending on the elapsed time since exposure. This temporal information aids in estimating the time of exposure and helps determine the urgency of medical interventions.

7.7. Intrachromosomal Exchange

Intrachromosomal exchange, also known as intra-chromosome rearrangements or intra-chromosome aberrations, is a type of chromosomal Aberration that involves structural rearrangements within a single chromosome [25]. This can result in alterations in the arrangement or order of genetic material within the affected chromosome. Various factors, including exposure to radiation, certain chemicals, or errors during DNA replication or repair processes, can cause intra-chromosomal exchanges. These aberrations can significantly affect gene expression, disrupting the normal functioning of genes or altering gene activity regulation.

There are several types of intrachromosomal exchanges:

- *Inversion:* An inversion happens when a chromosomal segment splits and reattaches into the opposite orientation. This results in rearranging the genetic sequence within that segment, but the genetic material remains within the same chromosome.

- *Insertion:* An insertion occurs when a portion of one chromosome splits off and inserts itself into another section of an identical chromosome. This can lead to a disruption or rearrangement of the genetic sequence at the insertion site.
- *Deletion:* A deletion happens when a chromosomal fragment splits and is lost. This may result in genetic material loss inside the afflicted chromosomal region.
- *Amplification:* Amplification refers to the duplication of a specific chromosome segment, resulting in increased copies of that segment within the chromosome [26]. This can lead to an overabundance of certain genes or genetic material.

7.8. Interchromosomal Exchanges

Inter-chromosomal exchanges, also known as inter-chromosomal rearrangement or inter-chromosomal aberrations, are chromosomal aberrations that involve structural rearrangements between different chromosomes [27]. Unlike intrachromosomal exchanges, which occur within a single chromosome, interchromosomal exchanges involve the exchange of genetic material between two distinct chromosomes. This can lead to alterations in the arrangement or distribution of genetic material among the involved chromosomes. Inter-chromosomal exchanges can be spontaneous but induced by exposure to certain mutagens, such as ionizing radiation or certain chemicals. These exchanges can have significant consequences on gene expression, as they can disrupt gene function, alter regulatory elements, or lead to the formation of fusion genes.

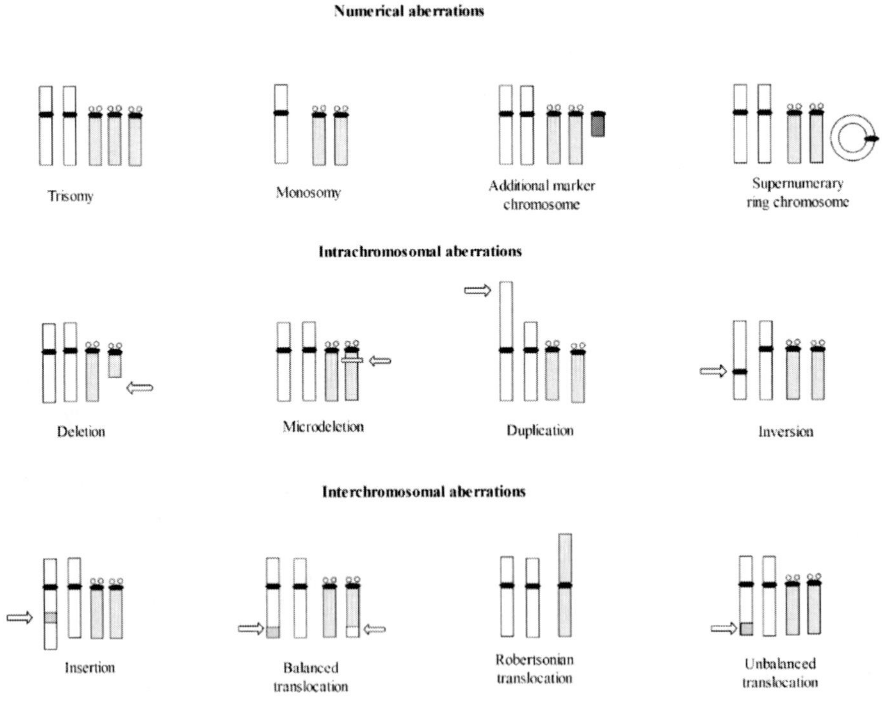

Figure 7.3. Schematic representation of the principal types of chromosomal aberration observed under the microscope.

There are several types of inter-chromosomal exchanges:

- *Translocation:* When a section of one chromosome falls off and attaches to another, this is referred to as translocation. There are two main types of translocations.
  - *Reciprocal Translocation:* Two non-homologous chromosomes exchange portions in reciprocal translocation, resulting in a balanced rearrangement [28]. Thus, no genetic material loss or gain exists, but the chromosomes involved have been architecturally altered.
  - *Robertsonian Translocation:* Robertsonian translocation occurs when two acrocentric chromosomes (chromosomes with the centromere near one end) fuse at their centromeres, resulting in a single, large chromosome and a smaller chromosome fragment [29].
- *Insertion:* In an inter-chromosomal insertion, a segment of one chromosome splits and becomes inserted into a different chromosome. This can lead to a disruption or rearrangement of genetic material at the insertion site.
- *Transposition* involves the movement of genetic material from one chromosome to a non-homologous chromosome or a different location within the same chromosome [30]. This can occur through mechanisms such as transposable elements or DNA recombination processes.

7.9. Genetic Disorder

Genetic issues are far more common than many individuals realize. In their lifetime, 670 persons are expected to be affected by genetic disorders [31]. These 670 person includes not only "classic" hereditary disorders but also cancer and cardiovascular disease, the Western world's two leading causes of death. Both have substantial genetic components. Cardiovascular diseases, such as atherosclerosis and hypertension, are caused by complex interactions between genes and the environment, and most cancers are now assumed to be generated by the Accumulation of mutations in somatic cells [32]. The genetic illnesses encountered in medical practice are merely the tip of the iceberg, with less severe genotypic abnormalities allowing full embryonic development and live birth. It is believed that 50% of spontaneous abort uses during the first few months of pregnancy have a chromosomal defect; there are also several minor identifiable mistakes and many others that are yet beyond our ability to identify. Approximately 1% of all new-borns have a significant chromosomal defect, and 5% of people under the age of 25 acquire a severe disease with a vital hereditary component. Although genomes and proteomics reveal a wealth of information, our capacity to organize and mine such a massive amount of data is still in its infancy. Analyzing patterns of expression containing thousands of genes and proteins simultaneously has necessitated the creation of computer-based systems capable of managing massive amounts of data. As a result, an intriguing new discipline known as bioinformatics has emerged. This has included biologists, computer scientists, physicists, and mathematicians, demonstrating the actual value of a multidisciplinary approach in current medical practice.

The fantastic advances in molecular biology, utilizing recombinant DNA technologies, have fueled most of the progress in medical genetics. The specifics of these approaches are well-known and will not be recounted here. However, several examples of the impact of recombinant DNA technology on medicine are worth mentioning.

7.9.1. The Molecular Basis of Human Disease

Two broad techniques have been utilized to isolate and characterize relevant genes. The functional cloning, or classic, strategy has been used successfully to explore a range of inborn metabolic abnormalities, including phenylketonuria and hemoglobin synthesis problems [33]. These genetic disorders share knowledge of the aberrant gene product and the related protein. When the damaged protein is identified, various techniques can be used to isolate the normal gene, clone it, and eventually establish the molecular modifications that impact the gene in patients with the condition. Because there was no clue as to the nature of the defective gene product in many common single-gene illnesses, such as cystic fibrosis, an alternate procedure known as positional cloning or the "candidate gene" approach had to be used. This technique first disregards biochemical indications from the phenotypic in favor of mapping the disease phenotype to a specific chromosome position. Linkage analysis achieves this mapping if the disease is associated with a specific chromosomal alteration (e.g., fragile-X syndrome) [34]. In the latter case, the gene's approximate position is identified by linkage to known "marker genes" or SNPs around the illness locus. Once the location of the mutant gene has been narrowed down, the next step is to clone multiple bits of DNA from the relevant part of the genome. The abnormal protein encoded by the mutant genes can subsequently be identified by expressing the cloned DNA in vitro and identifying the protein products. This method has been used successfully in the treatment of a variety of disorders, including cystic fibrosis, neurofibromatosis, Duchenne muscular dystrophy (a genetic ailment characterized by progressive muscle weakness), polycystic kidney disease, and Huntington's disease. Once the location of the mutant gene has been narrowed down, the next phase is to clone multiple bits of DNA from the relevant part of the genome. The abnormal protein encoded by the mutant genes can subsequently be identified by expressing the cloned DNA in vitro and identifying the protein products. This method has been used successfully in treating various disorders, including cystic fibrosis, neurofibromatosis, Duchenne muscular dystrophy (a genetic ailment characterized by progressive muscle weakness), polycystic kidney disease, and Huntington's disease [35].

7.9.2. The Production of Human Biologically Active Agents

By putting the necessary gene into bacteria or other compatible cells in tissue culture, various ultrapure biologically active agents can now be produced in nearly endless quantities. Soluble TNF receptor for blocking TNF in the treatment of rheumatoid arthritis (RA), the activator of tissue plasminogen for the treatment of thrombotic states, growth hormone for the treatment of deficiency states, erythropoietin to reverse several types of anemia, and myeloid growth and differentiation factors (granulocyte-macrophage colony-stimulating factor, granulocyte colony-stimulating factor) for improving.

1. *Gene therapy:*
   Although the goal of curing genetic illnesses by transferring somatic cells transfected with the normal gene is straightforward in theory, it has yet to be realized broadly. Designing adequate vectors to deliver the gene is a problem, as are unforeseen difficulties caused by random insertion of the normal gene into the host genome. Gene therapy in individuals with x-linked SCID who lack the standard chain of cytokine receptors had to be halted in recent well-publicized cases because the transduced gene was inserted close to a host gene that controls cell proliferation [36]. The patient developed T-cell leukemia as a result of the dysregulation.
2. *Disease diagnosis:*
   Molecular probes have proven to be incredibly beneficial for genetic and non-genetic (e.g., infectious) disease diagnosis. The first step in functional cloning is to link the clinical condition to biochemical-protein abnormalities, followed by the isolation of the mutant gene. Positional cloning, commonly known as the candidate gene technique, begins by using linkage analysis to map and clone the disease gene despite having any understanding of the gene product [37]. Following the isolation of the mutated gene, the gene product, and the mechanism by which it causes the disease are identified. With this background in human genetics, we can proceed to the time-honored classification of human disorders into three groups:
   - Those determined by environmental factors
   - Those determined by genetic factors
   - Those in which both environmental and genetic variables play a role.

Obesity may appear to be a representation of the first group; nevertheless, given the discovery of genes that govern satiety and energy metabolism, it is clear that overnutrition—and, to a lesser or greater extent, all disorders—is conditioned by the genotype. Many essential human diseases, such as peptic ulcer, diabetes mellitus, atherosclerosis, schizophrenia, autoimmune disorders, and most malignancies, fall into the third group just indicated, in which both nature and nurture play substantial roles.

7.10. Mutation

A mutation is an irreversible alteration in the DNA sequence. Mutations affecting germ cells are passed down to children and can result in genetic disorders. While not causing inherited disorders, somatic cell mutations are significant in developing malignancies and some congenital abnormalities [38]. Mutations are divided into three types based on the level of genetic alteration. Genome mutations result in the loss or acquisition of entire chromosomes, resulting in monosomy or trisomy. Chromosome mutations originate from genetic material rearrangement and cause observable structural alterations in the chromosome. Mutations involving alterations in the number or arrangement of chromosomes are only seldom transferred because the majority are incompatible for survival [39]. The overwhelming majority of inherited illness mutations are sub-microscopic gene alterations. These can result in a gene's partial or total deletion or, more commonly, the deletion of a single nucleotide. A single nucleotide base, for example, could be replaced by an alternative base, resulting in a point mutation. Less frequently, one or two base pairs may be inserted or deleted from the DNA, causing changes in the reading frame of the DNA strand; these are known as frameshift mutations [40]. The effects of mutations vary based on several parameters, particularly the type of Mutation and the chromosomal location affected. This article discusses specific mutations and their effects in conjunction with the related illnesses. In this section, we will go over some general principles concerning the impact of gene mutations.

- *Point mutations throughout coding sequences:* Point mutations (single base substitution) can change the code in a triplet of bases, causing one amino acid in the gene product to be replaced by another. Missense mutations are so-called because they change the significance of the genetic code [41]. A "conservative" missense mutation occurs when the substituted amino acid has little effect on the protein's function. A "nonconservative" missense mutation, on the other hand, substitutes the typical amino acid with a radically different one. The sickle Mutation, which affects the -globin chain of hemoglobin, is an outstanding example of this type. CTC (or GAG in messenger RNA [mRNA]), a code for glutamic acid, is converted to CAC (or GUG in mRNA), a code for valine. This single amino acid alteration alters the physicochemical properties of hemoglobin, resulting in sickle cell anemia. A point mutation can alter an amino acid codon to a chain terminator or stop codon in addition to causing an amino acid substitution (nonsense mutation) [42]. Using -globin as an example, a point mutation affecting the glutamine (CAG) codon results in a stop codon (UAG) if U is substituted for C. This Mutation causes early termination of -globin gene translation, resulting in a short peptide that is rapidly destroyed. Individuals affected lack -globin chains and acquire a severe type of anemia called β0-thalassemia.
- *Non-coding sequence mutations:* Mutations that do not include exons can also have negative consequences [43]. As is well known, promoter and enhancer regions located downstream or upstream of the gene initiate and regulate DNA transcription. Point mutations or deletions involving certain regulatory regions may interfere with transcription factor binding, resulting in a significant reduction or complete lack of transcription. This is true in some cases of hereditary hemolytic anaemia. Furthermore, point mutations inside introns result in incorrect splicing of intervening regions. As a result, the usual processing of the early mRNA transcripts is disrupted, resulting in the failure to produce mature mRNA transcripts. As a result, translation cannot occur, and the resulting gene product is not produced.
- *Deletions and insertions:* minor deletions or insertions impacting the coding region resulted in changes to the reading frame of the DNA strand, resulting in frameshift mutations. Frameshift does not occur if the number of base pairs involved is three or a multiple of three; instead, an aberrant protein lacking one or more amino acids is synthesized.
- *Trinucleotide repeated mutations:* Trinucleotide repeating mutations are unique in that they are characterized by the amplification of a three-nucleotide sequence [44]. Although the particular nucleotide sequence amplified varies per disease, practically all impacted sequences contain the nucleotides guanine (G) and cytosine (C). In fragile-X syndrome, the classic condition in this category, there are between 250 to

4000 repeated tandems of the pattern CGG within a gene termed as FMR-1(fragile X messenger ribonucleoprotein, or FMRP). The average number of repeats in typical populations is 29. Such trinucleotide sequence expansions hinder normal expression of the FMR-1 gene, resulting in mental impairment. Another property that distinguishes trinucleotide repeat mutations is their dynamic nature (the degree of amplification rises throughout gametogenesis). These characteristics, which will be addressed in more detail later, influence the pattern of inheritance as well as the phenotypic manifestations of the diseases induced by this class of mutations.

A three-base deletion in the common cystic fibrosis (CF) genotype leads to the production of a protein lacking amino acid 508 (phenylalanine) [45]. This is not a frameshift mutation since the deletion is a multiple of three. To summarise, mutations can disrupt protein production at multiple levels. Gene deletions and point mutations in promoter sequences can inhibit transcription. Mutations affecting introns, splice junctions, or both might cause abnormal mRNA processing. A stop codon (chain termination mutation) within an exon affects translation. Ultimately, at some point, mutations can create an aberrant protein while not interfering with any phase of protein synthesis. Finally, it should be mentioned that, in rare cases, mutations might be beneficial. The human immunodeficiency virus (HIV) enters cells via a chemokine receptor, CCR5, and a deletion in the CCR5 gene protects against HIV infection [46].

In light of this, researchers now turn our focus to the three major types of genetic disorders:

1. Disorders caused by large-effect mutant genes
2. Diseases with multifactorial aetiology
3. Chromosomal abnormalities.

The first category comprises numerous uncommon illnesses, such as storage disorders and inborn metabolic abnormalities, all caused by large-effect single-gene mutations. Because the majority of them follow traditional Mendelian inheritance patterns, they are often known as Mendelian disorders. The second category comprises some of the most common human ailments, such as hypertension and diabetes. They are called multifactorial because genetic and environmental factors influence them. The genetic component consists of the additive effect of several genes with little effects; the environmental contribution might be tiny or significant, and in some situations, it is necessary for disease expression. The third category comprises disorders that are caused by genomic or chromosomal alterations and are thus linked with numerical or structural changes in chromosomes [47].

7.11. Mendelian Disorder

Expressed mutations in single large-effect genes cause all Mendelian illnesses. Going into depth regarding Mendel's rules here is optional because every biology student is familiar with them. Only a few medically relevant comments are offered. The number of Mendelian illnesses now known has reached epic proportions. Every person is thought to carry five to eight harmful genes. The majority of them are recessive and so have no significant phenotypic consequences. Approximately 80% to 85% of these mutations are hereditary. The remaining mutations are novel mutations acquired by an affected individual. Some autosomal mutations result in heterozygote partial expression and homozygote complete expression. Sickle cell anemia is caused by the replacement of hemoglobin S (HbS) for normal hemoglobin (HbA) [48]. When a person is homozygous for the mutant gene, all of the hemoglobin is of the aberrant HbS type, and the condition is wholly expressed even with normal oxygen saturation (i.e., sickling deformity of all red cells and hemolytic anemia). Because only a fraction of the hemoglobin in the heterozygote is HbS (the remainder is HbA), red cell sickling and probably hemolysis occur only when exposed to low oxygen tension. It is also called the sickle cell trait, distinguishing it from full-blown sickle cell anemia. Although gene expression is typically classified as dominant or recessive, codominance occurs when both alleles of a gene pair are entirely expressed in the heterozygote. Codominant inheritance can be seen in histocompatibility and blood group antigens.

Pleiotropism occurs when a single mutant gene produces many end effects; conversely, genetic heterogeneity occurs when mutations at multiple genetic loci create the same feature [49]. Pleiotropism can be seen in the case of sickle cell anemia. Besides the point mutation in the gene creating HbS, which predisposes red cells to haemolysis, the aberrant red cells also cause a logjam in tiny capillaries, causing splenic fibrosis, organ infarctions, and bone abnormalities in this hereditary condition. The various end-organ abnormalities are all linked to the main flaw in hemoglobin production. In contrast, profound infantile deafness, which appears to be a homogeneous clinical entity, is caused by any of 16 autosomal recessive mutations. Recognizing genetic variability is crucial in genetic counseling and understanding the pathophysiology of several common illnesses, such as diabetes mellitus.

7.12. Single-Gene Disorders Transmission Patterns

Single-gene mutations often follow one of three inheritance patterns: autosomal dominant, autosomal recessive, or X-linked [50]. The general rules governing the transmission of single-gene diseases are well established and will not be repeated here. Only a few key points are highlighted. Later, single-gene disorders with non-classical inheritance patterns are discussed.

7.13. Autosomal Dominant Disorders

Because autosomal dominant disorders present in the heterozygous state, no less than a single parent of an index case typically has been affected; both males and females have been impacted, and both can transmit the condition [51]. When an affected individual marries an unaffected person, every child has a one in two risk of inheriting the condition. Some patients with autosomal dominant disorders have no affected parents. These patients' disorders result from novel mutations in the egg or sperm from which they were formed. Their siblings are not afflicted and are not at increased risk of contracting the disease. The proportion of people who get the disease due to a novel mutation is proportional to the condition's influence on fertility. Most disease cases significantly decreasing reproductive fitness would be expected to arise from new mutations. Many new mutations appear to arise in the germ cells of older fathers.

Reduced penetrance and varied expressivity can alter clinical characteristics. Some people inherited the mutant gene yet have normal phenotypes. This is known as reduced penetrance. Penetrance is stated numerically: 50% penetrance means that 50% of the individuals who possess a particular gene express the trait. In contrast to penetrance, variable expressivity occurs when a trait is exhibited in all individuals inheriting the mutant gene but is expressed variably among individuals. Neurofibromatosis type 1 symptoms, for example, range from brownish patches on the skin to many skin tumors and skeletal abnormalities [52]. The processes driving lower penetrance and varied expressivity are unknown. However, they are most likely caused by the influence of additional genes or environmental variables on the mutant allele's phenotypic expression. For example, the genotype at the -globin locus affects the overall quantity of hemoglobin generated, which influences the phenotype of an individual with sickle cell anemia (due to Mutation at the -globin locus). Familial hypercholesterolemia exemplifies the impact of environmental influences. The daily consumption of lipids influences the disease's manifestation as atherosclerosis.

The molecular mechanisms of autosomal dominant illnesses are best understood in the context of the kind of protein affected and the nature of the Mutation [53]. Most mutations result in decreased gene product output or the formation of an inactive protein. The type of the protein impacted determines the impact of such loss of functional mutations. Heterozygotes usually are expected if the Mutation affects an enzyme protein. Mutations in genes that encode enzyme proteins do not exhibit an autosomal dominant inheritance pattern because up to 50% loss of enzyme function can be compensated for. In contrast, autosomal dominant diseases impact two essential types of non-enzyme proteins:

1. Those involved in regulating complicated metabolic pathways are subject to feedback inhibition. Membrane receptors such as the LDL receptor are one example of familial hypercholesterolemia. A 50% loss of LDL receptors results in a secondary elevation of cholesterol, predisposing affected heterozygotes to atherosclerosis.
2. Essential structural proteins, such as collagen and red cell membrane cytoskeletal components (e.g., spectrin): The molecular mechanisms by which a 50% decrease in such protein levels results in an aberrant phenotype are not entirely understood. In rare circumstances, mainly when the gene produces one subunit of a multimeric protein, the mutant allele's output can disrupt the assembly of a functionally normal multimer [54]. The collagen molecule, for example, is a trimer with three collagen chains organised in a helical form. Each of the three collagen chains in the helix must be regular for the collagen molecule to assemble and be stable. Normal collagen trimers cannot be produced with a single mutant collagen chain, resulting in a significant collagen shortage. The mutant allele is termed dominant negative in this case because it interferes with the function of a normal allele. Some osteogenesis imperfecta, characterized by a severe collagen shortage and skeletal deformities, demonstrate this impact.

The gain of function mutations is less prevalent than the loss of functional mutations. As the name implies, the protein product of the mutant allele gains features that are not generally associated with the wild-type protein in this type of Mutation. As Huntington's disease demonstrates, the transmission of diseases caused by gain of function mutations is virtually usually autosomal dominant [55]. The trinucleotide repeat mutation affecting the Huntington gene (see below) causes this disease by producing an aberrant protein. Because the mutant Huntington protein is neurotoxic, even heterozygotes have neurologic deficits. To summarise, autosomal dominant disorders are caused by two types of mutations and two categories of proteins. The most common loss of function mutations impacts regulatory proteins and multimeric protein subunits, with the latter having a dominant negative effect. Gain of function mutations are rare; they bestow normal proteins with hazardous qualities, affecting the functionality of other proteins produced by the mutant gene.

7.14. Autosomal Recessive Disorders

Autosomal recessive inheritance is the most common type of Mendelian disorder [56]. Because autosomal recessive illnesses occur only if both alleles at a specific gene locus are defective, they are distinguished by the following characteristics:

1. The trait does not usually affect the parents, but siblings may be affected;
2. siblings have one in four chances of being affected (i.e., the recurrence risk is 25% for each birth);
3. if the mutant gene occurs at a low frequency in the population, the proband is most likely the product of a consanguineous marriage.
4. The defect's expression is more uniform than autosomal dominant illnesses.
5. Total penetration is expected.
6. The onset is usually early in life.
7. Although novel recessive disease mutations can occur, these are rarely found clinically. Because the individual with the new Mutation is an asymptomatic heterozygote, multiple generations may pass before the offspring of such a person develops symptoms.

A decrease in function affects enzyme proteins in numerous circumstances. In heterozygotes, the standard and faulty enzymes are synthesized in equal amounts. Usually, the natural "margin of safety" guarantees that cells with half their normal enzyme complement usually operate.

7.14.1. X-Linked Disorders

All sex-linked illnesses are X-linked, and nearly all are recessive [56]. The "male-specific region of Y" encodes several genes, all of which are involved in spermatogenesis. Males with Y-linked gene mutations are frequently infertile; therefore, there is no Y-linked inheritance. A few more genes with homologues on the X chromosome have been mapped to the Y chromosome, but no illnesses caused by mutations in such genes have been described. A modest number of clinical disorders are caused by X-linked recessive inheritance. Because the Y chromosome is not similar to the X, mutant genes on the X are not linked with alleles on the Y. As a result, these illnesses manifest in him because the male is hemizygous for X-linked mutant genes. A father with the disease does not pass it on to his sons, but all daughters are carriers. Sons of heterozygous mothers have a one in two probability of inheriting the mutant gene.

Due to the paired normal allele, the heterozygous female frequently does not express the whole phenotypic change. Females, on the other hand, have a variable proportion of cells in which the mutant X chromosome is active due to the random inactivation of one of the X chromosomes. As a result, the normal allele may be inactivated in most cells, allowing full expression of heterozygous X-linked conditions in the female. Much more typically, the normal allele is inactivated in only a portion of the cells, causing the heterozygous female to display the condition only partially. Glucose-6-phosphate dehydrogenase (G6PD) deficiency is one example [57]. This enzyme deficiency, which predisposes to red cell hemolysis in individuals receiving specific types of medicines and is transmitted on the X chromosome, is primarily expressed in males. A fraction of the red cells in females may be produced from marrow cells due to the inactivation of the normal allele. These red cells are at the same danger of hemolysis as the red cells in the hemizygous male. As a result, not only is the female a carrier of this trait, but she is also prone to drug-induced hemolytic responses. Because the proportion of faulty red cells in heterozygous females is determined by the random inactivation of one of the X chromosomes, the severity of the hemolytic reaction in heterozygous women is nearly always smaller than in hemizygous men.

7.15. The Biochemical and Molecular Basis of Single-Gene (Mendelian) Disorders

Single gene mutations cause Mendelian disorders. The genetic flaw may result in the creation of an aberrant protein or a decrease in the gene product's output. As previously stated, mutations can interfere with protein synthesis by altering transcription, mRNA processing, or translation. A mutation's phenotypic effects might be caused directly by defects in the protein encoded by the mutant gene or indirectly by the interaction of the mutant protein with other normal proteins. For example, all kinds of Ehlers-Danlos syndrome (EDS) are associated with collagen anomalies [58]. Some types (e.g., vascular type) have a mutation in one of the collagen genes, whilst others (e.g., kyphoscoliosis type) have normal collagen genes but a mutation in the gene that encodes lysyl hydroxylase, an enzyme required for collagen cross-linking. A lack of lysis hydroxylase causes collagen to weaken in these patients.

7.16. Enzyme Defects and Their Consequences

Mutations can cause the creation of a faulty enzyme with decreased activity or a reduced quantity of a normal enzyme. The end result is a metabolic block in either situation. The biochemical repercussions of an enzyme deficiency in such a process can have three significant outcomes:

1. Depending on the block's location, the substrate's Accumulation may be accompanied by the Accumulation of one or both intermediates. Furthermore, an increase in intermediate concentration may promote the minor route. Tissue harm may occur under these settings if the precursor, intermediates, or products of alternate minor pathways are toxic in high doses. For example, a lack of galactose-1-phosphate uridyl-transferase causes galactose buildup and tissue damage in galactosemia. A lack of phenylalanine hydroxylase results in the buildup of phenylalanine in phenylketonuria [59,60]. Excessive buildup of the complex substrate within the lysosomes due to a lack of degradative enzymes causes a range of disorders known as lysosomal storage diseases.
2. An enzyme deficiency can cause a metabolic block and decrease the end product required for regular activity. A lack of melanin, for example, may occur from a lack of tyrosinase, which is required to produce melanin from its precursor, tyrosine. Albinism is the clinical term for this illness. Suppose the end product is a feedback inhibitor of the enzymes engaged in the early processes. In that case, its absence may allow for the overproduction of intermediate and their catabolic products, some of which may be toxic at high doses. The Lesch-Nyhan syndrome is a prime example of a disease having such an underlying mechanism [61].
3. The failure to inactivate a tissue-damaging substrate is best represented by a lack of 1-antitrypsin (AT). Patients with a hereditary lack of serum 1-AT cannot inactivate neutrophil elastase in their lungs [62]. The unchecked activity of this protease causes elastin degradation in the walls of lung alveoli, eventually leading to pulmonary emphysema.

7.17. Defects in Receptors and Transport Systems

Many physiologically active chemicals must be actively carried through the cell membrane. This transport is often accomplished by one of two mechanisms: receptor-mediated endocytosis or transport protein. Familial hypercholesterolemia is an example of a genetic defect in a receptor-mediated transport system, in which decreased production or function of low-density lipoprotein (LDL) receptors leads to defective transport of LDL into cells and, secondarily, excessive cholesterol synthesis via complex intermediary mechanisms [63]. The transport pathway for chloride ions in exocrine glands, sweat ducts, lungs, and pancreas is faulty in cystic fibrosis. Impaired chloride transport causes substantial damage to the lungs and pancreas through poorly understood mechanisms.

7.17.1. Alterations in Structure, Function, or Quantity of Non-Enzyme Proteins

As sickle cell disease demonstrates, genetic abnormalities that frequently result in non-enzyme protein changes have broad downstream effects. This category is best exemplified by hemoglobinopathies, such as sickle cell disease, which are all characterised by flaws in the molecular makeup of the globin molecule. Unlike hemoglobinopathies, thalassemias are caused by mutations in globin genes that influence the number of globin chains synthesised

[64]. Thalassemia is characterised by low structurally normal -globin or ß-globin chains. Collagen, sceptrin, and dystrophin are genetically faulty structural proteins that cause osteogenesis imperfecta, hereditary spherocytosis, and muscular dystrophies, respectively.

7.17.2. Genetically Determined Adverse Reactions to Drugs

Particular genetically determined enzyme deficits become apparent only when the sick individual is exposed to particular medicines. This subject of genetics, known as pharmacogenetics, is vital in clinical practice. A deficit of the enzyme glucose-6-phosphate dehydrogenase (G6PD) is a typical example of drug-induced damage in the genetically vulnerable individual. G6PD deficiency does not cause disease under normal conditions, but when the antimalarial drug primaquine is administered, it causes severe hemolytic anaemia. Recently, polymorphisms in genes encoding drug-metabolizing enzymes, transporters, and receptors have been found [65]. These genetic variables can significantly impact drug sensitivity and destructive reactions in some circumstances. Pharmacogenetic improvements will lead to patient-tailored therapy, or "personalised medicine."

7.17.3. Multifactorial Inheritance Disorder

Multifactorial disorders are caused by the combined actions of environmental factors and two or more mutant genes that have cumulative effects. The genetic component has a dosage effect—the more detrimental genes that are inherited, the more severe the disease's manifestation. The term polygenic inheritance is inappropriate because environmental influences considerably influence the development of certain genetic illnesses [66]. Several regular phenotypic features, including hair color, eye color, skin color, height, and IQ, are influenced by multifactorial inheritance. These features vary continuously among demographic groupings, resulting in the conventional bell shaped distribution curve. Environmental factors, on the other hand, have a substantial impact on the phenotypic expression of multifactorial features. Type II diabetes mellitus, for example, has many of the characteristics of a complex illness [67]. Clinically, it is well understood that individuals frequently show this disease after gaining weight. Obesity, together with other environmental factors, thereby reveals the diabetic genetic characteristic. Even monozygotic twins can have varied heights due to nutritional effects. The culturally impoverished youngster is unable to reach his or her entire intellectual potential.

The following characteristics define multifactorial inheritance. Such were established for the multifactorial inheritance of congenital abnormalities and will almost certainly apply to other multifactorial disorders.

1. The number of inherited mutant genes influences the likelihood of a multifactorial illness. As a result, the risk is higher among siblings of patients with severe manifestations of the illness. For example, the probability of cleft lip in siblings of an index case is 2.5% if the cleft lip is unilateral but 6% if it is bilateral. Similarly, the bigger the danger for other relatives, the greater the quantity of affected relatives.

2. The rate of recurrence of the disorder (in the range of 2% to 7%) is the same for all first-degree relatives (i.e., the affected individual's parents, siblings, and kids). As a result, if a parent has had one affected child, the probability of the next child being affected is between 2% and 7%. Similarly, one of the parents has the same chance of being afflicted.
3. The chances of both identical twins being harmed are much less than 100%, but far greater than the chances of both nonidentical twins being affected. For identical twins, for example, experience has shown that the rate of concordance ranges from 20% to 40%.
4. The likelihood of both identical twins being harmed is much less than 100% but much greater than the likelihood of both nonidentical twins being affected. For identical twins, for example, experience has shown that the incidence of concordance ranges between 20% and 40%.

The expression of a multifactorial trait might be continuous (no unique phenotype, such as height) or discontinuous (specific phenotype, such as diabetes mellitus) [68]. Disease is only manifested in the latter when the combined impacts of genes and environment exceed a particular threshold. In the case of diabetes, for example, when blood glucose levels rise above a particular threshold, the chance of phenotypic expression rises.

Assigning an illness to this mode of inheritance requires prudence. It is determined by a number of criteria, the most important of which are familial clustering and the exclusion of Mendelian and chromosomal modes of transmission. A variation of illness severity suggests multifactorial inheritance, but as previously stated, varying expressivity and reduced penetrance of single mutant genes may also account for this phenomenon. Because of these issues, distinguishing between Mendelian and multifactorial inheritance can be challenging at times.

7.17.4. Cytogenetic Disorder

Cytogenetic disorders are caused by chromosome mutations, which might be a disproportionate number of chromosomes or changes in the molecular makeup of one or more chromosomes [69]. The female chromosome complement is 46, XX, whereas the male chromosome complement is 46, XY. Euploid refers to any precise multiple of the haploid number. Aneuploidy occurs when a cell gets a chromosomal complement that is not an exact multiple of 23 due to a mistake in Meiosis or Mitosis. Nondisjunction and anaphase lag are the most common causes of aneuploidy [70]. The former happens when a homologous pair of chromosomes fail to separate during the first meiotic division, when the two chromatids fail to separate during the second meiotic division, or during somatic cell divisions, resulting in two aneuploid cells. Nondisjunction during gametogenesis results in gametes with either an additional chromosome (n+1) or one fewer chromosome (n-1). Fertilization of such gametes by regular gametes results in either trisomic (2n+1) or monosomic (2n-1) zygotes. Anaphase lag occurs when one homologous chromosome in Meiosis or one chromatid in Mitosis lags and is excluded from the cell nucleus. As a result, there is one normal cell and one with monosomy. Monosomy or trisomy involving the sex chromosomes, or more unusual aberrations, are compatible with life and are frequently linked with varying degrees of phenotypic abnormalities, as seen below. Monosomy, including an autosome, typically signifies too much genetic information loss to allow for live delivery or even development, but a few autosomal trisomies do allow for life [71]. With the exception of trisomy 21, all result in profoundly disabled infants who nearly always die at a young age.

Mitotic mistakes in early development can occasionally result in two or more populations of cells in the same individual, a situation known as mosaicism [72]. Mosaicism can occur as a result of mitotic mistakes during ovum cleavage or in somatic cells. Mosaicism of the sex chromosomes is rather prevalent. A mistake during the division of the fertilized ovum may result in one of the daughter cells obtaining three sex chromosomes while the other receives only one, resulting in, for example, a 45, X/47, XXX mosaic. As a result, all descendant cells from each of these precursors have either a 47, XXX complement or a 45, X complement. This is a mosaic variety of Turner syndrome, with the extent of phenotypic expression determined by the patient [73]. If the error occurs later in the cleavage, the mosaic includes three populations of cells, some of which have the typical 46, XX complement (i.e., 45, X/46, XX/47, XXX). Repeated mitotic mistakes can result in a large number of cell populations.

Autosomal mosaicism appears to be significantly less common than sex chromosomal mosaicism [74]. An early mitotic division mistake affecting the autosomes usually results in a nonviable mosaic with autosomal monosomy. Rarely embryogenesis tolerates the loss of a nonviable cell line, resulting in a mosaic (e.g., 46, XY/47, XY+21). A trisomy 21 mosaic patient has varying expression of Down syndrome based on the fraction of cells displaying the trisomy.

A second type of chromosomal Aberration is connected with alterations in chromosome structure. Routine banding approaches require a pretty substantial amount of DNA (about 4 million base pairs), including numerous genes, to be involved. FISH has a lot greater resolution. Chromosome structural alterations are often caused by chromosome breaking, followed by material loss or rearrangement. Such changes occur naturally at a modest pace, accelerated by exposure to environmental mutagens such as chemicals and ionizing radiation.

Furthermore, certain rare autosomal recessive genetic illnesses, including Fanconi anemia, Bloom syndrome, and ataxia-telangiectasia, are associated with such high levels of chromosomal instability called chromosome-breakage syndromes. All of these syndromes have a significantly elevated risk of malignancy. In the next part, we will review the most prevalent types of chromosomal structural changes and the symbols used to represent them.

A translocation is the transfer of a section of one chromosome to another. In one variant, balanced reciprocal translocation, single breaks exist in each of the two chromosomes, resulting in material exchange [75]. Without banding procedures, such a translocation may go undetected. A balanced reciprocal translocation across chromosome 2's extended arm and chromosome 5's short arm would be written 46, XX. This person has 46 chromosomes, with one chromosome 2 and one chromosome 5 having abnormal morphology. Because no genetic material has been lost, the individual is expected to be phenotypically normal. A balanced translocation carrier, on the other hand, is more likely to produce aberrant gametes. A gamete with one normal chromosome 2 and one translocated chromosome 5 may be created in the preceding scenario. Because it lacks the usual complement of genetic material, such a gamete would be imbalanced. Following fertilization by a normal gamete, an abnormal (unbalanced) zygote would form, leading to spontaneous abortion or the birth of a deformed kid. A Robertsonian translocation (or centric fusion) is a translocation between two acrocentric chromosomes that is also crucial [76]. The breaks typically occur at the centromeres of each chromosome. The transfer of the segments results in one very large and one tiny chromosome. The tiny product is usually lost, but because it only contains highly redundant genes (e.g., ribosomal RNA genes), this loss is consistent with a normal phenotype. One in every 1000 apparently ordinary people has a Robertsonian translocation between two chromosomes. The relevance of this type of translocation is also found in the development of defective offspring, as mentioned subsequently in relation to Down syndrome.

Several numerical and structural anomalies are detailed in specialized texts, and the number of aberrant karyotypes seen in genetic illnesses grows by the month. As previously stated, clinically detectable chromosomal abnormalities are simply the "tip of the iceberg." It is believed that 7.5% of all conceptions contain a chromosomal defect, the majority of which are incompatible with survival or live birth. Thus, chromosomal abnormalities are seen in 50% of early spontaneous abortions and 5% of stillbirths and newborns who die shortly after birth. Even in live-born infants, the frequency ranges from 0.5% to 1.0%. Most clinically recognizable chromosomal diseases are beyond the scope of this work. As a result, we concentrated on the handful that were most common.

7.18. Autosome-Related Cytogenetic Disorders

7.18.1. Trisomy 21 (Down Syndrome)

Down syndrome is the most common genetic condition and a leading cause of mental disability [77]. As previously stated, meiotic nondisjunction is the most common cause of trisomy and, thus, Down syndrome. Both parents of such offspring possess a normal karyotype and are otherwise normal. The extra chromosomal material results from a Robertsonian translocation of chromosome 21's extended arm to another acrocentric chromosome (e.g., 22 or 14). Because the fertilized ovum already has two normal autosomes 21, the translocated material gives the identical trisomy 21 triple gene dosage. Such situations are commonly (but not always) familial, with the translocated chromosome inherited from one of the parents (usually the mother) who carries a Robertsonian translocation, such as a mother with karyotype 45, XX. The carrier parent has a one in three chance of having a live kid with Down syndrome; however, the observed frequency is lower. The causes for this disparity remain unknown. When neither parent is a translocation carrier, the rearrangement occurs during gametogenesis. Around 1% of Down syndrome patients have mosaics, meaning they have a mix of cells with 46 and 47 chromosomes. This mosaicism is caused by chromosome 21's nondisjunction during the early stages of embryogenesis [78]. Symptoms vary and are milder in such cases, depending on the number of aberrant cells. Maternal age is irrelevant in cases of translocation or mosaic Down syndrome.

Even at birth, the definitive clinical signs of this condition—flat facial profile, oblique palpebral fissures, and epicanthic folds—are frequently visible. Down syndrome is a leading cause of severe mental impairment, with 80% of individuals affected having an IQ ranging from 25 to 50. These highly challenged youngsters, however, may have a soft, modest demeanor and be more easily directed than their more fortunate siblings who are not burdened with additional chromosomes. It should be noted that some Down syndrome mosaics have minimal phenotypic alterations and may even have average or near-normal intellect [79].

Aside from the phenotypic anomalies and mental retardation already mentioned, certain other clinical aspects are worth mentioning.

Although the karyotype and clinical symptoms of trisomy 21 have been recognized for decades, the molecular basis of Down syndrome is still unknown. Fortunately, all of the sequence of human chromosome 21 has been finished, and roughly 300 genes have been discovered on this chromosome; this condition should change quickly [80]. Interestingly, numerous gene clusters are anticipated to be involved in the same physiological pathway. There are 16 genes involved in the mitochondrial energy route, several that are expected to influence central nervous system structure, and a group involved in folate metabolism, for example. How each of these groupings relates to Down syndrome needs to be clarified. Until recently, it was unclear whether the extra copy of chromosome 21 creates aberrant feedback systems to shut down some genes or causes overexpression of key genes. According to new research, there is a worldwide increase in chromosome 21 gene expression in the developing Down syndrome brain. Such research and mice models of Down syndrome bode well for furthering our understanding of this widespread but complex condition.

7.18.2. Sex Chromosome-Related Cytogenetic Disorders

Sex chromosome-related cytogenetic disorders, also known as sex chromosome aneuploidies or sex chromosome abnormalities, are genetic conditions caused by an atypical number of sex chromosomes. Typically, humans have two sex chromosomes: females have two X chromosomes (XX), and males have one X and Y chromosome (XY). However, variations in the number of sex chromosomes can lead to different disorders [81].

7.18.2.1. Klinefelter Syndrome

Genetic illnesses caused by karyotypic alterations in the sex chromosomes are significantly more common than those caused by autosomal abnormalities [82, 83]. Furthermore, sex chromosomal imbalances (excess or loss) are far better tolerated than autosome abnormalities. This latitude is mostly due to two features unique to the sex chromosomes: (1) lyonization or inactivation of all but one X chromosome and (2) the small quantity of genetic material carried by the Y chromosome. These characteristics are briefly discussed to help us comprehend sex chromosomal abnormalities. Eunuchoid bodily habitus with abnormally long legs; small atrophic testes generally linked with a small penis; and lack of secondary masculine features such as deep voice, beard, and male distribution of pubic hair are also characteristics. Gynecomastia is possible. The average IQ is slightly lower than average, but mental impairment is unusual. The sole consistent result is hypogonadism, which is not present in all patients. Plasma gonadotropin levels, especially follicle-stimulating hormone, persistently increase, although testosterone levels vary. An unidentified process raises mean plasma estradiol levels. In each case, the ratio of estrogens to testosterone determines the degree of feminization. Klinefelter syndrome is the most common cause of male infertility and decreased spermatogenesis [84]. Some individuals' testicular tubules have completely atrophied and have been replaced by pink, hyaline, collagenous ghosts. In others, normal tubules appear to be mixed with atrophic tubules. In some cases, all tubules resemble embryonic, consisting of cords of cells that never established a lumen or advanced to full spermatogenesis. Because of tubule atrophy and crowding, Leydig cells are more visible.

Breast cancer (20 times more likely than in normal males), extragonadal germ cell tumors, and autoimmune diseases like systemic lupus erythematosus (probably connected to low testosterone and high estrogen levels) are also common in Klinefelter syndrome patients. A 47, XXY karyotype is related to the classic form of Klinefelter syndrome (82% of cases). This complement results from a nondisjunction during one of the parents' meiotic divisions. A bit more than half of the instances are due to maternal nondisjunction at the first meiotic division. Most of the remainder is the outcome of nondisjunction during the first paternal meiotic division. There is no difference in phenotype between those who inherit the extra X chromosome from their father and those who inherit it from their mother. Maternal age is raised in situations related to oogenesis defects. In addition to this conventional karyotype, around 15% of Klinefelter syndrome patients have a mosaic pattern, the majority of which are 46, XY/47, XXY. 47, XXY/48, XXXY, and variations on this subject are also available. Rare people have been discovered to have 48, XXXY or 49, XXXXY karyotypes. Individuals with polysomic X suffer additional anatomical abnormalities such as cryptorchidism, hypospadias, more severe hypoplasia of the testes, and skeletal alterations such as prognathism and radioulnar synostosis [85].

7.18.2.2. Turner Syndrome

Turner syndrome, also known as Monosomy X, is a genetic disorder that affects females and is characterized by the partial or complete absence of one of the two X chromosomes. Instead of having 46 chromosomes in each cell, individuals with Turner syndrome typically have 45 chromosomes, with only one X chromosome. Girls with Turner syndrome often have shorter-than-average height, with adult heights typically falling below the average range. Turner syndrome is associated with ovarian insufficiency, which can lead to delayed or incomplete puberty. This can result in a lack of breast development, absence or incomplete development of secondary sexual characteristics, and infertility. Other physical features that may be present in Turner syndrome include a webbed neck, low hairline at the back of the neck, drooping eyelids(ptosis), widely spaced nipples, a high-arched palate, and a characteristic facial appearance. Swelling of the hands and feet, known as lymphedema, can occur in individuals with Turner syndrome, particularly during infancy.

Some individuals with Turner syndrome may have heart defects, such as coarctation of the aorta, which is a narrowing of the main blood vessel that carrier blood from the heart. Kidney abnormalities, including structural abnormalities or an increased risk of urinary tract infection, may also be present. Turner syndrome occurs randomly and is not typically inherited from parents. However, in some cases, it can be caused by the presence of a structurally abnormal X chromosome inherited from one of the parents. Diagnosis is usually made through a chromosome analysis (karyotype) conducted on a blood sample [86, 87].

- **Non-classical inheritance of a single gene disease**

While most single-gene disorders follow classical patterns of inheritance (autosomal dominant, autosomal recessive, or X-linked), there are instances where non-classical patterns of inheritance can occur. These non-classical patterns deviate from the typical Mendelian inheritance patterns and involve more complex mechanisms. In genomic imprinting, the expression of a gene depends on the parent of origin. This means that the functioning of a particular gene is influenced by whether it is inherited from the mother or the father. For example, in Angelman syndrome, the disease results from the loss of function of the maternally inherited allele of the UBE3A gene, while in Prader-Willi syndrome, the disease results from the loss of function of the paternally inherited allele of the same gene [88]. Anticipation refers to a phenomenon where the severity or age of onset of a genetic disorder tends to increase with each successive generation. It is commonly observed in certain trinucleotide repeat disorders, such as Huntington's disease and myotonic dystrophy. In these disorders, the length of a repeated DNA sequence increases in subsequent generations, leading to more severe symptoms or earlier disease onset. Germline mosaicism occurs when a genetic alteration is present in some but not all germ cells (sperm or eggs) of an individual. This can result in a parent who appears unaffected but has a child with a genetic disorder. The genetic alteration is not present in the parent's somatic cells (non-reproductive cells).

Germline mosaicism is seen in conditions like neurofibromatosis type 1 and osteogenesis imperfecta. Uniparental disomy refers to the inheritance of two copies of a chromosome or a chromosome segment from a single parent rather than one copy from each parent [89]. This can occur when there is an error in Meiosis, leading to the loss of one parental chromosome and the duplication of the other. Depending on the chromosome involved, UPD can have varying effects. For example, Prader-Willi syndrome and Angelman syndrome can result from the UPD of the chromosomes. These non-classical inheritance patterns highlight the complexity of genetic inheritance and the influence of epigenetic factors and genetic mechanisms beyond simple Mendelian genetics. Understanding these patterns is important for accurate diagnosis, genetic counselling, and appropriately managing individuals and families affected by these disorders.

7.18.2.3. Factors Producing Chromosomal Aberration

- *Endogenous Factors:*
  - *DNA Replication Errors*: Errors that occur during DNA replication can lead to chromosomal aberrations [90]. These errors can result in DNA strand breaks, insertions, deletions, or duplication, which can subsequently lead to structural abnormalities in the chromosomes.
  - *DNA Repair Deficiencies*: Defects or deficiencies in DNA repair mechanisms can increase the likelihood of chromosomal Aberration. If DNA damage is not properly repaired, it can lead to incorrect re-joining of broken DNA strands, resulting in rearrangements or loss of genetic material.
  - *Genetic Predisposition*: Some individuals may have inherent genetic factors that make them more prone to chromosomal aberrations. These genetic predispositions can affect the stability and integrity of chromosomes, increasing the risk of aberrations.
- *Exogenous Factors:*
  - *Ionizing Radiation*: Exposure to ionizing radiation, such as X-rays, gamma rays, or cosmic rays, is a well-known cause of chromosomal aberrations. Ionizing radiation can directly induce DNA strand breaks or create reactive oxygen species that cause DNA damage, leading to chromosomal aberrations.
  - *Chemical Mutagens*: Certain chemicals, known as mutagens, can cause chromosomal aberrations by directly damaging DNA or interfering with DNA

repair mechanisms. Examples of chemical mutagens include certain industrial chemicals, environmental pollutants, and some chemotherapy drugs.

- *Viral Infections*: Some viral infections can contribute to chromosomal aberrations. Viruses can integrate into the host cell's DNA, disrupting or rearranging the chromosomes.
- *Environmental Factor*: Various environmental factors, such as certain heavy metals, pesticides, and radiation from sunlight (UV radiation), can also contribute to chromosomal aberrations.
- *Medications and therapies*: Certain medications, such as certain anticancer drugs, can induce chromosomal aberrations as a side effect. Additionally, therapies such as radiation therapy used for cancer treatment can also cause chromosomal damage in healthy cells.

Conclusion

This chapter provides a comprehensive overview of the structure, function, and inheritance of genetic material, as well as the mechanisms and consequences of chromosomal aberrations and gene mutations. It explained how errors in DNA replication, repair, or chromosomal segregation can lead to structural and numerical abnormalities that cause a wide spectrum of genetic disorders, ranging from Mendelian and multifactorial diseases to cytogenetic syndromes like Down syndrome and Turner syndrome. The discussion of classical and non-classical inheritance patterns, molecular techniques for genetic diagnosis, and the impact of mutations on health underscores the importance of genetics in modern medicine. By understanding these principles, clinicians and researchers are better equipped to diagnose genetic conditions, counsel families, and develop targeted therapies to manage and potentially correct genetic defects.

References

[1] Baitsell GA. The cell is a structural unit. *American Scientist.* 1955 Jan 1;43(1):133-47.

[2] James HM. *Overview of Deoxyribonucleic Acid* (DNA).

[3] Crick FH, Watson JD. The complementary structure of deoxyribonucleic acid. Proceedings of the Royal Society of London. *Series A. Mathematical and Physical Sciences.* 1954 Apr 7;223(1152):80-96.

[4] Carrasco-Ramiro F, Peiró-Pastor R, Aguado B. Human genomics projects and precision medicine. *Gene therapy.* 2017 Sep;24(9):551-61.

[5] Blackburn EH, Szostak JW. The molecular structure of centromeres and telomeres. *Annual review of biochemistry.* 1984 Jul;53(1):163-94.

[6] Harper JC, Coonen E, Handyside AH, Winston RM, Hopman AH, Delhanty JD. Mosaicism of autosomes and sex chromosomes in morphologically normal, monospermic preimplantation human embryos. *Prenatal diagnosis.* 1995 Jan;15(1):41-9.

[7] Moser H. Duchenne muscular dystrophy: pathogenetic aspects and genetic prevention. *Human genetics.* 1984 Mar;66:17-40.

[8] Johannsen W. The genotype conception of heredity. *The American Naturalist.* 1911 Mar 1;45(531):129-59.

[9] Kohler JN, Turbitt E, Biesecker BB. Personal utility in genomic testing: a systematic literature review. *European Journal of Human Genetics*. 2017 Jun;25(6):662-8.
[10] Gray JW, Coffino P. [19] Cell cycle analysis by flow cytometry. In *Methods in enzymology* 1979 Jan 1 (Vol. 58, pp. 233-248). Academic Press.
[11] Sclafani RA, Holzen T. Cell cycle regulation of DNA replication. *Annu. Rev. Genet.*. 2007 Dec 1;41:237-80.
[12] Dixon DC, Seagull RW, Triplett BA. Changes in the Accumulation of [alpha]-and [beta]-Tubulin Isotypes during Cotton Fiber Development. *Plant physiology*. 1994 Aug 1;105(4):1347-53.
[13] Nasmyth K. Putting the cell cycle in order. *Science*. 1996 Dec 6;274(5293):1643-5.
[14] Darzynkiewicz Z, Sharpless T, Staiano-Coico L, Melamed MR. Subcompartments of the G1 phase of cell cycle detected by flow cytometry. *Proceedings of the National Academy of Sciences*. 1980 Nov;77(11):6696-9.
[15] Karp G. *Cell and molecular biology: concepts and experiments*. John Wiley & Sons; 2009 Oct 19.
[16] Hughes RN. *Functional biology of clonal animals*. Springer Science & Business Media; 1989 Oct 31.
[17] Oliver T. Meiosis and the Embryo. *Early Pregnancy*. 2017 Feb 2:54.
[18] Wassink TH, Piven J, Patil SR. Chromosomal abnormalities in a clinic sample of individuals with autistic disorder. *Psychiatric genetics*. 2001 Jun 1;11(2):57-63.
[19] Rozgaj R, Kašuba V, Šentija K, Prlić I. Radiation-induced chromosomal aberrations and haematological alterations in hospital workers. *Occupational medicine*. 1999 Aug 1;49(6):353-60.
[20] Huang L, Snyder AR, Morgan WF. Radiation-induced genomic instability and its implications for radiation carcinogenesis. *Oncogene*. 2003 Sep;22(37):5848-54.
[21] Shakoori AR, Aftab S, Al-Ghanim K. Structural changes in chromosomes. *Chromosome Structure and Aberrations*. 2017:245-74.
[22] Pantelias GE, Maillie HD. Directly analysis of radiation-induced chromosome fragments and rings in unstimulated human peripheral blood lymphocytes using the premature chromosome condensation technique. *Mutation Research/Fundamental and Molecular Mechanisms of Mutagenesis*. 1985 Mar 1;149(1):67-72.
[23] Blakely WF, Salter CA, Prasanna PG. Early-response biological dosimetry—recommended countermeasure enhancements for mass-casualty radiological incidents and terrorism. *Health physics*. 2005 Nov 1;89(5):494-504.
[24] Müller I, Geinitz H, Braselmann H, Baumgartner A, Fasan A, Thamm R, Molls M, Meineke V, Zitzelsberger H. Time-course of radiation-induced chromosomal aberrations in tumor patients after radiotherapy. *International Journal of Radiation Oncology* Biology* Physics*. 2005 Nov 15;63(4):1214-20.
[25] Hada M, Wu H, Cucinotta FA. mBAND analysis for high-and low-LET radiation-induced chromosome aberrations: a review. Mutation Research/Fundamental and Molecular *Mechanisms of Mutagenesis*. 2011 Jun 3;711(1-2):187-92.
[26] Kim H, Nguyen NP, Turner K, Wu S, Gujar AD, Luebeck J, Liu J, Deshpande V, Rajkumar U, Namburi S, Amin SB. Extrachromosomal DNA is associated with oncogene amplification and poor outcome across multiple cancers. *Nature genetics*. 2020 Sep;52(9):891-7.
[27] Vetro R, Farhoodi R, Kotla R, Haspel N, Weisman D, Rosen J, Simovici D. TIDE: Inter-chromosomal translocation and insertion detection using embeddings. In *2014 IEEE International Conference on Big Data* (Big Data) 2014 Oct 27 (pp. 64–70). IEEE.
[28] Ciccone R, Giorda R, Gregato G, Guerrini R, Giglio S, Carrozzo R, Bonaglia MC, Priolo E, Laganà C, Tenconi R, Rocchi M. Reciprocal translocations: a trap for cytogenetists?. *Human genetics*. 2005 Oct;117:571-82.
[29] Scriven PN, Flinter FA, Braude PR, Ogilvie CM. Robertsonian translocations—reproductive risks and indications for preimplantation genetic diagnosis. *Human Reproduction*. 2001 Nov 1;16(11):2267-73.
[30] Nagy Z, Chandler M. *Regulation of transposition in bacteria. Research in microbiology*. 2004 Jun 1;155(5):387-98.
[31] Milunsky A, Milunsky JM.. John Wiley & Sons; 2015 Nov 9. *Genetic disorders and the fetus: diagnosis, prevention, and treatment*

[32] Andreassi MG. Coronary atherosclerosis and somatic mutations: an overview of the contributive factors for oxidative DNA damage. *Mutation Research/Reviews in Mutation Research.* 2003 Jan 1;543(1):67-86.
[33] Sherman JD, Greenfield JB, Ingall D. Reversible bone-marrow vacuolizations in phenylketonuria. *New England Journal of Medicine.* 1964 Apr 16;270(16):810-4.
[34] Mazzocco MM. Advances in research on the fragile X syndrome. *Mental retardation and developmental disabilities research reviews.* 2000;6(2):96-106.
[35] Emery AE, Muntoni F, Quinlivan R. *Duchenne muscular dystrophy.* Oxford Monographs on Medical G; 2015.
[36] Fischer A. Severe combined immunodeficiencies (SCID). *Clinical & Experimental Immunology.* 2000 Nov;122(2):143-9.
[37] Yu CE, Oshima J, Fu YH, Wijsman EM, Hisama F, Alisch R, Matthews S, Nakura J, Miki T, Ouais S, Martin GM. Positional cloning of the Werner's syndrome gene. *Science.* 1996 Apr 12;272(5259):258-62.
[38] Erickson RP. Somatic gene mutation and human disease other than cancer. *Mutation Research/Reviews in Mutation Research.* 2003 Mar 1;543(2):125-36.
[39] Lyon MF, Morris T. Gene and chromosome Mutation after large fractionated or unfractionated radiation doses to mouse spermatogonia. *Mutation Research/Fundamental and Molecular Mechanisms of Mutagenesis.* 1969 Jul 1;8(1):191-8.
[40] Streisinger G, Okada Y, Emrich J, Newton J, Tsugita A, Terzaghi E, Inouye M. Frameshift mutations and the genetic code. In *Cold Spring Harbor Symposia on Quantitative Biology* 1966 Jan 1 (Vol. 31, pp. 77-84). Cold Spring Harbor Laboratory Press.
[41] Stefl S, Nishi H, Petukh M, Panchenko AR, Alexov E. Molecular mechanisms of disease-causing missense mutations. *Journal of molecular biology.* 2013 Nov 1;425(21):3919-36.
[42] Sakuraba H, Oshima A, Fukuhara Y, Shimmoto M, Nagao Y, Bishop DF, Desnick RJ, Suzuki Y. Identification of point mutations in the alpha-galactosidase A gene in classical and atypical hemizygotes with Fabry disease. *American journal of human genetics.* 1990 Nov;47(5):784.
[43] Osato M. Point mutations in the RUNX1/AML1 gene: another actor in RUNX leukemia. *Oncogene.* 2004 May;23(24):4284-96.
[44] Pearson CE, Sinden RR. Trinucleotide repeat DNA structures: dynamic mutations from dynamic DNA. *Current opinion in structural biology.* 1998 Jun 1;8(3):321-30.
[45] Nousia-Arvanitakis S. Cystic fibrosis and the pancreas: recent scientific advances. *Journal of Clinical Gastroenterology.* 1999 Sep 1;29(2):138-42.
[46] McNicholl JM, Smith DK, Qari SH, Hodge T. Host genes and HIV: the role of the chemokine receptor gene CCR5 and its allele. *Emerging infectious diseases.* 1997 Jul;3(3):261.
[47] Navashin M. Chromosome alterations caused by hybridization and their bearing upon certain general genetic problems. *Cytologia.* 1934 Jan 30;5(2):169-203.
[48] Wilson M, Forsyth P, Whiteside J. Haemoglobinopathy and sickle cell disease. Continuing Education in Anaesthesia, *Critical Care & Pain.* 2010 Feb 1;10(1):24-8.
[49] McKusick VA. On lumpers and splitters, or the nosology of genetic disease. *Perspectives in biology and medicine.* 1969;12(2):298-312.
[50] Mahdieh N, Rabbani B. An overview of mutation detection methods in genetic disorders. *Iranian journal of paediatrics.* 2013 Aug;23(4):375.
[51] Caruso SM, Quinn PM, da Costa BL, Tsang SH. CRISPR/Cas therapeutic strategies for autosomal dominant disorders. *The Journal of Clinical Investigation.* 2022 May 2;132(9).
[52] Wilson BN, John AM, Handler MZ, Schwartz RA. Neurofibromatosis type 1: New developments in genetics and treatment. *Journal of the American Academy of Dermatology.* 2021 Jun 1;84(6):1667-76.
[53] Wilkie AO. The molecular basis of genetic dominance. *Journal of medical genetics.* 1994 Feb 1;31(2):89-98.
[54] Goodeve AC. The genetic basis of von Willebrand disease. *Blood reviews.* 2010 May 1;24(3):123-34.
[55] Bates GP, Dorsey R, Gusella JF, Hayden MR, Kay C, Leavitt BR, Nance M, Ross CA, Scahill RI, Wetzel R, Wild EJ. Huntington disease. *Nature reviews Disease primers.* 2015 Apr 23;1(1):1-21.

[56] Costa T, Scriver CR, Childs B, Opitz JM, Reynolds JF. The effect of Mendelian disease on human health: a measurement. *American journal of medical genetics*. 1985 Jun;21(2):231-42.
[57] Luzzatto L, Ally M, Notaro R. Glucose-6-phosphate dehydrogenase deficiency. Blood, *The Journal of the American Society of Hematology*. 2020 Sep 10;136(11):1225-40.
[58] Mao JR, Bristow J. The Ehlers-Danlos syndrome: on beyond collagens. *The Journal of Clinical Investigation*. 2001 May 1;107(9):1063-9.
[59] Tyfield L, Reichardt J, Fridovich-Keil J, Croke DT, Elsas LJ, Strobl W, Kozak L, Coskun T, Novelli G, Okano Y, Zekanowski C. Classical galactosemia and mutations at the galactose-1-phosphate uridyl transferase (GALT) gene. *Human Mutation*. 1999;13(6):417-30.
[60] Cacicedo ML, Weinl-Tenbruck C, Frank D, Limeres MJ, Wirsching S, Hilbert K, Pasha Famian MA, Horscroft N, Hennermann JB, Zepp F, Chevessier-Tünnesen F. Phenylalanine hydroxylase mRNA rescues the phenylketonuria phenotype in mice. *Frontiers in Bioengineering and Biotechnology*. 2022 Oct 7;10:993298.
[61] Bell S, Kolobova I, Crapper L, Ernst C. Lesch-Nyhan syndrome: models, theories, and therapies. *Molecular syndromology*. 2016 Nov 22;7(6):302-11.
[62] Shapiro SD, Goldstein NM, Houghton AM, Kobayashi DK, Kelley D, Belaaouaj A. Neutrophil elastase contributes to cigarette smoke-induced emphysema in mice. *The American journal of pathology*. 2003 Dec 1;163(6):2329-35.
[63] Brown MS, Goldstein JL. Receptor-mediated endocytosis: insights from the lipoprotein receptor system. *Proceedings of the National Academy of Sciences*. 1979 Jul;76(7):3330-7.
[64] Clarke GM, Higgins TN. Laboratory investigation of hemoglobinopathies and thalassemias: review and update. *Clinical chemistry*. 2000 Aug 1;46(8):1284-90.
[65] Elewa H, Wilby KJ. A review of pharmacogenetics of antimalarials and associated clinical implications. *European journal of drug metabolism and pharmacokinetics*. 2017 Oct;42:745-56.
[66] Mossey PA. The heritability of malocclusion: Part 1—Genetics, principles and terminology. *British journal of orthodontics*. 1999 May;26(2):103-13.
[67] Pickup JC, Crook MA. Is type II diabetes mellitus a disease of the innate immune system? *Diabetologia*. 1998 Sep;41:1241-8.
[68] Mossey PA. The heritability of malocclusion: Part 1—Genetics, principles and terminology. *British journal of orthodontics*. 1999 May;26(2):103-13.
[69] Renneville A, Roumier C, Biggio V, Nibourel O, Boissel N, Fenaux P, Preudhomme C. Cooperating gene mutations in acute myeloid leukemia: a review of the literature. *Leukaemia*. 2008 May;22(5):915-31.
[70] Delhanty JD. Mechanisms of aneuploidy induction in human oogenesis and early embryogenesis. *Cytogenetic and genome research*. 2005 Sep 21;111(3-4):237-44.
[71] Jacobs PA, Hassold TJ. 4 The origin of numerical chromosome abnormalities. *Advances in Genetics*. 1995 Jan 1;33:101-33.
[72] Biesecker LG, Spinner NB. A genomic view of mosaicism and human disease. *Nature Reviews Genetics*. 2013 May;14(5):307-20.
[73] Sybert VP, McCauley E. Turner's syndrome. *New England Journal of Medicine*. 2004 Sep 16;351(12):1227-38.
[74] Hsu LY, Perlis TE. United States survey on chromosome mosaicism and pseudo mosaicism in prenatal diagnosis. *Prenatal diagnosis*. 1984 Nov;4(7):97-130.
[75] Verdoni A, Hu J, Surti U, Babcock M, Sheehan E, Clemens M, Drewes S, Walsh L, Clark R, Katari S, Sanfilippo J. Reproductive outcomes in individuals with chromosomal reciprocal translocations. *Genetics in Medicine*. 2021 Sep;23(9):1753-60.
[76] Frydman N, Romana S, Le Lorc'h M, Vekemans M, Frydman R, Tachdjian G. Assisting reproduction of infertile men carrying a Robertsonian translocation. *Human Reproduction*. 2001 Nov 1;16(11):2274-7.
[77] Antonarakis SE, Skotko BG, Rafii MS, Strydom A, Pape SE, Bianchi DW, Sherman SL, Reeves RH. Down syndrome. *Nature Reviews Disease Primers*. 2020 Jan;6(1):9.

[78] Munné S, Sandalinas M, Escudero T, Márquez C, Cohen J. Chromosome mosaicism in cleavage-stage human embryos: evidence of a maternal age effect. *Reproductive biomedicine online*. 2002 Jan 1;4(3):223-32.

[79] Karmiloff-Smith A, Al-Janabi T, D'Souza H, Groet J, Massand E, Mok K, Startin C, Fisher E, Hardy J, Nizetic D, Tybulewicz V. *The importance of understanding individual differences in Down syndrome*. F1000Research. 2016;5.

[80] Antonarakis SE. Down syndrome and the complexity of genome dosage imbalance. *Nature Reviews Genetics*. 2017 Mar;18(3):147-63.

[81] Hassold TJ. Chromosome abnormalities in human reproductive wastage. *Trends in Genetics*. 1986 Jan 1;2:105-10.

[82] Lanfranco F, Kamischke A, Zitzmann M, Nieschlag E. Klinefelter's syndrome. *The Lancet*. 2004 Jul 17;364(9430):273-83.

[83] Smyth CM, Bremner WJ. Klinefelter syndrome. *Archives of internal medicine*. 1998 Jun 22;158(12):1309-14.

[84] Maiburg M, Repping S, Giltay J. The genetic origin of Klinefelter syndrome and its effect on spermatogenesis. *Fertility and sterility*. 2012 Aug 1;98(2):253-60.

[85] Nistal, M., Paniagua, R., González-Peramato, P. and Reyes-Múgica, M., 2016. Perspectives in pediatric pathology, chapter 16. Klinefelter syndrome and other anomalies in X and Y chromosomes. Clinical and pathological entities. *Pediatric and Developmental Pathology*, 19(4), pp. 259-277.

[86] Sybert VP, McCauley E. Turner's syndrome. *New England Journal of Medicine*. 2004 Sep 16;351(12):1227-38.

[87] Lippe B. Turner syndrome. *Endocrinology and metabolism clinics of North America*. 1991 Mar 1;20(1):121-52.

[88] Nicholls RD, Saitoh S, Horsthemke B. Imprinting in Prader–Willi and Angelman syndromes. *Trends in Genetics*. 1998 May 1;14(5):194-200.

[89] Biesecker LG, Spinner NB. A genomic view of mosaicism and human disease. *Nature Reviews Genetics*. 2013 May;14(5):307-20.

[90] Obe, G., Pfeiffer, P., Savage, J. R. K., Johannes, C., Goedecke, W., Jeppesen, P., Natarajan, A. T., Martınez-López, W., Folle, G. A. and Drets, M. E., 2002. Chromosomal aberrations: formation, identification, and distribution. *Mutation Research/Fundamental and Molecular Mechanisms of Mutagenesis*, 504(1-2), pp. 17-36.

Chapter 8

Cell Survival

Ashish Uke[1,*], MD
Ravishankar Patil[2], MD
Aakanksha Tiwari[3], MDS
and Shivali Kashikar[4], MD, PhD

[1]Department of Radiation Oncology, Datta Meghe Institute of Higher Education and Research, Wardha, India
[2]Department of Radiology, Datta Meghe Institute of Higher Education and Research, Wardha, India
[3]Department of Oral Medicine and Radiology, Datta Meghe Institute of Higher Education and Research, Wardha, India
[4]Department of Radio-diagnosis, Datta Meghe Institute of Higher Education and Research, Wardha, India

Abstract

This comprehensive review explores the concept of reproductive integrity and its relationship with radiosensitivity in mammalian cells. Reproductive integrity refers to a cell's ability to undergo infinite division and generate a multitude of progeny. The loss of reproductive integrity is a key indicator of cell death, which can be induced by radiation exposure. The review discusses the mechanisms of cell killing, including apoptosis, mitotic death, and autophagic cell death, and their relationship with radiation-induced damage. The shape of the survival curve, which describes the relationship between radiation dose and cell survival, is also examined. The review highlights the importance of understanding the underlying mechanisms of radiosensitivity and how they are influenced by genetic and environmental factors. Additionally, the review touches on the concept of the bystander effect, where cells that are not directly exposed to radiation can still experience biological consequences due to their proximity to irradiated cells. The review concludes by discussing the implications of these findings for cancer therapy and the potential for targeting radiosensitive cells to enhance treatment outcomes.

Keywords: apoptosis, cell survival curve, linear-quadratic model, mitotic death, radiosensitivity, reproductive integrity

* Corresponding Author's Email: ashishuke1@gmail.com

In: Fundamentals of Radiation Biology
Editors: Anurag Luharia, Ashish Uke, Gaurav Mishra et al.
ISBN: 979-8-89530-806-6

8.1. Introduction

Reproductive integrity is a fundamental concept in radiobiology, referring to the ability of cells to maintain their capacity for infinite division and generate a multitude of progeny. This concept is crucial in understanding the effects of radiation on living organisms, particularly in the context of cancer treatment. The loss of reproductive integrity is a key indicator of cell death, and understanding the mechanisms that govern this process is essential for developing effective cancer treatments.

Cell survival curves, which demonstrate the decline in reproductive capacity caused by exposure to radiation, provide valuable insights into the mechanisms of cell killing. The shape of the survival curve can vary depending on the type of radiation, the dose rate, and the cell type, but it generally exhibits a characteristic "shoulder" region at low doses, followed by a linear or exponential decline at higher doses. The mechanisms of cell killing are complex and multifaceted, involving various cellular processes such as apoptosis, mitotic death, and autophagic cell death. Genetic control plays a critical role in regulating radiosensitivity, with various genes contributing to the repair of DNA damage and the maintenance of genomic stability. Additionally, the bystander effect, where cells that are not directly exposed to radiation can still experience biological consequences, has significant implications for our understanding of radiation biology and the development of cancer treatments. In this chapter, we will explore the concept of reproductive integrity and its relationship to cell survival curves, examining the various mechanisms of cell killing and the role of genetic control in regulating radiosensitivity. By understanding the complex interactions between radiation, cells, and genetic factors, we can develop more effective cancer treatments and improve patient outcomes.

8.2. Reproductive Integrity

A cell survival curve demonstrates the relationship between radiation exposure and the proportion of viable cells. Death can be defined as the state in which differentiated cells, such as nerve, muscle, or secretory cells, cease to perform their specific functions and are no longer capable of undergoing multiplication. The term "loss of the capacity for persistent proliferation" or "loss of reproductive integrity" can be appropriately used to describe the phenomenon observed in proliferating cells, such as haematological system stem cells or intestinal epithelial cells [1]. This phenomenon is occasionally denoted as reproductive mortality. This outcome can be attributed to the measurements conducted through *in vitro* cell culture.

The cellular entity may persist in its physical form without visible damage, retain its ability to synthesize proteins or DNA, and potentially undergo one or two cycles of mitosis. Nevertheless, in the event that the cell loses its capacity for infinite division and the generation of a multitude of progeny, it can be deemed deceased and its survival compromised. The term "clonogenic" pertains to the capacity of an organism to perpetually reproduce and establish a substantial clone or colony while preserving its reproductive integrity [2].

The idea at hand generally encompasses the radiobiology of several organisms, including animals, plants, and their respective tissues. Tumor radiation holds significant importance in medical contexts. The sole cells that necessitate elimination for the total eradication of a tumour are those that undergo a state of functional impairment, rendering them incapable of multiplying and instigating the growth and dissemination of the tumour. As will be elaborated upon further, various methodologies can induce cellular death. After exposure to irradiation, the primary mechanism for most cells is cell death during the division process, known as mitotic death [3]. Apoptosis, also known as programmed cell death, is essential for some cellular processes. Regardless of the methodology employed, the outcome remains consistent. The cellular structure experiences a loss of reproductive integrity, resulting in the inability to undergo unlimited multiplication.

8.3. The *In Vitro* Survival Curve

A solitary cell has the capacity to proliferate into a collective of cells that may be seen discerned without the use of magnification. This indicates that the cell has successfully preserved its reproductive integrity. The radiation survival curve indicates the decline in reproductive capacity caused by exposure to radiation. Utilizing contemporary tissue culture methodologies, it is possible to extract a specimen from either a neoplastic growth or a substantial quantity of healthy regenerative tissues [4]. The sample may be subdivided into smaller fragments, and afterwards, the single-cell suspension can be generated with the use of trypsin, an enzymatic agent. Trypsin enzymatically degrades the cell membrane, facilitating the subsequent seeding of cells into a culture dish. Subsequently, the dish is enveloped with an appropriate intricate growth media and upheld at 37° C under sterile conditions. The cells adhere to the substrate of the culture dish, undergo proliferation, and undergo mitotic division.

Plating efficiency pertains to the proportion of cells that are introduced into a dish from an actively proliferating stock culture. Trypsin is employed to detach cells from the substrate of a culture medium. The quantification of cellular density inside a suspension is often achieved through a hemacytometer or an electronic counter. For example, when a dish is initially seeded with 100 individual cells and subsequently cultured for 1-2 weeks, each cell will undergo multiple rounds of division, resulting in the formation of a discernible colony that may be observed without the aid of magnification, particularly if the dish is subjected to fixation and staining techniques. Every cell comprising a colony is derived from a common progenitor. As an illustration, while inoculating a plate with 100 cells, the number of colonies observed is anticipated to range between 50 and 90 [5]. Ideally, one should be capable of enumerating a total of 100 colonies. Nevertheless, occurrences of this nature are few owing to a multitude of variables like the utilization of poor growing media, inaccuracies and ambiguities in the enumeration of cell suspensions, or the challenges associated with trypsinization and manipulation of the suspension.

8.4. The Shape of the Survival Curve

The conventional representation of the survival curve for mammalian cells involves a logarithmic-linear scale for the dosage plot and a logarithmic scale for the surviving fraction plot [6]. From a qualitative perspective, the curve can be succinctly summarized in Figure 8.1 (A) and Figure 8.1(B) as follows: At lower doses of low-level ionizing radiation, such as X-rays, the survival curve has a linear slope at the onset, with the fraction of organisms or cells that survive dependent on the dose received. As the dosage is increased, the curve tends to exhibit a bending or curving effect within a range of grayscale values. The surviving fraction has an exponential relationship with the dosage when administered in very high quantities, which is often observed only when the doses exceed those employed in routine radiation treatments.

Conversely, when considering highly ionizing radiations characterized by high linear energy transfer (LET), such as alpha particles or low-velocity neutrons, the cell survival curves exhibit linearity in relation to the radiation source [7]. In other words, the survival rate closely approximates an exponential function of the administered dosage.

Although the qualitative aspects of the cell survival curve can be readily elucidated, the explanation of the biological facts in terms of biophysical phenomena poses a more challenging task. Numerous models and theories exist to elucidate the underlying factors influencing the shape of the survival curve in mammalian populations. Most of these models can obtain a curved shape that aligns with the empirical data. However, selecting between several models or theories based solely on their fit to the experimental data is challenging. Furthermore, the accuracy of the biological data and the divergence of the prediction theory curves are significant enough to render it unfeasible.

Characterizing survival curves can be achieved using two distinct methods while minimizing the utilization of mathematical equations. The multitarget model, which has been extensively employed over an extended period, continues to retain a certain degree of validity. In the present model, the survival curve exhibits an initial gradient denoted as D_l, corresponding to the decline rate in survival for single event killing. Additionally, the survival curve demonstrates a final gradient represented as D_0, which signifies the rate of decline in survival for multiple event killing. The breadth or width of the curve's shoulder is denoted by a quantity (n or D_q) for each slope [8]. The numbers D_l and D_0 can be defined as the inverse of the initial and end slope, respectively. In both scenarios, the first gradient represents the dosage required to decrease the survival fraction to 37% (e^{-1}) on the initial linear segment of the survival curve ($D_l = 0.37$). The ultimate gradient ($D_0 = 0.037$) is the dosage required to decrease the survival fraction from 0.1/0.037 to 0.01/0.0037. The dosage necessary to decrease the cell population by a factor equivalent to e^{-1} (0.37) remains consistent across all levels of survival. This is attributed to the logarithmic relationship between the percentage of cells that survive and the linear nature of the survival curve at higher doses. This dosage is normally necessary to induce a single inactivation event in each cell.

The variable "n" represents the extrapolation number. If the value of n is either 10 or 12, the survival curve will exhibit a broad shoulder. However, when the value of n is equal to or less than 1.5, the width of the shoulder will be reduced. The quasithreshold dose denoted as D_q serves as an additional metric for assessing shoulder breadth [9].

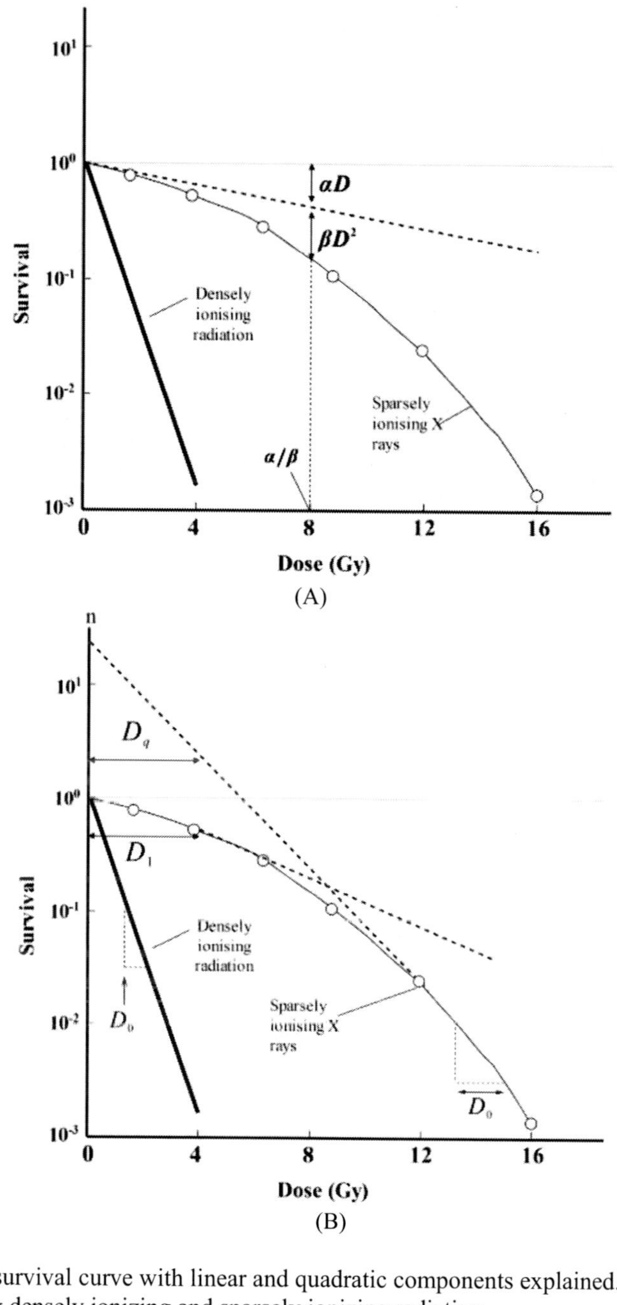

Figure 8.1. (A) cell survival curve with linear and quadratic components explained. (B) cell survival curves differentiating densely ionizing and sparsely ionizing radiation.

Basically, the "quasithreshold" dose is close to the "threshold" dose. It is defined as the point where the straight part of a survival curve, taken backwards, cuts off the dose axis drawn through the unit's survival fraction. The "threshold" is the dose with no effect since none is below that. So, there is no "true" threshold dose; the closest thing to it is D_q . n, D_0 and D_q are related by the following expression.

Formula:

$$D_q = D_0 \cdot \ln(n)$$

where:

Dq = quasithreshold dose (shoulder width)

D0 = the dose that reduces the surviving fraction by a factor of eee in the straight portion

n = extrapolation number

- The linear quadratic model has become the preferred model for survival curves. This is a direct evolution of the relationship used to describe exchange-type chromosome breaks that are unambiguously caused by an interaction between two distinct breaks [10].
- The linear quadratic model supposes two components to cell death by radiation: one proportional to the dose and one proportional to the quadratic dose. The idea that there is a component of cell inactivation that changes with the doubling of the dose gives rise to the concept of dual radiation action. The concept dates back to early work on chromosome aberrations, where many aberrations were the result of two separate breaks [11].

By this model, the expression for the cell survival curve is:

$$S = e^{-(\alpha D+\beta D^2)}$$

where:

S = fraction of surviving cells

D = dose

α = linear component coefficient (single-event damage)

β = quadratic component coefficient (two-event damage)

S, the fraction of cells surviving a dose D, and α and β are constants. The components of cell killing that are proportional to the dose and to the square of the dose are equal if

Or

$$D = \frac{\alpha}{\beta}$$

Notably, the linear and quadratic components of cell death exhibit equivalence at the dosage corresponding to the alpha-to-beta ratio [12]. One notable characteristic of the linear quadratic model is the absence of a final linear segment in the resulting cell survival curve since it consistently exhibits a bending pattern. The observed experimental results deviate from the statement, as survival curves obtained across a range of 7-10 decades of cell death demonstrate a dose-response relationship that closely resembles a linear plot (log-linear). In other words, cell killing is exponentially related to the dose administered. During the initial 10-20 years of cell death and up to the dosage of daily fractions employed in clinical radiation, the linear Quadratic model well captures the facts. One of its advantages is that it possesses only two adjustable parameters, alpha and beta.

8.5. Mechanisms of Cell Killing

Extensive evidence supports the notion that the primary locations of vulnerability to cell death caused by radiation are primarily situated within the nucleus, as opposed to the cytoplasm. The available evidence strongly supports the notion that chromosomal DNA is the major target of cell lethality. Although this evidence is largely anecdotal in nature, its cumulative weight is substantial. To provide a concise summary, the evidence can be outlined as follows:

1. Incorporating radioactive tritium (thymidine) into the DNA results in the fatal destruction of cells [13]. The generation of radiation dose is attributed to the emission of β particles with a limited range, resulting in a high degree of localization.
2. Certain structural analogues, such as thymidine and halogenated pyrimidines, exhibit a preferential propensity to be integrated into DNA rather than thymidine when substituted in cell cultures' growth medium. The insertion of this alteration significantly enhances the radiosensitivity of mammalian cells, exhibiting an exponential relationship with the extent of incorporation.
3. Various factors, including as the kind of radiation, oxygen content, and dosage rate, have been observed to influence both cell mortality and the generation of chromosomal damage in a comparable fashion.
4. The initial findings indicated a correlation between virus size and radiosensitivity, but subsequent research revealed a more robust association [14]. There exists a correlation between radiosensitivity and the average interphase chromosome volume, which refers to the ratio of nuclear volume to chromosomal number, in a diverse range of plant species. A positive correlation exists between the average volume of chromosomes and their sensitivity. The main focus of radiation-induced toxicity lies in the DNA of chromosomes. However, advanced tests utilizing microbeams have convincingly shown that α particles, which traverse the cell membrane without reaching the nucleus, can generate mutations at low levels.

8.6. The Bystander Effect

In the field of radiation biology, previous teachings to successive cohorts of students emphasized the necessity of direct DNA damage for the occurrence of heritable biological consequences. However, in the last decade, a series of tests have emerged, revealing the existence of what is now known as the bystander effect. The bystander effect refers to the phenomenon in which cells that are not directly exposed to a charged particle yet experience biological consequences due to their proximity to cells that have been exposed [15]. The study conducted by Nagasawa et al. in 1992 catalyzed the growing interest in the bystander effect. This research revealed that even a small amount of low-dose alpha particles could result in biological damage in cells that were not directly exposed to these particles.

Interestingly, approximately 30% of these cells exhibited an increase in the exchange of sister chromatids despite only 1% of cells being estimated to have experienced nuclear traversal. The number of affected cells was calculated based on the fluence of alpha particles and the cross-sectional area of cell nuclei. The observed result was deemed statistical due to the inherent difficulty in distinguishing the specific cells that were impacted from those that were unaffected on an individual basis.

The bystander effect is a phenomenon that has been further investigated through the utilization of improved single-particle micromachines [16]. These micromachines enable the controlled delivery of a certain quantity of particles into the nucleus of select cells, facilitating the examination of biological impacts on adjacent non-irradiated cells. Most microbeam investigations have employed α particles due to their comparatively simpler focusing capabilities. However, it is worth noting that a bystander effect has also been observed in the context of protons and soft X-rays. The utilization of single particle micromachines has demonstrated the occurrence of a bystander effect in various biological phenomena, such as chromosome aberrations, cell death, mutations, oncogenetic transformation, and gene expression [17]. The impact is particularly pronounced when the bystander cell engages in gap-junction contact with irradiation cells, resulting in a mortality rate of up to 30%. When cell monolayers are reduced in thickness to a range of a few hundred micrometres, it has been observed that only a small percentage, specifically 5-10%, of the surrounding bystander cells undergo cell death. This observation implies that the scope of radiation damage extends beyond the cellular level. The relevance of this phenomenon is primarily observed at lower dosage levels, where not all cells are specifically targeted. Additionally, it may have a substantial impact on the prediction of risks.

In addition to the aforementioned single particle microbeam investigations, a substantial body of research exists regarding media transmission from irradiated to non-irradiated cells, leading to a biological consequence characterized by cell death [18]. The investigations mentioned above, commonly known as the bystander effect, demonstrate that irradiated cells release a chemical into the surrounding medium, which can induce cell death when transferred onto uninfected cells. The majority of bystander medium transfer experiments have employed low-linear energy transfer (LET) x- or γ-rays.

8.7. Apoptotic and Mitotic Death

Kerr et al. initially characterized apoptosis as a distinct series of cellular alterations. The term "apoptosis" originates from the Greek word "apotheosis," denoting the concept of "falling," analogous to the shedding of petals from a flower or leaves from a tree [19]. Apoptosis, also known as programmed cell death, is a prevalent occurrence throughout embryonic development, wherein specific tissues undergo obsolescence. This process serves as the method via which many organisms, such as tadpoles, shed their tails. This particular form of cellular demise follows a characteristic progression of morphological occurrences. When a cell within a tissue undergoes commitment to apoptosis, an initial action is the termination of intercellular connection with neighbouring cells. As the cell undergoes rounding and detachment from adjacent cells, it experiences a reduction in size attributed to the condensation of chromatin on the nuclear membrane and the fragmentation of the nucleus. Ultimately, the cellular structure undergoes division, forming several pieces enclosed by membranes, known as apoptotic bodies [20]. These entities may consist only of cytoplasm or fragments of the nucleus. The characteristic morphological feature of apoptosis is the aggregation of nuclear chromatin, which occurs in crescents along the periphery of the nucleus or as a cluster of spherical fragments.

The dissociation of double-strand (DSB) sections located between nucleosomes leads to the generation of DNA fragments [21]. These fragments have a length that is a multiple of around 185 base pairs and are responsible for the observed ladder-like patterns on gel electrophoresis. In contrast, necrosis leads to a dispersed distribution of DNA throughout the gels. As previously stated, apoptosis is a phenomenon observed in healthy cells and can also be triggered by radiation in both normal tissues and some types of malignancies. The occurrence of apoptosis is heavily influenced by the specific cell type in which radiation is caused and typically relies on the presence of p53 (Bcl-2) for its execution [22]· Mitotic cell death, the prevailing form of cell death induced by radiation, exhibits a significant reliance on cell type and is notably expedited by radiation in most tumour cells. Mitotic death is characterized by cell death during cell division, which can occur either during the first or second division following radiation exposure. Previous studies have documented a strong quantitative correlation between cellular apoptosis and the occurrence of distinct chromosomal abnormalities.

The process of apoptosis has a significant reliance on the specific cellular phenotype. Hemopoietic cells and lymphoid cells exhibit a heightened susceptibility to prompt cell death induced by radiation through the apoptotic pathway [23]. In most tumour cells, mitotic cell death holds comparable significance to apoptosis, and in many instances, it represents the sole mechanism of cell demise. Multiple genes appear to be involved. Initially, it appears that the occurrence of cell death following radiation exposure is contingent upon the presence of p53, while Bcl-2 assumes a repressive function.

The most prevalent type of cell death resulting from radiation exposure is mitotic death. Cell death can occur due to unsuccessful attempts to undergo cell division, which can be attributed to damaged chromosomes. Mortality can manifest either in the initial or subsequent cellular divisions following exposure to radiation [24]. A strong quantitative relationship exists between the process of cell death and the occurrence of particular chromosomal abnormalities, such as rings or dicentrics. The tests done by Cornforth and Bedford were carried out using a cell line that lacked the occurrence of apoptosis.

8.8. Autophagic Cell Death

Autophagy is a cellular mechanism that involves the destruction of cellular components through lysosomal processes, serving to either repair or uphold cellular homeostasis [25]. The process in question is evolutionarily conserved and encompasses a series of dynamic phases. One of these steps entails the sequestration of cytoplasmic sections or organelles within a vesicle known as an autophagosome, which consists of a double membrane structure. The autophagosomes ultimately undergo fusion with lysosomes, leading to the degradation and processing of proteins and organelles. The acidification of lysosomes occurs during their maturation into autolysosomes, a phenomenon referred known as autophagy flux. The process of autophagy is a complex series of steps that is governed by a specific set of genes known as autophagy-related genes (Atgs). Autophagy-related genes (Atgs) were initially discovered in yeast, and it has been established that around 30 Atgs orthologs are present in mammals. Among these orthologs, two ubiquitin-type conjugation systems have been identified, namely Atg12-ATG5 and Atg8(LC-3)-phosphatidylthanolamine. These mechanisms play a crucial role in the elongation process of the autophagosomal membrane [26].

Initially, autophagy was perceived as a cellular mechanism employed for the sake of cellular survival and the generation of nutrients and energy. Nevertheless, recent research has indicated that extended periods of exposure to stress-inducing circumstances can also stimulate autophagy (specifically, planned type II autophagy), leading to cellular demise. Malfunctioning autoimmunity has been observed in a range of medical conditions, including infections, neuromuscular disorders, age-related disorders, Crohn's disease, cardiovascular diseases, and many forms of cancer [27]. The presence of autophagy in cells undergoing stress-induced death raises uncertainty regarding its role as a potential mechanism for cellular survival, such as self-digestion, or if it instead triggers cell death. Data exists supporting the presence of this phenomenon in several cell types. However, additional investigations are required to ascertain its specific role in cells exposed to radiation.

Antimicrobial agents, including ionizing radiation, are deliberately engineered to induce cell death in cancer cells. Nevertheless, many solid tumor cells exhibit deficiencies in their apoptotic mechanisms due to mutations in crucial regulatory proteins [28]. Consequently, these cells acquire resistance to apoptosis, rendering them less susceptible to cell death induced by chemotherapy and radiotherapy. Prior research has demonstrated that metabolic stress within human tumours induces a state of resistance to apoptosis in cancer cells while concurrently stimulating autophagy to sustain energy demands and prevent necrosis. Chemotherapy and radiotherapy have been observed to elicit autophagy, a process involving cellular self-degradation, as well as autophagy-mediated cell death. The precise mechanism underlying this particular type of cellular demise still needs to be completed and elucidated. However, the observed aggregation of cells in reaction to chemotherapy or radiation implies a plausible association with suppressing cellular proliferation and breakdown processes. The exploration of signalling pathways involved in the induction of radiation remains ongoing, with the potential involvement of signalling from the Endoplasmic Reticulum Kinase-like Protein Kinase (PERK) [29]. Therefore, the incorporation of autophagy as a novel target for anticancer therapy should be considered in managing cancer.

8.9. Senescence

Cellular senescence has been identified as a planned cellular stress response that serves as a distinctive reaction to the build-up of cellular damage [30]. The induction of senescence in primary cells can occur through various mechanisms, such as the shortening of telomeres due to frequent cell divisions, activation of oncogenes, or DNA damage caused by oxidative stress. This process leads to a permanent halt in the cell cycle, consistently marked by activating the p53 and retinoblastoma (Rb) proteins. Additionally, chromatin modifications occur, resulting in the suppression of genes that are crucial for facilitating the transition from the G1 to the S phase of the cell cycle. Senescence has been categorized as a tumour suppressor mechanism due to its ability to hinder excessive cellular divisions in response to improper growth signals or cell division that has accumulated DNA damage. The loss of senescence in response to DNA damage can be attributed to the genetic regulation of this process, which involves the p53 and Rb proteins [31]. It is reasonable to expect that the disruption of p53 and Rb control, caused by gene mutations, will lead to the loss of senescence.

Nevertheless, while tumour cells commonly experience a loss of their capacity to undergo senescence due to DNA damage resulting from mutations in the p53 and Rb pathways, normal cells retain this ability. In contrast, tumour cells retain their capacity to undergo senescence even in DNA damage due to mutations in the p53 and Rb signalling pathways. Acknowledging the induction of senescence in normal tissues is crucial, given that these cells retain metabolic activity while experiencing reproductive inhibition. For instance, fibroblasts in cell culture demonstrate prolonged attachment to plates over the course of weeks without undergoing division [32]. Nevertheless, these cells release growth factors, mitogens, and various other substances that facilitate the proliferation of tumour cells. Therefore, senescence results in an irreversible cessation of the cell cycle, although it does not eliminate the mitogenic and cytokine effects exerted by the halted cell, potentially facilitating the resurgence of tumour growth.

8.10. Survival Curves in Cell Culture

The surival curves have been determined for many well-established cell lines that have been grown in culture. The cell lines are derived from human or mammalian tissues (e.g., small rodents). In some cases, the parent tissue is neoplastic, while in others, it is normal [33, 34].

The first *in vitro* survival curve for mammalian cells irradiated with x-rays is shown in Figure 8.2.

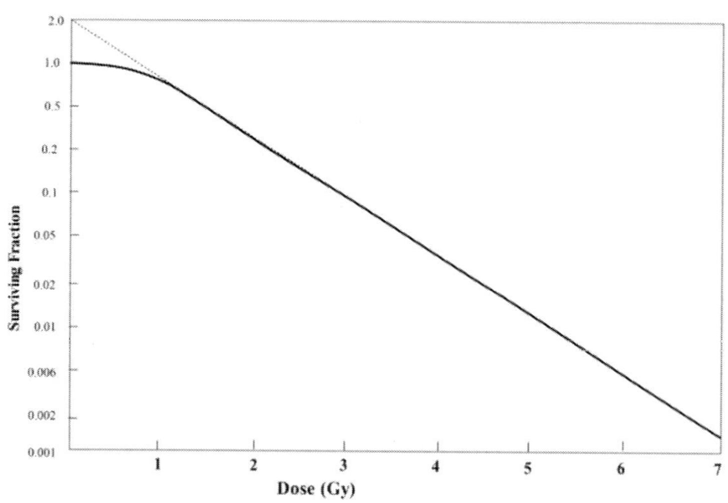

Figure 8.2. *In vitro* cell survival curve for mammalian cell.

An initial "shoulder" is followed by a "straight-line" portion on the log-log linear plot. The size of the "first" shoulder is highly variable. Some cell lines appear to have a continuous survival curve, resulting in a better fit between linear and quadratic relationships and n having no meaning. The D0 for the x-ray survival curves for most cell lines cultured *in vitro* is in the 1-2 Gy range. The exceptions are cells in patients with cancer risk syndromes, such as AT; these cells are susceptible to ionizing radiations, with an *in vitro* D0 for X-rays of approximately 0.5Gy. This sensitivity correlates to these patients' lack of radiotherapy sensitivity [35].

The initial *in vitro* survival curve was documented in 1956, generating enthusiasm in radiobiology [36]. Establishing a quantitative framework for assessing the relationship between absorbed dose and the survival rate of cells will enable significant progress in comprehending the impact of ionizing radiation on biological substances. Specifically, this study aims to make major advances to the existing body of knowledge regarding the practice of radiation. Nevertheless, this enthusiasm was limited. Certain experts expressed scepticism regarding the potential therapeutic applicability of *in vitro* methodologies, wherein cells are cultivated in a controlled environment within a petri dish that does not accurately replicate natural conditions, for radiotherapy.

According to David Gould, a professor of radiology at the University of Colorado, the appropriate answer suggests that the *in vitro* culture method assessed reproductive integrity [37]. It is reasonable to assume that Robinson's reproductive integrity on the desert island would not have differed from that in York. The sole distinction lies in the fact that, if Robinson had been cultured in a petri dish with optimal temperature and humidity regulation and abundant nutrients, he would have had the opportunity to reproduce to the best of his abilities. During that period, it was necessary to possess a certain level of faith and optimism to accept the extrapolation of survival curves determined through *in vitro* methods to the intricate *in vivo* scenario. Nevertheless, this faith and optimism were entirely shattered when *in vivo* cell survival techniques were introduced, revealing that the parameters for dose-response relationships were comparable to those observed *in vitro* [38].

8.11. Survival Curve Shape and Mechanisms of Cell Death

A notable variation exists in the vulnerability of mitotic cells derived from several mammalian cell lines cultivated *in vitro*, when subjected to radiation-induced cell death. The mammalian cell line known as asynchronous EMT6 has the highest degree of radioresistance, followed by the Glioblastoma cell line of human origin [39]. Subsequently, the radiosensitivity progressively increases, with two neuroblastoma cell lines identified as the most susceptible among the tested cell lines. The sensitivity to radiation varies significantly across asynchronous cells. However, it is noteworthy that mitotic cells from various mammalian cell lines have a consistent amount of sensitivity to radiation. Hence, it can be observed that when chromosomes undergo condensation in the process of mitosis, all mammalian cell lines demonstrate equivalent levels of radiosensitivity, primarily determined by the DNA content [40]. However, during interphase, radiosensitivity varies due to distinct DNA conformations.

Characteristic laddering indicates programmed cell death, also known as apoptosis, when the DNA undergoes fragmentation into distinct lengths, as previously elucidated. Cell lines that exhibit high sensitivity to radiation, as indicated by broad shoulders on their survival curves, do not exhibit any indications of apoptosis. Conversely, highly radiosensitive cells and demonstrate survival as an exponential function of radiation dose exhibit distinct DNA laddering [41]. The intensity of this DNA laddering is directly correlated with increasing radiosensitivity, as evidenced by the diminishing size of the shoulders on the survival curve. Most well-established cell lines, which have been extensively utilized *in vitro* to establish fundamental principles of radiation biology over an extended period, do not exhibit apoptotic death or demonstrate any impairment of p53 function. Prolonged cultivation *in vitro* frequently leads to the preferential survival and proliferation of cells possessing this particular property. Mitotic death primarily occurs due to chromosome abnormalities, particularly those of the exchange type [42]. Consequently, the cell survival curve exhibits a log-linear pattern with a wide initial shoulder, indicating a notable dose-rate effect.

The underlying mechanisms responsible for apoptotic death remain incompletely elucidated. However, it is seen that the corresponding cell survival curve exhibits a linear log-linear pattern, indicating that an exponential relationship concerning dosage governs survival. Moreover, dosage's impact seems minimal or inconsequential, but with limited available data. Cell lines can exhibit varying amounts of mitotic death and apoptosis. While certain cell lines mostly undergo mitotic death, and others primarily undergo apoptosis, most cell lines lie somewhere in between [43]. These cell lines experience a combination of mitotic and post-exposure apoptotic death, with the relative contributions of each varying. There has been a proposal to characterize the dose-response connection in the following manner:

$$S = e^{-(\alpha_M D+\beta_M D^2+\alpha_A D)}$$

In which S is the fraction of cells surviving a dose D, αM and αA describe the contributions to cell killing from mitotic and apoptotic death that are linear functions of dose, and βM describes the contribution to mitotic death that varies with the square of the dose [44].

8.12. Genetic Control of Radiosensitivity

Extensive research has been conducted on the molecular biology of repair mechanisms in lower organisms such as yeast and bacteria. In certain instances, a very radiosensitive mutation can be attributed to a mutation in a single gene that functions as a repair or checkpoint gene [45]. Nevertheless, in mammalian cells, evidence suggests that numerous genes may contribute to regulating radiosensitivity. Additionally, laboratory cell lines have identified several mutations associated with increased radiosensitivity, particularly those derived from rodents. In numerous instances, although not universally applicable, the vulnerability of cells to radiation-induced cell death is associated with their limited capacity to effectively repair DNA double-strand breaks (DSBs). As an illustration, the DNA-dependent Kinase activity is influenced by two genes, namely Ku 80 and Ku 70 [46]. The two genes in question exhibit binding affinity towards the unattached terminus of a DNA double-strand break (DSB), potentially influencing the repair process of DSBs if they are malfunctioning. In mice exhibiting severe combined immune dysfunction syndrome, a third gene is responsible for encoding a malfunctioning protein that displays sensitivity to radiation.

Individuals who display an abnormally intense normal tissue reaction to radiation therapy share certain traits reminiscent of specific hereditary conditions. One prominent illustration is the medical condition known as Ataxia-telangiectasia (AT). Individuals diagnosed with this particular syndrome exhibit fibroblasts that display a heightened sensitivity to radiation, about two to three times more than those found in individuals without the disease [47]. Patients diagnosed with ataxia telangiectasia (AT) who undergo radiation therapy exhibit notable adverse effects on normal tissue integrity if the administered dosages are not suitably decreased. Individuals diagnosed with ataxia-telangiectasia (AT) exhibit an elevated susceptibility to the development of malignancies. Cells derived from heterozygous individuals for the AT gene have a somewhat heightened sensitivity compared to cells from individuals with the normal genotype. There exists a certain degree of controversy on whether individuals with AT-tumour-related heterozygosity possess a susceptibility to developing cancer.

The gene associated with Ataxia-Telangiectasia has undergone characterization and sequencing and is commonly known as the ATM (Ataxia-Telangiectasia Mutated) gene [48]. The ATM protein is hypothesized to participate in signal transduction pathways that have a role in numerous physiological functions. Nevertheless, the precise mechanism through which the genetic mutation in AT cells leads to increased susceptibility to radiation remains uncertain.

In order to conduct individual tumour radiosensitivity experiments, it is important to cultivate cells derived from recently obtained human tumour samples. The growth of these cells in conventional clonogen assays is comparatively inferior to that of the connected cells. However, enhanced outcomes can be achieved by utilizing the Courtenay assay, wherein cells are cultivated within a semi-solid agar gel supplemented with growth agents. Numerous nonclonogenic tests have also been devised, utilizing cell proliferation in a multiwell plate [49]. The quantification of cell growth is determined through the cells' capacity to decrease the visibility of a substance via staining or by assessing the overall DNA/RNA content within the multwell plate. The endpoints above serve as surrogate indicators for clonogenicity and reproductive integrity.

The phenomenon of cell radiosensitivity altering during the process of cellular differentiation is generally acknowledged in the scientific community [50]. In the hypothetical scenario presented, cell death in tumours exposed to ionizing radiation would be linked to the depletion of tumour stem cells. In contrast, the relatively differentiated tumour cells that have forfeited their capacity for regeneration would exhibit higher chances of survival. However, the findings presented in recent literature do not align with this assertion. Indeed, there is the possibility that cancer stem cells exhibit a higher degree of sensitivity towards ionizing radiation than their more differentiated counterparts. The underlying mechanism can be attributed to the possibility that cancer stem cells exhibit reduced levels of reactive oxygen species due to heightened amounts of free radicals. If this hypothesis is correct, it can be inferred that the heightened quantities of free radicals shield cancer stem cells from the metabolic effects of reactive oxygen species during growth and provide protection against the harmful effects of ionizing radiation [51]. The radiosensitivity of cancer stem cells can be enhanced by pretreating them with free radical inhibitors before radiation exposure.

The phenomenon of cell radiosensitivity altering during the process of cellular differentiation is generally acknowledged in the scientific community. In the hypothetical scenario presented, cell death in tumours exposed to ionizing radiation would be linked to the depletion of tumour stem cells. In contrast, the relatively differentiated tumour cells that have forfeited their capacity for regeneration would exhibit higher chances of survival [52]. However, the findings presented in recent literature do not align with this assertion. Indeed, there is the possibility that cancer stem cells exhibit a higher degree of sensitivity towards ionizing radiation than their more differentiated counterparts. The underlying mechanism can be attributed to the possibility that cancer stem cells exhibit reduced levels of reactive oxygen species due to heightened amounts of free radicals. If this hypothesis is correct, it can be inferred that the heightened quantities of free radicals shield cancer stem cells from the metabolic effects of reactive oxygen species during growth and provide protection against the harmful effects of ionizing radiation. The radiosensitivity of cancer stem cells can be enhanced by pre-treating them with free radical inhibitors before radiation exposure.

Conclusion

This chapter provided an in-depth examination of how ionizing radiation affects cell survival, highlighting the concept of reproductive integrity as a critical measure of cellular viability. It explored the development and interpretation of cell survival curves, including the multi-target and linear-quadratic models that describe the relationship between radiation dose and the fraction of surviving cells. The chapter detailed various mechanisms of radiation-induced cell death, such as mitotic death, apoptosis, autophagy, and senescence, emphasizing their dependence on cellular context and genetic factors. The bystander effect was also discussed, illustrating how unirradiated cells can be indirectly affected by signals from irradiated neighbors. By integrating knowledge of these processes, radiobiology informs the optimization of radiotherapy and enhances our understanding of radiosensitivity, ultimately contributing to more effective and targeted cancer treatments.

References

[1] Smith SK, Abel MH, Kelly RW, Baird DT. The synthesis of prostaglandins from persistent proliferative endometrium. *The Journal of Clinical Endocrinology & Metabolism*. 1982 Aug 1;55(2):284-9.

[2] Munshi A, Hobbs M, Meyn RE. *Clonogenic cell survival assay. Chemosensitivity: Volume 1 In Vitro Assays*. 2005:21-8.

[3] Erenpreisa J, Cragg MS. Mitotic death: a mechanism of survival? A review. *Cancer cell international*. 2001 Dec;1:1-7.

[4] Pusztai L, Lewis CE, Lorenzen J, McGee JO. Growth factors: regulation of normal and neoplastic growth. *The Journal of pathology*. 1993 Feb;169(2):191-201.

[5] Garry DJ, Olson EN. A common progenitor at the heart of development. *Cell*. 2006 Dec 15;127(6):1101-4.

[6] Sinclair WK. The shape of radiation survival curves of mammalian cells cultured *in vitro*. *Biophysical aspects of radiation quality*. 1966 Jul 1:21-43.

[7] Kraft G. Radiobiological effects of highly charged ions. *The Physics of Multiply and Highly Charged Ions*. 2003 Sep 30:149-96.

[8] Deacon J, Peckham MJ, Steel GG. The radioresponsiveness of human tumours and the initial slope ofthe cell survival curve. *Radiotherapy and Oncology*. 1984 Dec 1;2(4):317-23.

[9] Scheim D. *Ivermectin for COVID-19 treatment: clinical response at quasi-threshold doses via hypothesized alleviation of CD147-mediated vascular occlusion*. Available at SSRN 3636557. 2020 Jun 26.

[10] Goodhead DT, Thacker J, Cox R. Effects of radiations of different qualities on cells: molecular mechanisms of damage and repair. *International journal of radiation biology*. 1993 Jan 1;63(5):543-56.

[11] Bender MA. Somatic chromosomal aberrations: Use in the evaluation of human radiation exposures. *Archives of Environmental Health: An International Journal*. 1968 Apr 1;16(4):556-64.

[12] Nunes MD, Nunes MD. Modelling Heavy Ion Radiation Effects. *Protontherapy Versus Carbon Ion Therapy: Advantages, Disadvantages and Similarities*. 2015:69-76.

[13] Baserga R, Lisco H, Kisieleski WE. Tumor induction in mice by radioactive thymidine. *Radiation Research*. 1966 Dec 1;29(4):583-96.

[14] Jiao Y, WANG HC, FAN SJ. Growth suppression and radiosensitivity increase by HMGB1 in breast cancer 1. *Acta Pharmacologica Sinica*. 2007 Dec;28(12):1957-67.

[15] Marín A, Martín M, Liñán O, Alvarenga F, López M, Fernández L, Büchser D, Cerezo L. Bystander effects and radiotherapy. *Reports of practical oncology and radiotherapy*. 2015;20(1):12-21.

[16] Prise KM. Studies of bystander effects in human fibroblasts using a charged particle microbeam. *International journal of radiation biology*. 1998 Jan 1;74(6):793-8.

[17] Hall EJ. *The bystander effect. Health physics*. 2003 Jul 1;85(1):31-5.

[18] Nuta O. *The influence of telomerase on induction and repair of targeted and non-targeted radiation effects*.

[19] Serres M. *The incandescent*. Bloomsbury Publishing; 2018 Jul 26.

[20] Xu X, Lai Y, Hua ZC. Apoptosis and apoptotic body: disease message and therapeutic target potentials. *Bioscience reports*. 2019 Jan;39(1):BSR20180992.

[21] Schipler A, Iliakis G. DNA double-strand–break complexity levels and their possible contributions to the probability for error-prone processing and repair pathway choice. *Nucleic acids research*. 2013 Sep 1;41(16):7589-605.

[22] Jiao Y, Cao F, Liu H. Radiation-induced cell death and its mechanisms. *Health Physics*. 2022 Nov 1;123(5):376-86.

[23] Brown JM, Wouters BG. Apoptosis, p53, and tumor cell sensitivity to anticancer agents. *Cancer research*. 1999 Apr 1;59(7):1391-9.

[24] Failla G. *The aging process and cancerogenesis*.

[25] Yin X, Zhou C, Li J, Liu R, Shi B, Yuan Q, Zou S. Autophagy in bone homeostasis and the onset of osteoporosis. *Bone research*. 2019 Oct 3;7(1):28.

[26] Noda T, Suzuki K, Ohsumi Y. Yeast autophagosomes: de novo formation of a membrane structure. *Trends in cell biology*. 2002 May 1;12(5):231-5.

[27] Wen X, Yang Y, Klionsky DJ. Moments in autophagy and disease: Past and present. *Molecular Aspects of Medicine*. 2021 Dec 1;82:100966.

[28] Fogal V, Richardson AD, Karmali PP, Scheffler IE, Smith JW, Ruoslahti E. Mitochondrial p32 protein is a critical regulator of tumor metabolism via maintenance of oxidative phosphorylation. *Molecular and cellular biology*. 2010 Mar 1;30(6):1303-18.

[29] Fogal V, Richardson AD, Karmali PP, Scheffler IE, Smith JW, Ruoslahti E. Mitochondrial p32 protein is a critical regulator of tumor metabolism via maintenance of oxidative phosphorylation. *Molecular and cellular biology*. 2010 Mar 1;30(6):1303-18.

[30] Baraibar MA, Ladouce R, Friguet B. Proteomic quantification and identification of carbonylated proteins upon oxidative stress and during cellular aging. *Journal of proteomics*. 2013 Oct 30;92:63-70.

[31] Rayess H, Wang MB, Srivatsan ES. Cellular senescence and tumor suppressor gene p16. *International journal of cancer*. 2012 Apr 15;130(8):1715-25.
[32] Reynolds BA, Weiss S. Clonal and population analyses demonstrate that an EGF-responsive mammalian embryonic CNS precursor is a stem cell. *Developmental biology*. 1996 Apr 10;175(1):1-3.
[33] Pickard MR, Mourtada-Maarabouni M, Williams GT. Long non-coding RNA GAS5 regulates apoptosis in prostate cancer cell lines. *Biochimica et Biophysica Acta (BBA)-Molecular Basis of Disease*. 2013 Oct 1;1832(10):1613-23.
[34] Gown AM, Vogel AM. Monoclonal antibodies to human intermediate filament proteins. II. Distribution of filament proteins in normal human tissues. *The American journal of pathology*. 1984 Feb;114(2):309.
[35] Morgan WF. Non-targeted and delayed effects of exposure to ionizing radiation: II. Radiation-induced genomic instability and bystander effects *in vivo*, clastogenic factors and transgenerational effects. *Radiation research*. 2003 May 1;159(5):581-96.
[36] Hall EJ. Radiation and the single cell: the physicist's contribution to radiobiology. *Physics in Medicine and Biology*. 1976 May 1;21(3):347-59.
[37] Hall EJ. The Janeway Lecture 1992. Nine decades of radiobiology: is radiation therapy any the better for it?. *Cancer*. 1993 Jun 1;71(11):3753-66.
[38] Olds WJ, McKinley AR, Moore MR, Kimlin MG. *In vitro* model of vitamin D3 (cholecalciferol) synthesis by UV radiation: dose–response relationships. *Journal of Photochemistry and Photobiology B: Biology*. 2008 Nov 13;93(2):88-93.
[39] Khaitan D, Chandna S, Arya MB, Dwarakanath BS. Establishment and characterization of multicellular spheroids from a human glioma cell line; Implications for tumor therapy. Journal of translational medicine. 2006 Jun;4:1-3.
[40] Rothkamm K, Krüger I, Thompson LH, Lübrich M. Pathways of DNA double-strand break repair during the mammalian cell cycle. *Molecular and cellular biology*. 2003 Aug 1;23(16):5706-15.
[41] Xu H, Balakrishnan K, Malaterre J, Beasley M, Yan Y, Essers J, Appeldoorn E, Thomaszewski JM, Vazquez M, Verschoor S, Lavin MF. Rad21-cohesin haploinsufficiency impedes DNA repair and enhances gastrointestinal radiosensitivity in mice. *PloS one*. 2010 Aug 12;5(8):e12112.
[42] Bedford JS. Sublethal damage, potentially lethal damage, and chromosomal aberrations in mammalian cells exposed to ionizing radiations. *International Journal of Radiation Oncology* Biology* Physics*. 1991 Nov 1;21(6):1457-69.
[43] Dewey WC, Ling CC, Meyn RE. Radiation-induced apoptosis: relevance to radiotherapy. *International Journal of Radiation Oncology* Biology* Physics*. 1995 Nov 1;33(4):781-96.
[44] Conte M, Dzierma Y, Knobe S, Surulescu C. Mathematical modeling of glioma invasion and therapy approaches. *arXiv preprint arXiv*:2203.11578. 2022 Mar 22.
[45] Taylor AM, Lam Z, Last JI, Byrd PJ. Ataxia telangiectasia: more variation at clinical and cellular levels. *Clinical genetics*. 2015 Mar;87(3):199-208.
[46] Jin S, Weaver DT. Double-strand break repair by Ku70 requires heterodimerization with Ku80 and DNA binding functions. *The EMBO journal*. 1997 Nov 15;16(22):6874-85.
[47] Paterson MC, Sell BM, Smith BP, Bech-Hansen NT. Impaired colony-forming ability following γ irradiation of skin fibroblasts from tuberous sclerosis patients. *Radiation Research*. 1982 May 1;90(2):260-70.
[48] Platzer M, Rotman G, Bauer D, Uziel T, Savitsky K, Bar-Shira A, Gilad S, Shiloh Y, Rosenthal A. Ataxia-telangiectasia locus: sequence analysis of 184 kb of human genomic DNA containing the entire ATM gene. *Genome research*. 1997 Jun 1;7(6):592-605.
[49] Lecault V, VanInsberghe M, Sekulovic S, Knapp DJ, Wohrer S, Bowden W, Viel F, McLaughlin T, Jarandehei A, Miller M, Falconnet D. High-throughput analysis of single hematopoietic stem cell proliferation in microfluidic cell culture arrays. *Nature methods*. 2011 Jul;8(7):581-6.
[50] Olive PL. The role of DNA single-and double-strand breaks in cell killing by ionizing radiation. *Radiation research*. 1998 Nov 1;150(5s):S42-51.
[51] Grieve S, Biswas D. Targeting reactive oxygen species homeostasis and metabolism in cancer stem cells. InHandbook of oxidative stress in cancer: *Mechanistic aspects* 2022 Jan 31 (pp. 2385-2405). Singapore: Springer Nature Singapore.

[52] Frey B, Rubner Y, Wunderlich R, Weiss EM, G Pockley A, Fietkau R, S Gaipl U. Induction of abscopal anti-tumor immunity and immunogenic tumor cell death by ionizing irradiation-implications for cancer therapies. *Current medicinal chemistry*. 2012 Apr 1;19(12):1751-64.

Chapter 9

Pathophysiology of Radiobiology in Normal Cells and Tissues and Normal Tissue Toxicity

Ashish Uke[1,*], MD
Umang Jajoo[2], MD
Jaishriram Rathored[3], PhD
and Gautam Kumar Sharan[4], MD
[1]Department of Radiation Oncology, Datta Meghe Institute of Higher Education and Research, Wardha, India
[2]Department of Radio-diagnosis, Datta Meghe Institute of Higher Education and Research, Wardha, India
[3]Department of Molecular Diagnostics, Datta Meghe Institute of Higher Education and Research, Wardha, India
[4]Department of Radiotherapy, Jawaharlal Nehru Cancer Hospital and Research Centre, Bhopal, India

Abstract

The cell is the smallest unit of life, and it is the structural and operational unit of a living thing. Cells have various characteristics, including the need for nutrition and oxygen, the production of energy, and the elimination of waste products. The cell membrane, cytoplasm, and nucleus are the three main components of a cell. The cell membrane is a semipermeable membrane that regulates the movement of substances in and out of the cell. The cytoplasm is a jelly-like substance that makes up 80% of a cell's volume, and it contains various organelles, including the endoplasmic reticulum, Golgi apparatus, lysosomes, and mitochondria. The nucleus is the control center of the cell, and it contains the genetic material in the form of DNA.

Cells can adapt to changes in their environment through various mechanisms, including atrophy, hypertrophy, hyperplasia, dysplasia, and metaplasia. Cell death can occur through two distinct processes: apoptosis and necrosis. Apoptosis is a genetically controlled process of cell death, while necrosis is an uncontrolled process of cell death caused by external factors.

Radiation dermatitis is a common side effect of radiation therapy, and it can cause skin reactions, including erythema, dry desquamation, and moist desquamation. The severity of radiation dermatitis depends on various factors, including the dose of radiation, the size of the treatment field, and the individual's skin type. Prevention and management of

* Corresponding Author's Email: ashishuke1@gmail.com

In: Fundamentals of Radiation Biology
Editors: Anurag Luharia, Ashish Uke, Gaurav Mishra et al.
ISBN: 979-8-89530-806-6

radiation dermatitis include the use of topical corticosteroids, moisturizers, and dressings, as well as the avoidance of skin irritants and extreme temperatures.

Keywords: apoptosis, cell adaptation, necrosis, radiation dermatitis, skin toxicity

9.1. Introduction

The human body is composed of trillions of cells, each with unique characteristics and functions. The cell is the smallest unit of life, and it is the structural and operational unit of a living thing. Cells are the building blocks of tissues, and tissues are the building blocks of organs. Understanding the structure and function of cells is essential to understanding the human body and its various systems. Cells are incredibly diverse, with different types of cells performing different functions. For example, muscle cells are responsible for movement, nerve cells are responsible for transmitting signals, and epithelial cells form the lining of organs and glands. Despite their diversity, all cells share certain characteristics, such as the need for nutrition and oxygen, the ability to produce energy, and the ability to respond to stimuli. The cell membrane is a critical component of the cell, separating the cell from its environment and regulating the movement of materials in and out of the cell. The cell membrane is composed of lipids, proteins, and carbohydrates, and it is semi-permeable, allowing certain substances to pass through while keeping others out. Inside the cell, there are various organelles, each with its own unique function. The nucleus is the control center of the cell, containing the genetic material that determines the cell's characteristics and functions. The mitochondria are the powerhouses of the cell, generating energy through the process of cellular respiration. The endoplasmic reticulum is involved in protein synthesis and transport, while the Golgi apparatus is responsible for processing and packaging proteins and lipids for transport out of the cell.

Radiation dermatitis is a common side effect of radiation therapy, and it can have a significant impact on a patient's quality of life. Radiation dermatitis is characterized by skin changes, including erythema, dry desquamation, and moist desquamation, which can lead to skin necrosis or ulceration. The severity of radiation dermatitis can vary depending on the dose and duration of radiation therapy, as well as individual patient factors. Prevention and management of radiation dermatitis are crucial to minimizing its impact on patients. Topical steroids, such as mometasone furoate and hydrocortisone, have been shown to be effective in reducing the severity of radiation dermatitis. Other protective options, such as intensity-modulated radiation therapy (IMRT), low-level laser therapy, and amifostine, have also been studied for their potential to prevent and manage radiation dermatitis. In addition to these treatments, patients can take steps to care for their skin during radiation therapy. This includes gently washing the skin with mild soap and water, applying a water-based moisturizer, and avoiding skin irritants. Patients should also be advised to avoid temperature extremes, refrain from being in the sun, and wear sunscreen with at least SPF 30.

9.2. The Cell

The smallest unit that includes all the characteristics of life is the cell. The structural and operational unit of a living thing is referred to as a cell.

General characteristics of each cell in the body:

- Needs nutrition and oxygen
- Produces its own energy necessary for its growth, repair and other activities
- Eliminates carbon dioxide and other metabolic wastes
- Maintains the medium, i.e., the environment for its survival
- Shows immediate response to the entry of invaders like bacteria or toxic substances into the body
- Reproduces by division. There are some exceptions like neuron, which do not reproduce [1].

9.2.1. Tissue

The definition of a tissue is a collection of cells with a common purpose. There are four major categories of tissues, referred to as the primary tissues. The primary tissues include:

- Muscle tissue (skeletal muscle, smooth muscle and cardiac muscle)
- Nervous tissue (neurons and supporting cells)
- Epithelial tissue (squamous, columnar and cuboidal epithelial cells)
- Connective tissue (connective tissue proper, cartilage, bone and blood) [2].

9.2.2. Structure of the Cell

A cell body and the membrane cover the cell body, known as the cell membrane, make up each individual cell. The nucleus and the cytoplasm that surrounds it make up the two components of the cell body. As a result, three categories are used to study the structure of a cell:

1. Cell membrane
2. Cytoplasm
3. Nucleus.

9.2.3. Cell Membrane

A protective sheath that encloses the cell body is the cell membrane. Other names for it include plasma membrane and plasmalemma. This membrane divides the intracellular fluid (ICF) from the extracellular fluid (ECF) that surrounds each individual cell. Semipermeable membranes make up cell membranes. Consequently, certain substances can be exchanged freely between ECF and ICF [3].

- **Composition of Cell Membrane**

Cell membrane is composed of three types of substances:

- Proteins (55%)
- Lipids (40%)
- Carbohydrates (5%).

1. Structure of Cell Membrane

The term "unit membrane" or "three-layered membrane" refers to the structure of the cell membrane. The cell membrane is found to be composed of three layers: one central layer that is electron-lucent and two outer layers that are electron-dense. The central layer is surrounded by one each of the two electron-dense layers. Lipid compounds form the lipid layer that makes up the central layer. The two additional layers are made up of layers of proteins [4]. Carbohydrate molecules are also present in the cell membrane.

2. Functions of Cell Membrane

- The cytoplasm and its organelles are shielded by the cell membrane.
- The cell membrane functions to be a semipermeable membrane that serves as a barrier for some substances and as a conduit for others.
- The cell membrane allows nutrients to enter the cell.
- Through the cell membrane, metabolites as well as other waste products inside the cell is excreted.
- The cell receives oxygen from the blood, and carbon dioxide exits the cell and passes through the blood via the cell membrane.
- The maintenance of the cell's size and shape is handled by the cell membrane.

9.2.4. Cytoplasm

The jelly-like substance that makes up 80% of a cell's cytoplasm is water [5]. In addition to various particles of various sizes and shapes, it also consists of a clear liquid component called cytosol. These specks are naturally occurring electrolytes, proteins, carbohydrates, or lipids. There are numerous organelles with unique structures and functions in cytoplasm as well.

Cytoplasm is divided into two zones:

- Ectoplasm: located just below the cell membrane, the periphery of the cytoplasm
- Endoplasm: The inner portion of cytoplasm, interposed in between ectoplasm and the cell's nucleus.

- **Organelles in Cytoplasm**

The cellular components that are enmeshed in the cytoplasm are called cytoplasmic organelles. Small organs of a cell are referred to as organelles. There are some organelles that are bound by a limiting membrane whereas there are others that do not. Each organelle has a distinct structure and serves a specific purpose.

9.2.5. Endoplasmic Reticulum

The endoplasmic reticulum is an interconnected network of tubular and microsomal vesicular structures. A limiting membrane that is made of proteins and bilayered lipids covers it. Endoplasmic matrix is a fluid medium that is present in the endoplasmic reticulum lumen [6]. The lumen's diameter ranges from 400 to 700. The endoplasmic reticulum joins the nuclear membrane to the cell membrane to create the connection between the nucleus and cell membrane.

- *Types of Endoplasmic Reticulum:* There are two types of endoplasmic reticulum smooth endoplasmic reticulum and rough endoplasmic reticulum. Both types are connected to and continue one another. Rough endoplasmic reticulum transforms into smooth endoplasmic reticulum, and vice versa, depending on the activities of the cells.

1. Rough Endoplasmic Reticulum: Endoplasmic reticulum is what has the bumpy, rough, or bead-like appearance. The presence of granular ribosomes on its outer surface accounts for its rough appearance. It is also known as the granular endoplasmic reticulum because of this. Structure-wise, the rough endoplasmic reticulum is the vesicular or tubular [7].

- **Functions of Rough Endoplasmic Reticulum**

- *Synthesis of proteins*
  The synthesis of proteins within the cell is a concern of the rough endoplasmic reticulum. The amino acids are organised by ribosomes into tiny protein building blocks before being transported through the rough endoplasmic reticulum. Here, the protein building blocks are combined with the carbohydrates to create glycosylated proteins, also known as glycoproteins, which are organised in the shape of reticular vesicles [8]. These vesicles are primarily transported to the Golgi apparatus for additional processing and modification.
- *Degradation of worn-out organelles*
  The worn-out organelles are encircled by rough endoplasmic reticulum, which then forms a vacuole that is frequently referred to as the autophagosome. Lysosomal enzymes break down autophagosomes.

2. Smooth Endoplasmic Reticulum

It has the smooth appearance of the endoplasmic reticulum. The agranular reticulum is another name for it. It is made up of numerous connected tubules. The tubular endoplasmic reticulum is another name for it [9].

- **Functions of Smooth Endoplasmic Reticulum**

- *The synthesis for non-protein substance*
  The smooth endoplasmic reticulum is in charge of producing non-protein compounds like cholesterol and steroids. Cells which play a role in the synthesis of lipids, phospholipids, lipoprotein substances, steroid hormones, sebum, etc. have a lot of this type of endoplasmic reticulum. The smooth endoplasmic reticulum has less prevalent rather than the rough endoplasmic reticulum in the majority of the other cells.
- *Function in cellular metabolism*
  There are numerous enzymes on the smooth endoplasmic reticulum's outer surface that are involved in the cell's various metabolic processes.
- *Storage and metabolism of the calcium*
  The main location for calcium storage and metabolism is the smooth endoplasmic reticulum. It causes the release of calcium in skeletal muscle fibres, which is essential for inducing muscle contraction.
- *Catabolism and detoxifying*
  The liver's smooth endoplasmic reticulum also participates in the catabolism and detoxification of harmful substances, including some drugs and carcinogens (substances that cause cancer).

9.2.6. Golgi Apparatus

Golgi apparatus is an organelle bound to the membrane, involved in the processing of proteins. All cells, with the exception of red blood cells, contain it. It bears Camillo Golgi's name, the discoverer. Typically, there is one Golgi apparatus per cell. There could be multiple Golgi apparatuses present in some of the cells. The cisternae, or five to eight flattened membranous sacs, make up each Golgi apparatus. The Golgi apparatus is found close to the nucleus [10]. The cis face and the trans face are its two ends or faces. The endoplasmic reticulum is situated not far from the cis face. Through the cis face, reticular vesicles from the endoplasmic reticulum enter the Golgi apparatus. Around the cell membrane is where you'll find the trans face. Through the trans face, the processed materials leave the Golgi apparatus.

- **Functions of Golgi Apparatus**

- *Processing of materials:*
  Vesicles containing lipids and glycoproteins are transported into the Golgi apparatus. Here, lipids and glycoproteins are altered and processed.

- *Packaging of materials:*
  Secretory granules, secretory vesicles and lysosomes, that are transported either outside the cell or to another area inside the cell, are used to pack all the processed materials. The Golgi apparatus is referred to as the "post office of the cell" as a result.
- *Labelling and delivery of materials:*
  The Golgi apparatus finally separates the processed and packaged materials into groups according to their chemical composition before labelling them (for example, phosphate group) and distributing them to the correct locations. The Golgi apparatus is referred to as the "shipping department of the cell" as a result [11].

9.2.7. Lysosomes

The membrane-bound vesicular organelles known as lysosomes are present throughout the cytoplasm. The Golgi apparatus creates the lysosomes. The Golgi apparatus processes and stores the enzymes created in the rough endoplasmic reticulum in the form of tiny vesicles. The lysosomes are the cytoplasmic organelles with the thickest membranes. Lipid bilayers are what make up the membrane [12].

There are two types of lysosomes:

1. A primary lysosome that is severed from the Golgi apparatus. Despite having hydrolytic enzymes, it is inactive.
2. The active lysosome, or secondary lysosome. A primary lysosome and a phagosome or endosome fuse to form it.

- **Functions of Lysosomes**

Two mechanisms are involved in lysosomal functions:

- Heterophagy: The breakdown of extracellular substances that cells endocytose.
- Autophagy: The breakdown of cytoplasmic organelles that have lost their functionality.

Specific lysosome functions:

- Macromolecule degradation: The cell engulfs macromolecules through endocytosis. Phagosomes or vacuoles are the names for the macromolecules, such as bacteria, that are engulfed by the cell during phagocytosis.
- Organelle degradation from worn-out state
- Elimination of extra secretory products from cells
- Secretory lysosomes have a secretory function.

9.2.8. Peroxisomes

Like lysosomes, peroxisomes as well as microbodies are membrane-restricted vesicles. Peroxisomes, unlike lysosomes, are detached from endoplasmic reticulum rather than the Golgi apparatus. Some oxidative enzymes, including catalase, urate oxidase, and D-amino acid oxidase, are found in peroxisomes.

- **Functions of Peroxisomes:**

1. Degrade the fatty acids using beta-oxidation
2. Through detoxification, degrade harmful substances like hydrogen peroxide as well as other metabolic byproducts.
3. Function as the primary site of oxygen uptake in cells
4. Accelerate the production of glucose from fats.
5. Purine degradation to uric acid
6. Contribute to the production of myelin
7. Contribute to the production of bile acids.

9.2.9. Centrosome and Centrioles

The centrosome is a membrane-bound cellular organelle located close to the cell's nucleus. It is composed of two protein-based centrioles, which are cylinder-shaped structures. During cell division, chromosome movement is controlled by centrioles [13].

9.2.10. Secretory Vesicles

Organelles with a limiting membrane that house secretory materials are known as secretory vesicles. The endoplasmic reticulum produces these vesicles, which are then processed and packaged in the Golgi apparatus. There are secretory vesicles all over the cytoplasm. These vesicles can be ruptured when necessary, releasing secretions into the cytoplasm.

9.2.11. Mitochondrion

An organelle in the cytoplasm that is membrane-bound and involved in energy production is called a mitochondrion (plural = mitochondria). It has an oval or rod-shaped shape and a diameter of 0.50 to 1. It has a bilayer membrane covering it. The mitochondrion's contents are enclosed by a smooth outer membrane. Several enzymes, including glycerophosphate acetyltransferase and acetyl-CoA synthetase, are present in this membrane. The inner membrane covers the inner matrix space and is folded into cristae, which are shelf-like inward projections [14]. Numerous enzymes and other protein molecules that are essential for respiration and ATP synthesis can be found in cristae.

- **Functions of Mitochondrion**

- *Production of energy*
  The mitochondria, also known as the "powerhouse" or "power plant," produces the energy needed for cellular activities. The oxidising enzymes in the cristae produce the energy while digested food components like proteins, carbohydrates, and lipids are being oxidised. Water and carbon dioxide are produced along with the release of energy during the oxidative process. The energy that is released is stored in the mitochondria and used to create ATP later.
- *ATP synthesis*
  The respiratory chain in the mitochondrion uses oxidative phosphorylation to generate energy, which is used to synthesise ATP. From the mitochondrion, ATP molecules spread throughout the entire cell [15]. The ATP molecules are disassembled whenever cellular activity requires energy.
- *Apoptosis*
  Apoptosis occurs by cytochrome C and the second mitochondria-derived activator of caspases (SMAC)/diablo secreted by mitochondria.

Additional liver functions include calcium storage and ammonia detoxification.

- **Organelles without Limiting Membrane**

- *Ribosomes*
  The membranous organelles without restrictions are ribosomes. These organelles have a 15 nm diameter and resemble small, granular dots. 35% of the proteins along with 65% of the ribonucleic acid (RNA) in ribosomes. Ribosomal RNA (rRNA) refers to the RNA found in ribosomes. The synthesis of proteins within the cell is a concern for ribosomes.

Ribosome Subtypes

There are two types of ribosomes:

- Ribosomes connected to the rough endoplasmic reticulum
- Distributed free ribosomes in the cytoplasm.

- **Functions of Ribosomes**

Ribosomes are referred to as 'protein factories' because of their role in protein synthesis. From the nucleus to the ribosomes, messenger RNA (mRNA) transports the genetic instructions for protein synthesis. The amino acids are then organised by the ribosomes into tiny protein building blocks [16].

Rough endoplasmic reticulum-attached ribosomes play an important role in the synthesis of a variety of proteins, including those needed for enzyme activity, hormone production, lysosomal function, and cell membrane proteins.

The synthesis of proteins in haemoglobin, peroxisomes, and mitochondria is carried out by free ribosomes.

9.3. Cytoskeleton

The cytoskeleton is a cellular organelle found throughout the cytoplasm. It establishes the cell's shape and provides stability. Additionally, it is necessary for cellular motion and the way a cell reacts to outside stimuli [17].

There are three main protein parts that make up the cytoskeleton:

1. Microtubules

The cytoskeleton's straight, hollow, and tubular components are known as microtubules. These organelles are organised into various bundles without the limiting membrane. The diameter of each tubule ranges from 20 to 30 nm.

In terms of structure, tubulin protein bundles make up the microtubules. There are two subunits of tubulin: subunit and subunit [18]

- **Functions of microtubules:**

- Establish the cell's shape.
- Give the cell structural sturdiness
- Act like conveyer belts to move granules, vesicles, protein molecules, and some organelles, like mitochondria, to various locations within the cell.
- Create the spindle fibres necessary for mitosis, which separates the chromosomes.
- Control the motion of complex cellular structures like cilia and centrioles.

- **Intermediate Filaments**

The networks of structures that surround a nucleus and extend outside of the cell are called intermediate filaments. Each filament has a diameter of about 10 nm [19]. Rope-like polymers made of fibrous proteins are used to create the intermediate filaments.

Subclasses of intermediate filaments:

- Keratins (in epithelial cells)
- Glial filaments (in astrocytes)
- Neurofilaments (in nerve cells)
- Vimentin (in many types of cells)
- Desmin (in muscle fibers).

- **Functions of intermediate filaments**

The cell's shape is kept stable by intermediate filaments. Through desmosomes, these filaments also link the adjacent cells.

2. Microfilaments

Microfilaments are long, thin, structures resembling threads with a diameter of between 3 and 6 nm. Actin and myosin, two non-tubular contractile proteins, are the building blocks of these filaments. Myosin is less common than actin [20].

Microfilaments have the following functions:

- They give the cell structural strength;
- They protect the cell from pulling forces;
- They are in charge of cellular movements like contraction, gliding, and cytokinesis (division of cytoplasm during cell division).

3. Nucleus

The nucleus is the most noticeable and largest cellular organelle. It is between 10 μ and 22 μ in diameter and takes up about 10% of the cell's overall volume. Except for red blood cells, every cell in the body has a nucleus [21]. Eukaryotes are cells that contain a nucleus, and prokaryotes are cells that do not. For cells to divide, a nucleus must be present. In most cells, the nucleus is found in the cell's middle. Its shape is mostly spherical. However, different cells have different nuclei in terms of location and shape.

- **Structure of Nucleus**

The nuclear membrane, which encloses the nucleus, is made up of numerous parts. Nucleoplasm, chromatin, and nucleolus are the three main parts of the nucleus.

A. *Nuclear Membrane*

   The nuclear membrane has double layers and is porous in nature. This enables communication between the cytoplasm and nucleoplasm. The endoplasmic reticulum membrane and the outer layer of the nuclear membrane are one membrane. The endoplasmic reticulum lumen is continuous with the gap among the two nuclear membrane layers [22].

   Protein molecules line the pores of the nuclear membrane. The pores have a diameter of between 80 and 100 nm. However, due to protein molecules adhering to the pores' edges, it is reduced to between 7 and 9 nm. Through these pores, materials are exchanged between the cytoplasm and nucleoplasm.

B. *Nucleoplasm*

   The base material of the nucleus is made up of the extremely viscous fluid known as nucleoplasm. It resembles the cytoplasm that is found outside of the nucleus. The nuclear matrix, a dense fibrillar network of proteins, as well as numerous chemicals like nucleotides and enzymes, are all present in it. Nuclear hyaloplasm is the name for the liquid, soluble portion of the nucleoplasm.

C. *Chromatin*

   Large DNA molecules make up the material known as chromatin, which resembles a thread. With the aid of a specialised basic protein called histone, the DNA molecules are closely packed. Thus, the term "chromatin" refers to the DNA-histone complex. It makes up the bulk of the nuclear material.

The basic packing unit of chromatin known as the nucleosome is made up of 8 histone molecules and a double helix of DNA [23]. A histone molecule assists in the tightly packed assembly of nucleosomes to create a chromatin fibre. Chromosomes are formed when chromatin gathers just prior to cell division.

D. *Chromosomes*

A chromosome is a rod-shaped nuclear structure which includes an exhaustive description of all the hereditary characteristics of that species. A single molecule of DNA coils around histone molecules to form a chromosome. Many genes can be found in each DNA. Under a microscope, the chromosomes are typically not visible in the nucleus. Under a microscope, the chromosomes are only visible during cell division. This is due to the fact that just before cell division, DNA becomes more densely packed, making the chromosome visible. Except for reproductive cells, the body's dividing cells all have twenty-three pairs of chromosomes. One chromosome from the mother along with one from the father make up each pair. Diploid cells are defined as having 23 chromosome pairs [24]. There are only twenty-three single chromosomes in the reproductive cells known as gametes or sex cells. They are known as haploid cells.

E. *Nucleolus*

The nucleus contains a tiny, granular structure called a nucleolus. As many as three nucleoli can be found in each nucleus. RNA and a few proteins that are equivalent to those in ribosomes can be found in the nucleolus. Five different sets of chromosomes work together to create the RNA, which is then stored inside the nucleolus. Later, it is compressed to create the ribosome subunits. Through the pores in the nuclear membrane, all the subunits created in the nucleolus get carried to the cytoplasm. These fragments combine in the cytoplasm to create ribosomes, which are crucial for the production of proteins [25].

- **Functions of Nucleus**

- Regulation of all cellular functions, such as metabolism, protein synthesis, growth, and division (cell division);
- RNA synthesis
- Creation of ribosomal subunits
- Using messenger RNA (mRNA) to deliver genetic instructions through the cytoplasm for protein synthesis
- Genetic regulation of cell division
- The preservation of genetic information and its transmission from one generation of a species to another.

9.4. Deoxyribonucleic Acid

Deoxyribonucleic acid (DNA) is a nucleic acid which transmits an organism's genetic code to its progeny. Hereditary traits are chemically based on DNA. It contains the instructions needed for ribosomes to produce proteins. DNA molecules contain a gene. The mitochondria and chromosomes in a cell both contain DNA. The RNA is created by the DNA that is found in the nucleus [26]. Ribosomes' production of proteins is controlled by RNA. Non-chromosomal DNA refers to the DNA found in mitochondria.

- **Gene**

Genes are portions of DNA that contain the instructions or codes needed to synthesise particular proteins from amino acids. It functions as a book-like repository for the knowledge required for protein synthesis. The basic hereditary unit of a cell is the gene. A triplet or codon is the collective name for three consecutive base pairs that make up a DNA nucleotide. For one amino acid, each codon creates a code word (information). There are twenty amino acids, and each amino acid has its own unique code [27].

9.5. Ribonucleic Acid

A nucleic acid called ribonucleic acid (RNA) has a lengthy chain of nucleotide units. It resembles DNA but instead of deoxyribose, it contains ribose. RNA performs a variety of tasks that are encoded in the genes in the cell's cytoplasm. DNA is the source of RNA.

- **Types of RNA:**

RNA is of three types.

- *The messenger RNA (mRNA):* Messenger RNA transports from the DNA to the cytoplasm the genetic code for the amino acid sequence needed to synthesise proteins.
- *Transfer RNA (tRNA):* Transfer RNA decodes the genetic information contained in mRNA.
- *Ribosomal RNA (rRNA):* Ribosomal RNA is a component of the ribosome's structure and is found inside of it. It is in charge of assembling proteins in the ribosome from amino acids [28].

- **Gene Expression**

Gene expression involves two steps:

1. Transcription.
2. Translation.

9.6. Transcription of Genetic Code

It denotes the transfer of genetic information from DNA to RNA. The ribosomes, which are found in the cytoplasm, are where proteins are made. However, the information (sequence of codons) encoded in the genes of the DNA that are present in the nucleus determines how various proteins are synthesised. The gene needs to be copied (transcribed) into mRNA, which is created from DNA. Thus, transcription of genetic code, that takes place inside the nucleus, is the first step in the production of proteins. It entails the synthesis of mRNA and the concurrent copying or as transfer of data from DNA to mRNA [29]. Protein synthesis is triggered when mRNA from the nucleus enters the cytoplasm and activates the ribosome. The RNA polymerase enzyme aids in the production of mRNA from DNA.

9.6.1. Translation of Genetic Code

The process of translation is how genetic instructions carried by mRNA from DNA are used to direct protein synthesis in the cell's ribosome. Alternately, it could be the procedure by which the ribosome reads the mRNA to create a protein. Other two RNA types, namely tRNA and rRNA, play a part in this.

The mRNA exits the nucleus and travels to the cytoplasm. Now, mRNA is joined by a polysome, a collection of ribosomes. The complementary base sequence in tRNA exposes and recognises the sequence of codons in mRNA. Anticodon is the name given to the base's complementary sequence. Different amino acids are carried by tRNA, which serves as a carrier, from the cytoplasm in the ribosome in accordance with the base order in the anticodon [30]. The amino acid building blocks of protein molecules are put together with the aid of rRNA. The ribosomes, which are connected to the rough endoplasmic reticulum, are where protein synthesis takes place.

9.6.2. Growth Factors

Similar to cytokines and hormones, growth factors are proteins that function as cell signalling molecules. These substances interact with certain surface receptors on the target cell to promote cell growth, differentiation, and/or maturation. The terms "cytokine" and "growth factor" are frequently used interchangeably. Growth factors, however, are different from cytokines. The cells of the developing tissues are affected by growth factors [31]. However, cytokines are focused on immune system as well as hemopoietic cells.

Many growth factors are identified. The known growth factors are:

- Platelet derived growth factor – PDGF
- Colony stimulating factors – CSF
- Nerve growth factors – NGF
- Neurotrophins
- Erythropoietin
- Thrombopoietin

- Transforming growth factors (TGF) – present in transforming cells (cells undergoing differentiation) and in large quantities in tumors and cancerous tissue.

9.7. Cell Death

Cell death occurs by two distinct processes:

1. Apoptosis
2. Necrosis.

1. Apoptosis

Apoptosis is characterised as a cell's genetically controlled natural or programmed death. Due to the fact that the cell's genes play a significant role in the death, it is also known as "cell suicide." It is common and necessary for the body to develop normally for this kind of programmed death of cells to occur [32]. Apoptosis, in contrast to necrosis, typically does not result in inflammatory responses in the surrounding tissues.

- **Functional Significance of Apoptosis:**

Apoptosis is used to eliminate cancerous cells without stressing or harming healthy cells nearby. The importance of apoptosis in terms of function

1. Essential for maintaining cellular homeostasis. The human body undergoes mitosis every day to produce about 10 million new cells. Apoptosis causes an equal number of cells to perish. This promotes the homeostasis of cells.
2. Effective for removing a cell that has been irreparably harmed by a virus or toxin.
3. A crucial occurrence both during development and in the adult stage [33].

- **Activation of Apoptosis:**

Apoptosis is triggered by either the withdrawal or arrival of positive signals (survival factors).

Positive signals are being withdrawn.

Positive signals are required for the long-term survival of the majority of cells. Other cells or chemical stimulants continuously produce positive signals [34]. The following are some of the most effective chemical stimulants:

1. Nerve growth factors (for neurons)
2. Interleukin-2 (for cells like lymphocytes).

The absence or withdrawal of the positive signals activates apoptosis.

- **Arrival of negative signals:**

Negative signals are the external or internal stimuli which initiate apoptosis. The negative signals are produced during various events like:

- Normal developmental procedures
- Cellular stress
- Increase in the concentration of intracellular oxidants 4. Viral infection
- Damage of DNA
- Exposure to agents like chemotherapeutic drugs, X-rays, ultraviolet rays and the death-receptor ligands.

- **Death-receptor ligands and death receptors:**

The substances known as death receptor ligands attach to particular cell membrane receptors and start the apoptotic process. Tumour necrosis factors (TNFs) and Fas ligands, which bind to the Fas receptor, are the most common death-receptor ligands.

The cell membrane receptors known as death receptors are the ones that bind to death receptor ligands. TNF receptor-1 (TNFR1) and TNF-related apoptosis inducing ligand (TRAIL) receptors DR4 and DR5 are well-known death receptors [35].

2. Necrosis

Necrosis is the unplanned and uncontrolled death of cells brought on by accidental and unforeseen damage. Because the cell dies by extracellular or external factors, it is also known as "cell murder." Following necrosis, the toxic chemicals released from dead cells harm and inflame the tissues in close proximity [37].

A. *Causes for Necrosis*
   Injury, infection, inflammation, infarction, and cancer are frequent causes of necrosis. Both physical and chemical factors, such as heat, radiation, trauma, hypoxia from a lack of blood flow, and exposure to toxins, can cause necrosis.
B. *Necrotic Process*
   Cell structure and activity are fatally disrupted as a result of necrosis. During the necrotic process, the cell experiences a number of distinctive changes, including:
   - Cell swelling damages the cell membrane and causes the membrane to develop numerous holes [38].
   - Intracellular materials spill out into the environment
   - Changes to the intracellular environment
   - A significant number of calcium ions are simultaneously released.
   - released by the compromised organelles and mitochondria
   - The organisation and functions of proteins in the intracellular components are significantly impacted by the presence of calcium ions.
   - Calcium ions also cause the release of toxic substances that cause the lysosomal enzymes to activate.

- Lysosomal enzymes degrade cellular components, completely disassembling the cell, and causing death.
- Neighbouring cells consume the breakdown products from the disassembled cell.

9.8. Cell Adaptation

Cell adaptation describes the alterations that occur within a cell as a result of environmental changes.

Numerous factors, including stress, chemical agents, diseases, and environmental dangers, pose a constant threat to a cell's ability to function normally. Nevertheless, the cell adapts to continue existing and functioning [39]. The cell can only withstand dangerous factors under extreme circumstances, which leads to cell death and destruction.

Cellular adaptation occurs by any of the following mechanisms.

1. Atrophy
2. Hypertrophy
3. Hyperplasia
4. Dysplasia
5. Metaplasia.

1. Atrophy

Atrophy refers to a cell's reduction in size. Increased cell atrophy causes the tissue, organ, or body part in question to shrink or waste away.

- **Causes of Atrophy Atrophy:**

- inadequate nutrition
- reduced blood flow
- lack of activity or exercise
- loss of nerve or hormonal control
- inherent disease in a tissue or organ.

- **Types of Atrophy**

There are two types of atrophy: pathological atrophy and physiological atrophy [40]. Thymus atrophy in childhood and tonsils atrophy in adolescence are two instances of physiological atrophy. Skeletal muscle atrophy, cardiac atrophy, sex organ atrophy, and brain atrophy are all common examples.

2. Hypertrophy

Cell hypertrophy refers to an increase in cell size. An organ or a portion of the body will enlarge or overgrow as a result of the hypertrophy of numerous cells. There are three types of hypertrophies.

- **Physiological Hypertrophy**

The growth in size brought on by more work or exercise is referred to as physiological hypertrophy. The widespread physiological hypertrophy consists of:

1. *Muscular hypertrophy*: An increase in the size of the skeletal muscles as a result of strength training.
2. *Ventricular hypertrophy*: Ventricular hypertrophy, an expansion of the heart's ventricular muscles, is only beneficial when it happens in response to exercise.
3. *Pathological Hypertrophy*: Pathological hypertrophy is an increase in cell size brought on by pathological changes. An illustration of this is the ventricular hypertrophy, in which the workload of the ventricles increases and is brought on by pathological conditions like high blood pressure.
4. *Compensatory Hypertrophy*: Increasing the size of an organ's cells to make up for the loss or dysfunctional functioning of a similar-type organ is known as compensatory hypertrophy [41]. Examples include the hypertrophy of a single kidney following the loss or dysfunction of the other kidney, and the development of stronger muscles in one arm following the loss or dysfunction of the other arm.

3. Hyperplasia

Hyperplasia is an increase in cell count brought on by more frequent cell division (mitosis). Additionally, it is described as abnormal or unusual cell proliferation (multiplication) brought on by ongoing cell division. The organ enlarges dramatically as a result of hyperplasia. Only normal cells undergo continuous cell division in hyperplasia. There are three types of hyperplasia.

- *Physiological Hyperplasia*
  The temporary adaptive response to regular physiological changes in the body is called physiological hyperplasia [42]. For instance, the number of endometrial cells in the uterus rises during the proliferative stage of every menstrual cycle.
- *Compensatory Hyperplasia*
  Increasing the number of cells in an organ to make up for lost or damaged cells is referred to as compensatory hyperplasia.
  The regeneration of tissues and organs is aided by compensatory hyperplasia. It is typical in the liver. There is an increase in the amount of liver cells following the surgical elimination of the damaged liver tissue, leading to regeneration. Additionally, frequent in intestine and epidermis epithelial cells is compensatory hyperplasia.
- *Pathological Hyperplasia*
  The growth in cell number brought on by an abnormal increase in the production of hormones is known as pathological hyperplasia. Additionally, known as hormonal hyperplasia. For instance, in gigantism, excessive growth hormone secretion causes the body to overgrow due to hyperplasia.

4. Dysplasia

The abnormal alteration in the size, shape, and organisation of the cell is what distinguishes dysplasia from other conditions [43]. Dysplasia is suggested to be related to hyperplasia and is not thought to be a true adaptation. It frequently occurs in respiratory tract and cervix epithelial cells.

5. Metaplasia

A particular kind of cell is replaced by another kind of cell in the condition known as metaplasia. There are two types.

- *Physiological Metaplasia*
  A normal process of replacing cells is known as physiological metaplasia. Examples include the conversion of monocytes into macrophages and cartilage into bone.
- *Pathological Metaplasia*
  The irreversible replacement of cells as a result of ongoing exposure to harmful stimuli is known as pathological metaplasia. For instance, long-term smoking causes the normal mucus-secreting ciliated columnar epithelial cells to change into non-ciliated squamous epithelial cells that cannot secrete mucus. If the stimulus (smoking) is kept up, these transformed cells might develop into cancerous cells.

9.9. Radiation Dermatitis

9.9.1. Mechanism

Skin exposure to radiation causes immediate cellular damage as well as an influx of inflammatory cells. After the initial dose of radiation, epidermal basal cells, endothelial cells, Langerhans cells, and vascular components suffer cellular damage; every subsequent fraction of radiation causes an inflammatory response in the epidermis and dermis.

Short-lived free-radical production and irreversible double-stranded breaks in nuclear and mitochondrial DNA cause the initial cellular damage [44]. Cellular damage results in direct cellular necrosis and apoptosis as well as nuclear chromatin clumping, nucleus swelling, nuclear disfiguration or loss of the nuclear membrane, mitochondrial distortion, and endoplasmic reticulum degeneration. Each fraction of treatment causes repetitive cellular damage that prevents cells from having time to repair DNA damage. Interleukins 1 and 6, tumour necrosis factor, and transforming growth factor are among the cytokines and chemokines that are produced as a result of the production of free radicals. These cytokines cause the migration of leukocytes and other immune cells from the circulation to the radioexposed skin by acting on the endothelial cells of local vessels, which express adhesion molecules in a constitutively active manner. The normal turnover of skin cells is altered as a result of radiation-induced reduction and impairment of functional stem cells.

After exposure, an immediate skin reaction that is linked to an inflammatory response, a discharge of histamine-like substances, capillary permeability and dilation, and ensuing dermal edoema may manifest. It begins with an early, transient skin erythema that appears shortly after radiation and goes away 24 to 48 hours later [45].

The later stage includes additional edoema, increased capillary dilation, and erythrocyte extravasation, leading to an erythematous reaction after the initial erythema has subsided. The epidermis thins, epithelial cells are damaged, glands degenerate, sebum production is reduced, sweat and clumps of exfoliated corneocytes (scales) form, which results in dry desquamation.

Epidermal necrosis, fibrinous exudates, and moist desquamation occur if damage to the basal cells and glands is more severe. Small blisters that can extend into the lower, more superficial parts of the epidermis form in and around the epidermis' basal layer, which is the result of moist desquamation. When these blisters burst and group together, the epidermis sloughs, denuding the dermis and resulting in permanent epilation. The most serious side effects from higher radiation doses may include skin necrosis or ulceration of the full thickness dermis [46].

9.9.2. Timing

As mentioned above, even after just a fraction of radiation (2 Gy), a transient early erythema can be observed within a few hours of radiation and goes away after 24-48 h. Within 1-4 weeks of radiation, the primary erythematous reaction starts to manifest around the second or third week. Patients with particularly sensitive skin might experience an earlier reaction. Effects typically continue to develop throughout treatment, and after the third week or a cumulative dose of 30 Gy, dry desquamation, which is clinically characterised by dryness, scaling, and pruritus, can emerge. Moist desquamation, which is characterised by serous oozing and dermal exposure, may happen after 4-5 weeks (45-60 Gy) of therapy. The severity of the symptoms increases in the first two weeks following the end of radiation therapy. Within one to three months (depending upon the severity of the reaction), the skin completely heals after radiation treatment, with epidermal regeneration starting about 3 to 5 weeks later. After radiation, post-inflammatory hyperpigmentation may last for 5-7 weeks or even longer [53]. Due to interindividual variation in how radiation damage manifests on the skin, patient skin type may also affect the timing and intensity of radiation reactions.

9.9.3. Signs and Symptoms

Erythematous skin, mild edoema, pruritus, or pain are the symptoms of mild dermatitis (Grade I). Adnexal structures may be involved, resulting in temporary epilation, dry, peeling skin, and desquamation.

Tender or edematous reactions and moist desquamation characterise moderate dermatitis Dermal integrity is compromised, and Staphylococcus aureus secondary infection could happen. Rarely seen, severe dermatitis (acute radionecrosis) can happen when superficial tumours that are extremely extensive are treated with high radiation doses over a very brief period of time. It appears as a deeply necrotizing, intensely painful inflammatory or hemorrhagic plaque that can expose the bones, muscles, and tendons [46].

9.9.4. Scoring

Numerous grading scales, including the Radiation Therapy Oncology Group (RTOG) toxicity scoring system, the Radiation Induced Skin Reaction Assessment Scale (RISRAS), and the Common Terminology Criteria for Adverse Event (NCI-CTCAE grading), are used to determine the severity of radiation dermatitis [47]. One of the most widely used is the Common Terminology Criteria for Adverse Event (NCI-CTCAE grading), and NCI-CTCAE v4.3 is displayed in the Table 9.1. The NCI-CTCAE grading system and RTOG scoring are very similar.

Table 9.1. Grading of radiation dermatitis

	Definition
Grade 1	Faint erythema or dry desquamation
Grade 2	Moderate to brisk erythema; patchy moist desquamation, mostly confined to skin folds and creases; moderate oedema
Grade 3	Moist desquamation in area other than skin folds and creases; bleeding induced by minor trauma or abrasion
Grade 4	Skin necrosis or ulceration of full-thickness dermis; spontaneous bleeding from involved site

9.10. Risk Factors

Various factors Related to Treatment Including The use of tissue expanders and bolus materials, concurrent systemic therapy with radiation, and radiation-sensitizing drugs like paclitaxel, docetaxel, anthracyclines, dactinomycin, methotrexate, 5-fluorouracil, hydroxyurea, bleomycin, and cetuximab are related to higher total dose, higher dose per fraction, reduced overall treatment time, beam energy (depending on the type and quality of the beam. Epidermal growth factor receptor (EGFR) plays a significant role in the regulation of numerous phases of epithelial biology, including cell cycle progression, differentiation, cell movement, and cellular survival; EGFR is highly expressed in the epidermis, particularly in the proliferative basal cell layers. Additionally, it plays a crucial role in the skin's inflammatory responses [48]. The effects of radiation and epidermal growth factors receptor inhibitors (such as cetuximab) on skin are inversely correlated.

Patients receiving radiation therapy along with cetuximab experience more severe radiation dermatitis than those receiving radiation therapy by itself or even concurrent chemoradiotherapy. When cetuximab is included in addition to radiation therapy, radiation dermatitis lasts slightly longer (11.1 compared to 9.4 weeks) and manifests sooner (week one or two compared with 3-5 weeks, respectively).

Following the completion of treatment with cetuximab plus radiation therapy, dermatitis typically shows quick healing without scarring. In patients receiving cetuximab and radiation therapy at the same time, a delayed rash resembling acne develops within the irradiated fields (approximately 3-5 weeks versus 7-10 days, respectively). It appears that there is no correlation between the severity of radiation dermatitis and the severity of the cetuximab-associated acne-like rash beyond radioactive fields.

9.10.1. Patient-Related Factors

Radiation-induced dermatitis incidence and severity can be influenced by comorbid diseases, inherited disorders, demographic and behavioural factors, and radiation therapy site. Smoking appears to hinder wound healing by constricting the blood vessels in the skin. The other factors are listed in Table 9.2.

Age-related changes in radiation dermatitis are correlated with slower epidermal turnover and longer healing times [49]. The severity and recovery of radiation dermatitis are influenced by coexisting conditions such as diabetes, obesity, high blood pressure, or malnutrition in older patients. According to reports, aspirating a seroma after breast surgery can harm the lymphatic system, impair wound healing, and trigger severe reactions to the skin during radiation treatment.

Table 9.2. Patient related factors related to radiation dermatitis

Demographic and behavioural factors	Comorbid disease	Inherited disorders	Site of radiation therapy
• Black race • Obesity • Female gender • Advanced age • Breast implant • Smoking • Poor nutrition	• Actinic skin lesions • Seroma aspiration after breast surgery • Systemic lupus erythematosus • Systemic sclerosis • Juvenile rheumatoid arthritis • HIV infection • Diabetes mellitus • Hypertension	• Basal cell nevus disease • Fanconi anemia • Bloom syndrome • Xeroderma • Pigmentosum • Ataxia-telangiectasia	• Anterior neck • Extremities • Submammary • Skin folds

Systemic sclerosis, juvenile rheumatoid arthritis, and systemic lupus erythematosus patients have significantly higher radiosensitivity and are more likely to experience radiation side effects. Radiation therapy is regarded as an approximate contraindication if that connective tissue illness is present. Patients with diabetes that is uncontrolled have more difficult time healing wounds because of poor macrophage function, which includes phagocytic activity, a protracted inflammatory phase, and a higher risk of infection. More research is required to determine how diabetes affects the normal tissue reaction to radiation therapy.

Rare genetic mutations, such as those in the ataxia-telangiectasia gene, can put patients at risk for developing severe radiation dermatitis. Unexpectedly severe radiation dermatitis has been theorised to be a sign of undiscovered genetic anomalies in the ATM gene (ataxia-telangiectasia mutated), which can put patients at risk for cutaneous complications [50]. The impact of haemoglobin levels on skin that is not exposed to radiation therapy has not been specifically studied.

9.10.2. Diagnosis

Acute radiation dermatitis is diagnosed clinically based on the discovery of skin changes that have a clear demarcation between them and the irradiated areas, as well as the course of radiation therapy. Typically, radiation dermatitis can be diagnosed without a skin biopsy.

Radiation recall and cellulitis are two significant possibilities for diagnosis of acute radiation dermatitis.

Following the administration of cytotoxic agents or other drugs, radiation recall is an acute inflammation skin reaction that is localised to the area that was previously exposed to radiation. It happens at least a week after radiation treatment and can happen weeks to years later [51]. Radiation recall has been linked to cytotoxic drugs like docetaxel, doxorubicin, and paclitaxel. Rash, dry desquamation, erythema, ulceration, haemorrhage, and necrosis are a few manifestations of radiation recall. After stopping the drug, radiation recall usually goes away in 1-2 weeks. A precise diagnosis will be made with the aid of the patient's medical history and skin reactions to radiation therapy. Skin and subcutaneous tissues can become infected with bacteria in cellulitis. Localised erythema, warmth, swelling, discomfort, tenderness, fevers, and even purulent drainage are some of its defining characteristics. Cellulitis and radiation dermatitis can be distinguished using these indicators. Radiation dermatitis, however, is a risk factor for secondary cellulitis, and it is possible for both conditions to coexist. Cellulitis may be diagnosed in this situation based on a wound culture [52]. Treatment with empiric antibiotics may be beneficial for these patients.

Eczema is a relapsing, chronic skin condition characterised by itchy, dry skin that is symmetrical and lasts for at least six months. Due to the fact both of these conditions are inflammatory in nature, chronic eczema may make radiation dermatitis worse. The symmetrical distribution of eczema can be used to distinguish it from radiation dermatitis. Radiation dermatitis, on the other hand, will only manifest itself in radiation fields.

If atypical plaques and nodules appear within the radiation field, recurrent or secondary tumours should be taken into consideration. A biopsy is helpful in this clinical scenario despite the fact that skin that has been exposed to radiation may have some healing issues. Atopic dermatitis, lichen planus, pemphigus, and dermatophyte infection are uncommon conditions that can be diagnosed as other conditions using the clinical course, lesion distribution, and laboratory tests.

9.10.3. Prevention

General Measures:

- Daily washing using water and mild soap (agents with a pH of zero) or normal saline, followed by drying and application of a water-based moisturiser.
- Dressing in baggy clothing.
- Steering clear of skin irritants like wax, lotions with alcohol as an ingredient, and perfumes.
- Steering clear of temperature extremes.
- Refraining from being in the sun and wearing sunscreen with at least SPF 30.
- The only type of prophylactic intervention for radiation dermatitis prevention that has been strongly recommended is the application of topical steroids. Topical steroids should always be used as a preventative measure because of their ability to reduce inflammation by inhibiting leukocyte migration and reducing the creation of IL-1, IL-2, IL-6, TNF, and histamine. After each radiotherapy treatment, the

treatment field is treated with low- to medium-potency topical corticosteroids (sets 4-6), such as mometasone furoate 0.1%, hydrocortisone 1% cream, methylprednisolone aceponate cream 0.1%, or beclomethasone dipropionate spray. If there is any exudate coming from the area that is affected or if a skin infection is thought to be present, treatment should be stopped.

Other protective options with primarily positive results that warrant further research on their efficacy in preventing and managing acute radiation dermatitis include:

A. *Intensity-Modulated Radiation Therapy (IMRT)*
According to some data, IMRT significantly reduces radiation dermatitis severity and duration when compared to standard conventional treatment.
B. *Low-Level Laser Therapy*
A type of phototherapy known as low-level laser therapy promotes the healing of wounds. Preventing radiation side effects like dermatitis, xerostomia, or oral mucositis has sparked a lot of interest. The main encouraging findings of these trials call for more investigation into its effectiveness in preventing and treating acute radiation dermatitis [53].

1. *Amifostine*
Amifostine is a thiol that, by selectively scavenging oxygen-derived free radicals, shields healthy cells from radiation damage. Patients receiving amifostine have been shown to have significantly less severe radiation dermatitis. The effectiveness as well as safety of amifostine as a cytoprotective agent against acute radiation-induced dermatitis require further research.
2. *Ascorbic Acid*
Ascorbic acid has the ability to fight free radicals and act as an antioxidant. For the prevention of radiation dermatitis, its topical application is not believed to be beneficial. Yet, oral ascorbic acid within breast cancer radiation therapy with a volume less than 500 mL and in patients who received radiation doses between 107% and 110% of the recommended dose demonstrated successful outcomes [54].
3. *Oral Zinc*
In studies on the protection of normal tissue against radiation injuries, zinc (Zn) has been examined as an antioxidant. Dermatitis has mostly encouraging results, but they still require more research.
4. *Silver Leaf Dressing*
Another suggestion for preventing radiation-induced dermatitis is the use of silver leaf dressing, which has antimicrobial properties. Positive outcomes regarding its efficacy need to be confirmed in additional research.
5. *MAS065D*
Hyaluronic acid, shea butter (emollient), glycyrrhetinic acid (licorice extract with anti-inflammatory properties), Vitis vinifera (antioxidant activity), and telmesteine (anti-elastase and anti-collagen activity *in vitro*) are all ingredients in the nonsteroidal water-in-oil cream known as MAS065D (Xclair). MAS065D appears to be useful in the treatment of radiation dermatitis, yet more research is required [55].

Further research is advised because oral proteolytic enzymes (such as those found in products that included papain, bromelain, trypsin, and chymotrypsin) appear to be effective in preventing radiation dermatitis.

6. *Soft Dressing or Barrier Film*

   In areas at risk, like the axilla, theneck and head region, perineum as well as skin folds, it appears that preventative usage of friction protections via soft dressings or barrier films may be an efficient intervention for reducing the severity of skin reactions.

7. *Hyaluronic Acid*

   Hyaluronic acid cream has been tested in radiation therapy studies as an adjunct therapy for radiation dermatitis and appears to decrease the inflammatory reaction and oxidative free radical damage. To fully understand hyaluronic acid's role as a treatment for radiation dermatitis, more research is necessary [56].

8. *Trolamine*

   This salicylate-based analgesic, which is used topically, has been shown to hasten wound healing by attracting macrophages and enhancing the formation of granulation tissue, which has therapeutic uses in dermatology. More research is needed to determine whether trolamine is effective in preventing radiation dermatitis because the evidence currently available does not support its use.

9. *Topical Sucralfate*

   Sucralfate is a topical medication that has been used to treat a variety of epithelial wounds, including burn wounds, ulcers, inflammatory dermatitis, and mucositis. With varying outcomes, some studies have looked at the effectiveness of sucralfate cream in preventing radiation dermatitis [57]. The prevention of radiation dermatitis is not supported by the available data.

10. *Theta Cream*

    It contains glucan, Hydroxyprolisilane, and matrixyl with the immune system-modulating effects and tissue regeneration properties [58]. Evidence from a limited number of randomized trials does not support theta cream in radiation dermatitis prevention.

11. *Dexpanthenol (Provitamin B5)*

    Dexpanthenol, the stable alcohol version of pantothenic acid, is transformed into pantothenic acid in tissues, which is necessary for healthy epithelial function and improves the regeneration of skin and wound healing. Dexpanthenol is not currently recommended for use in the treatment of radiation dermatitis.

12. *Calendula*

    Calendula is made from a plant in the marigold family called Calendula officinalis, and it has anti-inflammatory and antioxidant properties. Studies evaluating calendula's effectiveness in treating and preventing radiation dermatitis have produced conflicting findings that call for more research.

13. P*entoxifylline*

    Pentoxifylline, a helpful medication for a number of vaso-occlusive disorders, has anti-inflammatory properties. In carefully planned studies, the effects of pentoxifylline on acute reactions to the skin must be determined [59].

14. *Aloe Vera*
    The effectiveness of this traditional herbal remedy as well as natural product in preventing radiation dermatitis has yielded conflicting results, necessitating further study before its widespread use is advised.
15. *Laughter Therapy*
    Radiation dermatitis may be avoided with the help of laughter therapy. Large sample sizes in well-designed randomised studies are needed to confirm the impact of laughter therapy on radiation dermatitis [60].

9.10.4. Management

Throughout the course of radiation therapy, patients should be checked on at least once a week with regard to the skin's reaction. The degree of skin damage determines how radiation dermatitis should be treated.

- **Grade 1 Dermatitis**

The majority of patients appear to be able to reduce their symptoms with simple skin care techniques. As a supportive treatment for erythematous skin, patients should be instructed to gently wash their skin with mild soap and water (pH-neutral intermediaries) or normal saline solution. Washing lowers bacterial load and infection risk.

By applying a thin layer of nonscented, hydrophilic, lanolin-free ointment and cream to the affected area 2-4 times per day, dry desquamation can be controlled [61]. Patients should be advised not to use topical moisturisers right before radiation treatment because they may serve as a skin bolus and raise the radiation skin dose.

Mid-potency topical corticosteroids can reduce itching or pruritus.

The majority of practitioners are prescribing steroids for radiation-induced dermatitis, despite the fact that there is insufficient evidence to support their use of topical corticosteroids (corticosteroids Group IV and V). The topical steroids listed in Table 9.3 are typically prescribed for radiation-induced dermatitis.

Antihistamines do not appear to be helpful in reducing radiation dermatitis-related pruritus

Patients may benefit from using a normal saline compress up to four times per day to improve skin cleaning and reduce inflammation-related symptoms. Patients are instructed to gently apply moist gauze on the affected area for 10 to 15 minutes by moistening it with a warm or at room temperature saline solution. The wound's surface is gently irrigated via normal saline, dried, and the gauze is removed.

Table 9.3. Steroids used in radiation dermatitis

Group IV	Group V
• Fluocinolone acetonide 0.01-0.2% • Hydrocortisone valerate 0.2% • Hydrocortisone butyrate 0.1% • Flurandrenolide 0.05% • Triamcinolone acetonide 0.1% • Mometasone furoate 0.1%	• Fluticasone propionate 0.05% • Desonide 0.05% • Flucinolone acetonide 0.025%

- **Grade 2–3 Dermatitis**

A variety of topical applications, in combination with general skin care techniques, can help to alleviate symptoms in the second and third grades of radiation dermatitis. Patients who have moist desquamation are more susceptible to infection and must be watched out for fevers and purulent drainage.

Typically, wound dressings are used to treat moist desquamation. These dressings create the ideal moist environment for wound healing by absorbing wound secretions, phagocytosing bacteria, extracellular debris, and necrotic materials, reducing pain, and shielding the wound from infection.

The dressings need to be comfortable to boost the compliance of patients for prolonged use. They should additionally be able to absorb significant amounts of serious leakage from the wound in order to avoid maceration of the surrounding skin that is healthy [62]. Finally, they must be eliminated without disrupting granulation and new tissue. Various types of the dressing are available in clinical practise, but there is insufficient evidence to support any one type within the management of moist desquamation. Simple dressings alone are not suff. However, a recent study comparing hydrogel versus a dry dressing on the healing duration of moist desquamation discovered that the hydrogel group's dressings significantly prolonged healing time without enhancing patient comfort. With encouraging initial results, a new line of silicon foam skin dressings (like Mepilex Lite) is now available commercially.

Patients should be advised to apply normal saline reduces several times daily, clean the wound before applying a dressing, and change the dressing frequently depending on how much is weeping. Topical as well as systemic antibiotics should be used to treat infections when they occur. Antibacterial silver-based dressings have been shown to be successful for this use. Beta glucan or silver sulfadiazine cream can be helpful, but they should only be used after radiation therapy along with cleaning the affected area. Patients with severe renal as well as hepatic impairment, as well as those who lack the enzyme G6PD, should also use caution when using these products. A full blood count should be checked in patients receiving concurrent chemotherapy or who are at higher risk of developing neutropenia. The cultures of blood should be taken from patients who exhibit neutropenia or indications of sepsis.

Nonsteroidal anti-inflammatory medications are frequently successful at treating pain and can also ease the discomfort brought on by itching and swelling around a skin reaction. Depending on the patient's performance status, the existence of sepsis or severe neutropenia, and the radiation oncologist's discretion, treatment interruption may be required for Grade 3 radiation dermatitis.

Biologic treatments are being researched for some types of radiation dermatitis, such as the use of calcineurin inhibitors (such as tacrolimus or pimecrolimus cream) or topical granulocyte-macrophage colony stimulating cream for vulvar radiation dermatitis [63].

The effects on a foam dressing that included human recombinant human epidermal growth factor (rhEGF) and granulocyte-colony stimulating factor (G-CSF) have been suggested for radiation dermatitis with moist desquamation. To establish the optimal dosage, plan treatments, and confirm the agents' mechanism of action, more research is required. More research is needed, but it has been claimed that a Chinese medicine known as Lianbai liquid can effectively treat Grade III acute radiation dermatitis.

- **Dermatitis of Grade 4**

Grade 4 radiodermatitis is a very uncommon complication. The mainstay of treatment is actually surgical interventions. Treatment for this grade should include surgical debridement, full-thickness skin grafting, or myocutaneous or pedicle flaps. Radiation therapy should also be stopped [64].

Conclusion

This chapter detailed the structural and functional aspects of cells and tissues, describing how ionizing radiation damages cellular components and disrupts tissue homeostasis. The mechanisms of radiation-induced injury—including DNA damage, inflammation, apoptosis, and necrosis—were explored to highlight their impact on normal tissue toxicity. Special emphasis was placed on radiation dermatitis, its pathophysiology, clinical manifestations, and grading. The text reviewed numerous risk factors that modulate tissue sensitivity to radiation and outlined preventive and therapeutic strategies, such as topical steroids, advanced dressings, and supportive care. By understanding these processes, clinicians can better predict, prevent, and manage radiation-related adverse effects, ultimately improving patient outcomes during radiotherapy.

References

[1] Norbury C, Nurse P. Animal cell cycles and their control. *Annual review of biochemistry*. 1992 Jul;61(1):441-68.

[2] Joiner MC, van der Kogel AJ, editors. *Basic clinical radiobiology*. CRC press; 2018 Aug 28.

[3] Yeagle PL. Cholesterol and the cell membrane. *Biochimica et Biophysica Acta (BBA)-Reviews on Biomembranes*. 1985 Dec 9;822(3-4):267-87.

[4] Porter KR, Kenyon K, Badenhausen S. Specializations of the unit membrane. In *Symposium on Biophysics and Physiology of Biological Transport:* Frascati, June 15–18, 1965 1967 Mar 1 (pp. 262-274). Vienna: Springer Vienna.

[5] Claude A. The constitution of protoplasm. *Science*. 1943 May 21;97(2525):451-6.

[6] Du Y, Ferro-Novick S, Novick P. Dynamics and inheritance of the en doplasmic reticulum. *Journal of cell science*. 2004 Jun 15;117(14):2871-8.

[7] Sembulingam K, Sembulingam P. Essentials of medical physiology. *JP Medical* Ltd; 2012 Sep 30.

[8] Berridge MJ. The endoplasmic reticulum: a multifunctional signaling organelle. *Cell calcium*. 2002 Nov 1;32(5-6):235-49.

[9] Palade GE. *The endoplasmic reticulum. The Journal of biophysical and biochemical cytology*. 1956 Jul 7;2(4):85.

[10] Griffiths G, Simons K. The trans Golgi network: sorting at the exit site of the Golgi complex. *Science*. 1986 Oct 24;234(4775):438-43.

[11] Beams HW, Kessel RG. The Golgi apparatus: structure and function. *International review of cytology*. 1968 Jan 1;23:209-76.

[12] Luzio JP, Pryor PR, Bright NA. Lysosomes: fusion and function. *Nature reviews Molecular cell biology*. 2007 Aug;8(8):622-32.

[13] Nigg EA, Stearns T. The centrosome cycle: Centriole biogenesis, duplication and inherent asymmetries. *Nature cell biology*. 2011 Oct;13(10):1154-60.

[14] Lehniger AL. *The mitochondrion*. Wa Benjamin; 1964.

[15] 15). Senior AE. ATP synthesis by oxidative phosphorylation. *Physiological reviews*. 1988 Jan 1;68(1):177-231.
[16] 16). Lafontaine DL, Tollervey D. The function and synthesis of ribosomes. *Nature Reviews Molecular Cell Biology*. 2001 Jul 1;2(7):514-20.
[17] Hall A. The cytoskeleton and cancer. *Cancer and Metastasis Reviews*. 2009 Jun;28:5-14.
[18] Dustin P. *Microtubules*. Springer Science & Business Media; 2012 Dec 6.
[19] Fuchs E, Weber K. Intermediate filaments: structure, dynamics, function and disease. *Annual review of biochemistry*. 1994 Jul;63(1):345-82.
[20] Spooner BS, Yamada KM, Wessells NK. Microfilaments and cell locomotion. *The Journal of cell biology*. 1971 Jun 1;49(3):595-613.
[21] Lamond AI, Earnshaw WC. Structure and function in the nucleus. *Science*. 1998 Apr 24;280(5363):547-53.
[22] Dingwall C, Laskey R. The nuclear membrane. *Science*. 1992 Nov 6;258(5084):942-7.
[23] Felsenfeld G. Chromatin. *Nature*. 1978 Jan 12;271(5641):115-22.
[24] Sumner AT. *Chromosomes: organization and function*. John Wiley & Sons; 2008 Apr 30.
[25] Boisvert FM, Van Koningsbruggen S, Navascués J, Lamond AI. The multifunctional nucleolus. *Nature reviews Molecular cell biology*. 2007 Jul;8(7):574-85.
[26] Watson JD, Crick FH. Genetical implications of the structure of deoxyribonucleic acid. *Jama*. 1993 Apr 21;269(15):1967-9.
[27] Pearson H. What is a gene?. *Nature*. 2006 May 25;441(7092):398-402.
[28] Holley RW, Apgar J, Everett GA, Madison JT, Marquisee M, Merrill SH, Penswick JR, Zamir A. Structure of a ribonucleic acid. *Science*. 1965 Mar 19;147(3664):1462-5.
[29] Mellor J. Dynamic nucleosomes and gene transcription. *Trends in genetics*. 2006 Jun 1;22(6):320-9.
[30] Yarian C, Townsend H, Czestkowski W, Sochacka E, Malkiewicz AJ, Guenther R, Miskiewicz A, Agris PF. Accurate translation of the genetic code depends on tRNA modified nucleosides. *Journal of Biological Chemistry*. 2002 May 10;277(19):16391-5.
[31] Hogan BL, Blessing M, Winnier GE, Suzuki N, Jones CM. Growth factors in development: the role of TGF-β related polypeptide signalling molecules in embryogenesis. *Development*. 1994 Jan 1;1994(Supplement):53-60.
[32] Meier P, Finch A, Evan G. Apoptosis in development. *Nature*. 2000 Oct 12;407(6805):796-801.
[33] Earnshaw WC, Martins LM, Kaufmann SH. Mammalian caspases: structure, activation, substrates, and functions during apoptosis. *Annual review of biochemistry*. 1999 Jul;68(1):383-424.
[34] Redza-Dutordoir M, Averill-Bates DA. Activation of apoptosis signalling pathways by reactive oxygen species. *Biochimica et Biophysica Acta (BBA)-Molecular Cell Research*. 2016 Dec 1;1863(12):2977-92.
[35] Ashkenazi A, Dixit VM. Death receptors: signaling and modulation. *Science*. 1998 Aug 28;281(5381):1305-8.
[36] Nagata S. Apoptotic DNA fragmentation. *Experimental cell research*. 2000 Apr 10;256(1):12-8.
[37] Vassalli P. The pathophysiology of tumor necrosis factors. *Annual review of immunology*. 1992 Apr;10(1):411-52.
[38] Golstein P, Kroemer G. Cell death by necrosis: towards a molecular definition. *Trends in biochemical sciences*. 2007 Jan 1;32(1):37-43.
[39] Di Nicolantonio F, Mercer SJ, Knight LA, Gabriel FG, Whitehouse PA, Sharma S, Fernando A, Glaysher S, Di Palma S, Johnson P, Somers SS. Cancer cell adaptation to chemotherapy. *BMC cancer*. 2005 Dec;5(1):1-6.
[40] Ebert AD, Yu J, Rose Jr FF, Mattis VB, Lorson CL, Thomson JA, Svendsen CN. Induced pluripotent stem cells from a spinal muscular atrophy patient. *Nature*. 2009 Jan 15;457(7227):277-80.
[41] Goldberg AL, Etlinger JD, Goldspink DF, Jablecki C. Mechanism of work-induced hypertrophy of skeletal muscle. *Medicine and science in sports*. 1975 Jan 1;7(3):185-98.
[42] Wennbo H, Kindblom J, Isaksson OG, Törnell J. Transgenic mice overexpressing the prolactin gene develop dramatic enlargement of the prostate gland. *Endocrinology*. 1997 Oct 1;138(10):4410-5.
[43] Malkinson FD, Keane JT. Radiobiology of the skin: review of some effects on epidermis and hair. *Journal of Investigative Dermatology*. 1981 Jul 1;77(1):133-8.

[44] Sklar LR, Almutawa F, Lim HW, Hamzavi I. Effects of ultraviolet radiation, visible light, and infrared radiation on erythema and pigmentation: a review. *Photochemical & Photobiological Sciences*. 2012 Jan;12:54-64.

[45] Ferreli C, Gasparini G, Parodi A, Cozzani E, Rongioletti F, Atzori L. Cutaneous manifestations of scleroderma and scleroderma-like disorders: a comprehensive review. *Clinical reviews in allergy & immunology*. 2017 Dec;53:306-36.

[46] Trotti A, Byhardt R, Stetz J, Gwede C, Corn B, Fu K, Gunderson L, McCormick B, Morris M, Rich T, Shipley W. Common toxicity criteria: version 2.0. an improved reference for grading the acute effects of cancer treatment: impact on radiotherapy. *International Journal of Radiation Oncology* Biology* Physics*. 2000 Apr 1;47(1):13-47.

[47] Molina JR, Yang P, Cassivi SD, Schild SE, Adjei AA. Non-small cell lung cancer: epidemiology, risk factors, treatment, and survivorship. In *Mayo clinic proceedings* 2008 May 1 (Vol. 83, No. 5, pp. 584-594). Elsevier.

[48] De Ruysscher D, Niedermann G, Burnet NG, Siva S, Lee AW, Hegi-Johnson F. *Radiotherapy toxicity. Nature Reviews Disease Primers*. 2019 Feb 21;5(1):13.

[49] Sroussi HY, Epstein JB, Bensadoun RJ, Saunders DP, Lalla RV, Migliorati CA, Heaivilin N, Zumsteg ZS. Common oral complications of head and neck cancer radiation therapy: mucositis, infections, saliva change, fibrosis, sensory dysfunctions, dental caries, periodontal disease, and osteoradionecrosis. *Cancer medicine*. 2017 Dec;6(12):2918-31.

[50] Hymes SR, Strom EA, Fife C. Radiation dermatitis: clinical presentation, pathophysiology, and treatment 2006. *Journal of the American Academy of Dermatology*. 2006 Jan 1;54(1):28-46.

[51] Jelinek JA, Stelzer KJ, Conrad E, Bruckner J, Kliot M, Koh WJ, Laramore GE. The efficacy of radiotherapy as postoperative treatment for desmoid tumors. *International Journal of Radiation Oncology* Biology* Physics*. 2001 May 1;50(1):121-5.

[52] Ferreira EB, Ciol MA, Vasques CI, Bontempo PD, Vieira NN, Silva LF, Avelino SR, Dos Santos MA, Dos Reis PE. Gel of chamomile vs. urea cream to prevent acute radiation dermatitis in patients with head and neck cancer: a randomized controlled trial. *Journal of advanced nursing*. 2016 Aug;72(8):1926-34.

[53] Farivar S, Malekshahabi T, Shiari R. Biological effects of low level laser therapy. *Journal of lasers in medical sciences*. 2014;5(2):58.

[54] Washko PW, Welch RW, Dhariwal KR, Wang Y, Levine M. Ascorbic acid and dehydroascorbic acid analyses in biological samples. *Analytical biochemistry*. 1992 Jul 1;204(1):1-4.

[55] Primavera G, Carrera M, Berardesca E, Pinnaró P, Messina MG, Arcangeli G. A double-blind, vehicle-controlled clinical study to evaluate the efficacy of MAS065D (Xclair™), a hyaluronic acid-based formulation, in the management of radiation-induced dermatitis. *Cutaneous and Ocular Toxicology*. 2006 Jan 1;25(3):165-71.

[56] Pinnix C, Perkins GH, Strom EA, Tereffe W, Woodward W, Oh JL, Arriaga L, Munsell MF, Kelly P, Hoffman KE, Smith BD. Topical hyaluronic acid vs. standard of care for the prevention of radiation dermatitis after adjuvant radiotherapy for breast cancer: single-blind randomized phase III clinical trial. *International Journal of Radiation Oncology* Biology* Physics*. 2012 Jul 15;83(4):1089-94.

[57] Kochhar R, Sriram PV, Sharma SC, Goel RC, Patel F. Natural history of late radiation proctosigmoiditis treated with topical sucralfate suspension. *Digestive diseases and sciences*. 1999 May;44:973-8.

[58] Wong RK, Bensadoun RJ, Boers-Doets CB, Bryce J, Chan A, Epstein JB, Eaby-Sandy B, Lacouture ME. Clinical practice guidelines for the prevention and treatment of acute and late radiation reactions from the MASCC Skin Toxicity Study Group. *Supportive Care in Cancer*. 2013 Oct;21:2933-48.

[59] Samlaska CP, Winfield EA. Pentoxifylline. *Journal of the American Academy of Dermatology*. 1994 Apr 1;30(4):603-21.

[60] Erdman L. Laughter therapy for patients with cancer. *Journal of Psychosocial Oncology*. 1993 Dec 30;11(4):55-67.

[61] Hymes SR, Strom EA, Fife C. Radiation dermatitis: clinical presentation, pathophysiology, and treatment 2006. *Journal of the American Academy of Dermatology*. 2006 Jan 1;54(1):28-46.

[62] DeLand MM, Weiss RA, McDaniel DH, Geronemus RG. Treatment of radiation-induced dermatitis with light-emitting diode (LED) photomodulation. *Lasers in Surgery and Medicine: The Official Journal of the American Society for Laser Medicine and Surgery*. 2007 Feb;39(2):164-8.
[63] Hanifin JM. Secular change in the occurrence of atopic dermatitis. Acta dermato-venereologica. *Supplementum.* 1992 Jan 1;176:7-12.
[64] Singh M, Alavi A, Wong R, Akita S. Radiodermatitis: a review of our current understanding. *American journal of clinical dermatology*. 2016 Jun;17:277-92.

Chapter 10

Late Radiation Effects on Normal Tissues and Associated Syndromes

Ashish Uke[1,*], MD
Suvarna Dangore[2], MDS
Swapnil Mohod[3], MDS, PhD
and Shweta Dahake[4], MSc

[1]Department of Radiation Oncology, Datta Meghe Institute of Higher Education and Research, Wardha, India
[2]Department of Oral Medicine and Radiology, Datta Meghe Institute of Higher Education and Research, Wardha, India
[3]Department of Dentistry, Dr. Panjabrao Bhausaheb Deshmukh Memorial Medical College, Amravati, India
[4]Department of Radio physics and Radio safety, Datta Meghe Institute of Higher Education and Research, Wardha, India

Abstract

Radiation therapy is a crucial component of cancer treatment, but it can also lead to various toxicities that affect the central nervous system (CNS), endocrine system, eyes, ears, lungs, esophagus, urinary bladder, and rectum. This comprehensive review aims to summarize the current knowledge on radiation-induced toxicities, their pathophysiology, and management strategies. Radiation-induced CNS toxicity can manifest as cognitive decline, dementia, and radiation necrosis. The risk of CNS toxicity increases with radiation dose and time after treatment. Corticosteroids are the mainstay of treatment for many radiation-induced CNS toxicities. Radiation therapy can damage the hypothalamic-pituitary axis, leading to endocrine disorders such as growth hormone deficiency, central hypothyroidism, and adrenal insufficiency. The risk of endocrine toxicity increases with radiation dose and time after treatment. Hormone replacement therapy is the standard treatment for endocrine deficiencies. Radiation therapy can cause eye toxicity, including cataracts, retinopathy, and optic neuropathy. The risk of eye toxicity increases with radiation dose and time after treatment. Artificial teardrops and lubricating agents can help manage dry eye symptoms. Radiation therapy can also cause ear toxicity, including otitis externa, hearing loss, and tinnitus. Radiation therapy can cause lung toxicity, including pneumonitis and fibrosis. The risk of lung toxicity increases with radiation dose and time after treatment. Corticosteroids and pentoxifylline can help manage lung

* Corresponding Author's Email: ashishuke1@gmail.com

In: Fundamentals of Radiation Biology
Editors: Anurag Luharia, Ashish Uke, Gaurav Mishra et al.
ISBN: 979-8-89530-806-6

toxicity. Radiation therapy can cause esophageal toxicity, including esophagitis and stricture. The risk of esophageal toxicity increases with radiation dose and time after treatment. Dietary modifications, antacids, and endoscopy with dilatation can help manage esophageal toxicity. Radiation therapy can cause urinary bladder toxicity, including hemorrhagic cystitis and bladder contracture. The risk of urinary bladder toxicity increases with radiation dose and time after treatment. Hyperbaric oxygen therapy, medications, and surgical interventions can help manage urinary bladder toxicity. Radiation therapy can cause rectal toxicity, including proctitis and rectal bleeding. The risk of rectal toxicity increases with radiation dose and time after treatment. Hyperbaric oxygen therapy, laser coagulation, and sucralfate can help manage rectal toxicity.

Keywords: late effects, neuroendocrine complications, organ-specific toxicity, radiation toxicity, radiation necrosis

10.1. Introduction

Radiation-induced normal tissue toxicities are a significant concern in cancer treatment, as they can affect various organs and tissues, including the central nervous system, endocrine system, eyes, ears, lungs, oesophagus, urinary bladder, and rectum. These toxicities can manifest as acute or late effects, ranging from mild to severe, and can impact the quality of life of cancer survivors. Despite advances in radiation therapy techniques, radiation-induced normal tissue toxicities remain a major challenge in oncology. Radiation-induced normal tissue toxicities can be attributed to the damage caused by ionizing radiation to the DNA of normal cells, leading to cell death, genetic mutations, and epigenetic changes. The risk of radiation-induced normal tissue toxicities increases with radiation dose, fractionation, and volume of tissue irradiated. Additionally, individual patient factors, such as age, comorbidities, and genetic predisposition, can also influence the risk of developing radiation-induced normal tissue toxicities. Radiation-induced normal tissue toxicities are attributed to the damage caused by ionizing radiation to the DNA of normal cells, leading to cell death, genetic mutations, and epigenetic changes. The risk of radiation-induced normal tissue toxicities increases with radiation dose, fractionation, and volume of tissue irradiated. Individual patient factors, such as age, comorbidities, and genetic predisposition, can also influence the risk of developing radiation-induced normal tissue toxicities. The management of radiation-induced normal tissue toxicities is complex and requires a multidisciplinary approach. Treatment options vary depending on the type and severity of the toxicity, and may include medications, surgery, and supportive care. Recent advances in radiation oncology, such as IMRT and SBRT, have improved the delivery of radiation therapy and reduced the risk of radiation-induced normal tissue toxicities. However, further research is needed to develop effective strategies for preventing and managing radiation-induced normal tissue toxicities.

10.2. Radiation Induced CNS Toxicity

Brain radiation induces late cognitive changes in the adult brain and precise evaluation of these changes is complicated by a number of factors. Many patients with disorders (brain metastases, malignant glioma) requiring brain Radiotherapy (RT) have a limited lifespan, and do not survive long enough to develop late neurocognitive changes, which can develop years after cranial RT. Surgery, chemotherapy, medications, and disease recurrence also cause neurotoxicity, further complicating the precise evaluation of radiation's contribution to cognitive deficits [1].

Radiation-induced dementia associated with diffuse leukoencephalopathy is characterized by depression, emotional liability, and deficits in memory and attention which progress to gait disturbance and incontinence in approximately 80% of patients. The only available therapy is supportive care, and the time to death after developing symptoms of radiation-induced dementia ranges from 1 month to 2 years [2].

Historically, brain radiation has been frequently cited as the major cause of neurocognitive decline in patients treated for metastases. One of the most misinterpreted studies on this subject is the Memorial Sloan-Kettering experience from DeAngelis et al. who reported an 11% risk of radiation- induced dementia in patients undergoing WBRT for brain metastasis [3].

Recent studies that have used sophisticated neurocognitive testing are clearly demonstrating that the brain tumor itself (presence, recurrence, and progression) has the greatest effect on neurocognitive decline. In the large phase III motexafin gadolinium study, the neurocognitive battery examined memory recall, memory recognition, delayed recall, verbal fluency, pegboard hand coordination, and executive function. This study demonstrated that 21–65.1% of patients had impaired functioning at baseline before treatment with WBRT (30Gy in 10 daily fractions) [4].

Patients frequently present to the radiation oncologist already started on prophylactic anticonvulsants. This represents one of the most preventable causes of neurocognitive decline in brain tumor patients. Anticonvulsants are clearly known to adversely affect quality of life and neurocognition. Based on four negative randomized trials, the American Academy of Neurology recommends that prophylactic anticonvulsants not be initiated in newly diagnosed brain tumor patients who have not experienced a seizure [5].

Radiation Necrosis is a serious complication post radiation therapy and it develops months to years after RT. Total dose and fraction size clearly predict for the development of radio necrosis. It is a focal, well-circumscribed lesion that develops in regions of the brain near the primary tumor that have received high doses of radiation. Necrosis is typically associated with focal neurologic deficits that correspond to the lesion's location. The lesion is frequently associated with significant cerebral edema, which precedes the development of radiation necrosis. oedema and accompanying breakdown of the Blood Brain Barrier increase parenchymal susceptibility to radiation necrosis by facilitating a cascade of local inflammatory mediators [6]. Following Table 10.1 describes the grading for CNS toxicity clinically and radiologically.

Table 10.1. LENT–SOMA grading criteria for CNS toxicity

Brain	Grade 1	Grade 2	Grade 3	Grade 4
Subjective signs				
Headache	Occasional, minimal	Intermittent, tolerable	Persistent, intense	Refractory, and excruciating
Somnolence	Occasional, able to work or perform normal activity	Intermittent, interferes with work or normal activity	Persistent, needs some assistance for self-care	Refractory, prevents daily activity, coma
Intellectual deficit	Minor loss of ability to reason and judge	Moderate loss of ability to reason and judge	Major loss of ability to reason and judge	Complete loss of ability to reason and judge
Functional competence	Perform complex tasks with minor	Connot Perform complex tasks	Cannot Perform complex tasks	Incapable of selfcare/ supervision, coma
Memory	Decreased short term, difficulty with learning	Decreased short term, loss of short term	Loss of short and long term	Complete disorientation
Objective signs				
Neurologic deficit	Barely detectable neurologic signs, able to perform normal activities	Easily detectable neurologic abnormalities, interferes with normal activities	Focal motor signs, disturbances in speech, vision, etc. interfering with daily activities	Hemiplegia, hemisensory deficit, aphasia, blindness, etc. requires continuous care, coma
Cognitive functions	Minor loss of memory, reason and/or judgement	Moderate loss of memory, reason and/or judgement	Major intellectual impairment	Complete memory loss and/or incapable of rational thought
Mood and personality changes	Occasional and minor	Intermittent and minor	Persistent and minor	Total disintegration
Seizures	Focal, without impairment of consciousness	Focal with impairment of consciousness	Generalised, tonioclinic or absence attack	Uncontrolled with loss of consciousness >10 mn
Management				
Headache, somnolence	Occasional nonnarcotic medication	Persistent nonnarcotic medication intermittent low dose steroids	Intermittent high dose steroids	Parental high dose steroids, mannitol and/or surgery
Seizures	Behavioural modification	Behavioural modification and occasional oral medication	Permanent oral medication	Intravenous anticonvulsive medication
Cognition, memory	Minor adaption	Psychosocial + educational intervention	Occupational and physiotherapy	Custodial care
Analytic				
MRI	Focal white matter changes; dystrophic cerebral calcification	White matter changes affecting <1 cerebral lobe; limited perilesional necrosis	Focal necrosis with mass effect	Pronounced white matter changes, mass effect requiring surgical interventional
CT	Assessment of swelling, oedema, atrophy			

10.3. Management of Nervous System Toxicity

Corticosteroids are the mainstay of treatment for many radiation-induced CNS toxicities, including radiation necrosis, cranial nerve palsy, and peripheral neuropathy. Treatment with corticosteroids often affords significant symptomatic benefit. It may also alter the pathophysiology of radio necrosis by reducing local oedema and interrupting local inflammatory cascades.

However, the side effects of steroids are manifold, including worsening diabetic hyperglycaemia, immunosuppression, loss of muscle mass, osteoporosis, peripheral oedema, weight gain, skin changes, and psychosis [7].

A variety of psychoactive drugs have been utilized to treat post-RT cognitive dysfunction. Methylphenidate, a stimulant used to treat attention deficit disorder, may improve psychomotor slowing and arousal in patients with lassitude or lethargy following radiation. Because vascular injury plays a key role in the pathogenesis of radiation injury to the brain, memantine is an attractive therapeutic agent. Bevacizumab, as described above, has the potential to modulate post-RT vascular pathology as well and is under active investigation [8].

10.4. Neuroendocrine Complications of Radiation

The Hypothalamo pituitary axis (HPA) is the primary interface between the nervous system and the endocrine system. The actions and interactions of the endocrine and nervous systems constitute the major regulatory mechanisms for virtually all physiologic activities. The hypothalamus has extensive neural communications with other brain regions and regulates brain functions including temperature, appetite, thirst, sexual behavior, and fear. The hypothalamus contains two types of neurosecretory cells (1) neurohypophysial neurons, which transverse the hypothalamic–pituitary stalk and release vasopressin and oxytocin from their nerve endings in the posterior pituitary, and (2) hypophysiotropic neurons, which release hormones into the portal hypophysial vessels to regulate the secretion of tropic hormones from the anterior pituitary. The six anterior pituitary hormones and their major hypothalamic regulatory factors [9]. Table 10.2 shows various hormones secreted by pituitary gland along with their hypothalamic factors.

Table 10.2. Pituitary hormones with their hypothalamic factors

Pituitary hormone	Hypothalamic factor
• Growth hormone (GH)	• GH- releasing hormone (GHRH)(+) somatostatin (-)
• Prolactin (PRL)	• Dopamine (-)
• Luteinizing hormone (LH) and follicle- stimulating hormone (FSH)	• Gonadotropin- releasing hormone (GnRH)(+)
• Thyroid- stimulating hormone (TSH)	• Thyrotropin- releasing hormone (TRH)(+)
• Adrenocorticotropin (ACTH)	• Corticotropin- releasing hormone (CRH)(+)

RT is a significant contributor to neuroendocrine complications commonly observed after treatment for CNS tumors and tumors of the head and neck when the hypothalamus is subtended by the irradiated volume. Constine et al. reported on the radiation dose associations and frequency of HPA injury (other than GH) that occurred after treatment of CNS tumors, and demonstrated that the hypothalamus was the most sensitive component of the axis. HPA is incidentally irradiated in the treatment of nasopharyngeal cancer, retinoblastoma, Hodgkin lymphoma with involvement of Waldeyer's ring, and pediatric sarcomas of the head and neck (e.g., parameningeal and orbital rhabdo- myosarcoma) [10].

Growth hormone deficiency is the first and most common side effect of cranial irradiation in brain tumor survivors. The risk increases with radiation dose and time after treatment. GHD is the earliest hormone deficiency and sensitive to low doses. Altered GH secretion is an important and well-documented cause of poor growth in childhood cancer survivors, particularly in young children after surgery in the suprasellar region, cranial irradiation (>18 Gy), or total body irradiation (>12 Gy) [11]. In most patients with GHD, the deficiency occurs in the levels of hypothalamic GHRH and somatostatin, with a resulting loss of the circadian pulsatile pattern of GH secretion. Patients with GHD, both children and adults, are at increased risk for additional endocrine deficiencies. Roughly 35% of patients presenting with isolated GHD will eventually develop other endocrine deficiencies [12]. Current data suggest that nearly all children treated with doses in excess of 35 Gy will develop GHD, which generally occurs within the first 5 years after treatment. Standard therapy for GHD is synthetic recombinant human GH. The usual dose of GH in children is 0.15–0.3 mg/kg per week divided into daily doses and administered subcutaneously in the evening [13]. The use and timing of GH replacement is an individual decision. Safety data has allowed us to administer GH earlier and gain time of exposure. When gain in height is critical, delay to GH affects final height. During GH therapy, evaluation of the growth response and adjustment of GH dose should occur every 4–6 months and include measurement of height, weight, and arm span. Arm span is a surrogate measure of height, particularly in patients in whom height measurement may not fully reflect body growth [14].

Central hypothyroidism refers to thyroid hormone deficiency caused by a disorder of the pituitary, hypothalamus, or hypothalamic-pituitary portal circulation. Central hypothyroidism in many survivors of childhood cancer is characterized by blunted or absent nocturnal TSH surge, suggesting the loss of normal circadian variation in TRH release. In cancer survivors, mixed hypothyroidism reflects separate injuries to the thyroid gland and the hypothalamus (e.g., radiation injury to both structures) [15]. Standard treatment for TSH deficiency or for primary hypothyroidism is levothyroxine replacement therapy. Thyroid hormone replacement can precipitate clinical decompensation in patients with unrecognized adrenal insufficiency, because levothyroxine treatment may improve metabolic clearance of cortisol. Thus, it is necessary to evaluate patients for adrenal insufficiency, and if present, treat the patient with hydrocortisone before initiating thyroid hormone therapy. The typical thyroid hormone replacement dose for infants under 3 years of age is 5–10 mcg/kg per mouth daily. For healthy children and adolescents with TSH less than 30 mU/L, the typical thyroid replacement dose is levothyroxine 3 mcg/kg per mouth every morning [16].

ACTH deficiency is less common than other neuroendocrine deficits but should be suspected in patients who have a history of brain tumor (regardless of therapy modality), cranial irradiation, GH deficiency, or central hypothyroidism. The symptoms of central adrenal insufficiency can be subtle and include poor weight gain, anorexia, easy fatigability, and poor stamina. In patients who have ACTH deficiency, as opposed to primary adrenal insufficiency, symptoms of salt craving, electrolyte imbalance, vitiligo, and hyperpigmentation usually are not observed [17]. Clinically apparent ACTH deficiency is distinctly uncommon in patients receiving HPA irradiation <50 Gy. Following doses <50 Gy, the reported incidence of ACTH deficiency varies from 18 to 35% during follow- up periods ranging from 5 to >15 years. Patients with ACTH insufficiency require daily hydrocortisone replacement. Hydrocortisone is the preferred agent for glucocorticoid replacement in children because it is least likely to impair growth. The dose of hydrocortisone for replacement therapy is 7–10 mg/m2 per day, divided into two or three doses administered by mouth [18].

High doses of cranial radiation (<30 Gy) are more likely to cause hypothalamic GnRH deficiency and, therefore, gonadotropin deficiency (or in some patient's precocious onset puberty through loss of inhibition that later progresses to gonadotropin deficiency through loss of GnRH secretory cells) [19]. Lower doses of cranial radiation (18–24 Gy) are more likely to cause damage to gamma-aminobutyric acid secreting neurons alone (leading to disinhibition and pre- mature activation of GnRH neurons) and therefore, rapid tempo of puberty or precocious puberty. Patients with gonadotropin deficiency may have delayed, interrupted, or absent puberty [20]. Detailed information on the threshold dose for LH/FSH deficiency are lacking. Nonetheless, it appears to be quite rare following HPA doses <40 Gy. There is a progressive increase in incidence as the dose to the HPA exceeds 50 Gy. Full hormone replacement in adolescent girls who have reached their adult height is easily achieved with regular use of a standard oral contraceptive (28-day pill packet) or an adult regimen of estrogen patches plus progesterone. Boys who have attained their adult height can be treated with testosterone (200 mg injected intramuscularly every 2 weeks) with androgen by patch, or by topical gel [21].

Hyperprolactinemia has been described in patients who have received doses of radiation larger than 50 Gy to the hypothalamus, or surgery disrupting the integrity of the pituitary stalk. Hyperprolactinemia may result in delayed puberty. In adult women, hyperprolactinemia may cause galactorrhoea, menstrual irregularities, loss of libido, hot flashes, infertility, and osteopenia; in adult men, impotence and loss of libido [22]. Dopamine agonists such as bromocriptine and cabergoline are the treatment of choice to suppress PRL secretion and to restore normal gonadal function. Cabergoline is, in general, more potent, much longer acting, and better tolerated than bromocriptine. The usual starting dose is 0.25 mg twice a week [23].

10.5. Eye and Orbit

Radiation can cause a number of insults to the eyelids including pigment changes, telangiectasia, madarosis (or eyelash loss), lymphedema, and architectural alterations to the eyelids and nasolacrimal system. Table 10.3 shows various radiation induced eye and orbit related toxicities. Hyperpigmentation may follow the acute stages of erythema within a year of treatment. number of lid deformities may result from higher doses of radiation in the range of 60–75 Gy, such as ectropion (out- turning of lid margin) or entropion (in-turning of lid margin). However, these complications are rare and seldom seen today [24]. Destruction or occlusion of the puncta may occur when the medial portions of the eyelid are irradiated. Radiation induced canaliculitis leads to fibrosis and obstruction. typically to the lateral one-third of the nasolacrimal system. Lacrimal gland dysfunction can lead to a dry eye and associated chronic symptoms such as pain, and may result in corneal ulceration and visual loss. Radiation effects to the conjunctiva may occur via direct damage or through secondary effects on the ocular surface. At 1–2 years post-treatment, prolonged conjunctival injection may develop, particularly at exposures of 30–50 Gy [25]. The avascular property of sclera renders it relatively radioresistant. The sclera is able to tolerate doses of radiation up to 900 Gy from an iodine or cobalt plaque when administered over 4–7 days. However, scleral atrophy and necrosis has been documented in irradiated eyes, and is most common following the use of brachy- therapy. Radiation can disrupt many of the key structures that produce these tear film elements, and place the eye at risk for ocular surface damage (or dry eyes) via a number of mechanisms [26]. For example, radiation induced atrophy of the lacrimal gland, which occurs at 50–60 Gy, causes a decrease in aqueous tear substance. Furthermore, atrophy of meibomian glands at doses less than 30 Gy and damage to conjunctival goblet cells (which also have low radiation tolerance) cause reductions in the lipid and mucin constituent of tears, respectively. Artificial teardrops replace lost tear volume, dilute toxic chemotherapeutic metabolites, provide lubrication and thereby aid in relieving conjunctival irritation [27].

Radiation can cause a number of insults to the eyelids including pigment changes, telangiectasia, madarosis (or eyelash loss), lymphedema, and architectural alterations to the eyelids and nasolacrimal system. Hyperpigmentation may follow the acute stages of erythema within a year of treatment. number of lid deformities may result from higher doses of radiation in the range of 60–75 Gy, such as ectropion (out- turning of lid margin) or entropion (in-turning of lid margin) [28]. However, these complications are rare and seldom seen today. Destruction or occlusion of the puncta may occur when the medial portions of the eyelid are irradiated. Radiation induced canaliculitis leads to fibrosis and obstruction. typically to the lateral one-third of the nasolacrimal system. Lacrimal gland dysfunction can lead to a dry eye and associated chronic symptoms such as pain, and may result in corneal ulceration and visual loss [29]. Radiation effects to the conjunctiva may occur via direct damage or through secondary effects on the ocular surface. At 1–2 years post-treatment, prolonged conjunctival injec- tion may develop, particularly at exposures of 30–50 Gy. The avascular property of sclera renders it relatively radioresistant. The sclera is able to tolerate doses of radiation up to 900 Gy from an iodine or cobalt plaque when administered over 4–7 days. However, scleral atrophy and necrosis has been documented in irradiated eyes, and is most common following the use of brachy- therapy [30]. Radiation can disrupt many of the key structures that produce these tear film elements, and place the eye at risk for ocular surface damage (or dry eyes) via a number of mechanisms. For example, radiation induced atrophy of the lacrimal gland, which occurs at 50–60 Gy, causes a decrease in aqueous tear substance. Furthermore, atrophy of meibomian glands at doses less than 30 Gy and damage to conjunctival goblet cells (which also have low radiation tolerance) cause reductions in the lipid and mucin constituent of tears, respectively. Artificial teardrops replace lost tear volume, dilute toxic chemotherapeutic metabolites, provide lubrication and thereby aid in relieving conjunctival irritation [31].

Table 10.3. LENT–SOMA grading criteria for eye and orbital toxicity

EYES	Grade 1	Grade 2	Grade 3	Grade 4
Subjective				
Vision	indistinct colour vision	Blurred vision, loss of colour vision	Severe loss of vision, symptomatic vision field defect with decrease in central vision, some ability to perform daily living activities	Blind, inability to perform daily living activities
Light sensitivity	Photophobia, no change in vision	Increased photophobia, decreased vision	Photophobia, major loss of vision	
Pain/dryness	Occasional & minimal	Intermittent and tolerable	Persistent and intense	Refractory and excruciating
Tearing	Occasional	Intermittent	Persistent	
Objective				
Best corrected vision	>20/40	20/50-20/200	<20/200 count fingers at 1 m	Cannot count fingers at 1m
Cornea	Increased tearing on exam	Non- infectious keratitis	Infectious keratitis, corneal ulcer	Panophthalmitis, corneal scar, ulceration leading to perforation/ loss of globe
Iris	Rubeosis only	Rubeosis increased intraocular pressure	Neovascular glaucoma with ability to count fingers at 1m	Neovascular glaucoma without ability to count fingers at 1m, complete blindness
Sclera	loss of episcleral vessels	≤50% scleral thinning	>50% scleral thinning	Scleral or periosteal graft required due to perforation
Optic nerve	Afferent pupillary defect with normal appearing nerve	≤1/4 pallor with asymptomatic visual field defect	>1/4 pallor or central scotoma	Profound optic atrophy, complete blindness
Lens	Asymmetric lenticular opacities, no visual loss	Moderate lenticular changes with mild- moderate visual loss	Moderate lenticular changes with severe visual loss	Severe lenticular changes
Retina	Microaneurysms, non-foveal exudates, minor vessel attenuation, extrafoveal pigment changes	Cotton wool spots	Massive macular exudation, focal retinal detachment	Opaque vitreous hemorrhage , complete retinal detachment, blindness
Facial bones	Cosmetically undetachable facial asymmetry	Minimal cosmetic asymmetry	Moderate orbital contracture	Severe hypoplasia of orbital bones

Cataract is a well-known complication following radiation to the eye. An association between cataract formation and exposure to ionizing radiation was first recognized in 1897. A single dose of 2 Gy or a cumulative dose of 5.5 Gy given over longer than 3 months was enough to induce cataract formation. Subsequent studies have reported a slightly higher threshold of single dose of 5 Gy or lower [32]. In brachytherapy, eyes treated with doses less than 12 Gy of iodine 125 have a significantly lower rate of cataract and cataract surgery compared with doses greater than 24 Gy [33]. Dose rate is another known risk factor that affects cataract formation. Low exposure rates, ranging from less than 0.035–0.06 Gy/min, may have significant sparing effect in the form of lower incidence of cataracts and cataract surgery. The Schipper's lens sparing retinoblastoma treatment method, which involves positioning the radiation beam to pass lateral to the orbits and beneath the lens posterior pole, has been shown to prevent radiation cataracts in patients with uveal metastases treated with external beam radiation (Bajcsay et al. 2003). Lens shielding is another effective method and has been described to decrease the total dose of radiation to the lens by as much as 50% [34].

In 1933, Stallard was the first to describe radiation retinopathy, and it has since been extensively described following external bean radiation, proton beam radiation and brachytherapy. Retinopathy may develop as early as 3 weeks and as late as 15 years post-treatment, although it typically develops between 6 months and 3 years. The prevalence of radiation retinopathy at 5 years following plaque brachytherapy is close to 50% [35]. The risk for retinopathy is reported at exposures as little as 15 Gy, although the threshold is regarded at 40–50 Gy and others have suggested the threshold is higher. Irradiation to tumors in proximity to the optic nerve, chiasm, and retrogeniculate visual pathways can cause optic neuropathy and vision loss. DNA exposure to radiation is thought to generate free radicals, which induce vascular endothelial damage and result in white matter injury. The range of the reported prevalence of optic neuropathy is broad at 11–57%. At exposures greater than 60 Gy, the fractioned dose becomes influential in optic nerve injury, with more risk for injury with larger daily fraction size [36].

10.6. Ototoxicity

Many inherent defence mechanisms are associated with the external ear, including hair follicles that help prevent gross contamination. Radiation leads to progressive obliteration of vascular channels, inflammation and scaling of ear canal skin, and loss of adnexal structures, including the cerumen-producing glands. Radiation-induced acute external ear reactions are enlisted with its grading in Table 10.4 involve skin reactions including erythema and dry or moist desquamation. The eustachian tube connects the middle ear cavity and the nasopharynx. Post-RT eustachian tube dysfunction in nasopharyngeal carcinoma patients is caused by both tumor obstruction and functional impairment of the tube. Radiation-induced inner ear morbidity may include damage to the labyrinth (cochlea, otolithic organs, and semicircular canals), cochlear or vestibular nerves, and central auditory and vestibular pathways [37].

Table 10.4. LENT SOMA Scoring System of the Ear

EAR	Grade 1	Grade 2	Grade 3	Grade 4
Subjective				
Pain	Occasional and minimal	Intermittent and tolerable	Persistent and intense	Refractory and excruciating
Tinnitus	Occasional	Intermittent	Persistent	Refractory
Hearing	Minor loss, no impairment in daily activities	Frequent difficulties with faint speech	Frequent difficulties with loud speech	Complete deafness
Objective				
Skin	Dry desquamation	Otitis externa	Superficial ulceration	Deep ulceration, necrosis, and osteochondritis
Hearing	<10 decibel loss in one or more frequencies	10-15 decibel loss in one or more frequencies	>15-20 decibel loss in one or more frequencies	>20 decibel loss in one or more frequencies
Management				
Pain	Occasional non- narcotic	Regular nonnarcotic	Regular narcotic	Parenteral narcotics
Skin	Occasional lubrication/ointment	Regular eardrop or antibiotics	Eardrums	Parenteral narcotics
Hearing loss			Hearing aid	
Analytic				
Pure tone audiometry	Assessment of characteristics of sensorineural perception			
Speech audiometry	Assessment of characteristics of speech perception			

Both acute and chronic otitis externa increased significantly (above 5% in each dose bin of 5 Gy) as the dose received by the external ear increased above 50 Gy. The incidence of atrophy and canal stenosis was reported to increase significantly above 55 Gy to the external auditory canal. Incidence of both acute and chronic otitis externa as well as atrophy and canal stenosis increased with increases in the radiation dose received by the external auditory canal. Treatment of inflammation or infection generally involves topical application of corticosteroids and antimicrobials directly to the ear canal. Mild to moderate otitis externa can be treated with the combination of aural toilet and topical therapy including acidifying agents, antiseptics, steroids, and antibiotics [38].

Patients with pre-RT middle-ear effusion have been shown to be seven times more likely to have long-term post-RT middle ear effusion. Incidence of tympanic membrane perforation and otitis media has been observed to increase (above 5% in each dose bin of 5 Gy) above a total dose of 50 Gy to the middle ear. The incidences of chorda tympani dysfunction, middle ear fibrosis, and mastoiditis increase above the dose of 60 Gy to the middle ear, indicating an increase in the incidence of otitis media with increases in the dose received by the middle ear. Vasoconstricting agents (i.e., nasal spray) may be used episodically to manage complications due to eustachian tube dysfunction and its resultant negative middle ear pressure [39].

In a review of nine studies, when averaged over all frequencies (0.5, 1, 2, and 4 kHz), the incidence of SNHL was 18 ± 2%. About one-third of patients receiving a dose of 70 Gy in 2 Gy per fraction in close proximity to the internal ear developed hearing loss of at least 10 dB or more in the high-frequency region of 4 kHz. Corticosteroids have been shown to improve inflammation and edema in the inner ear after noise-induced damage. Fibroatrophic changes, localhypoxia, impaired cellular proliferation, and decreased vascularity are the commonly exhibited characteristics of tissue subjected to high doses of radiation. While using Hyperbaric oxygen (HBO) to treat or prevent hearing loss may elicit potential benefits in theory, there have not been any randomized trials conducted [40].

10.7. Late Oral Adverse Effects

1. Common oral complications will be presented, including oral mucosal alterations (late-mucosal injury and cGVHD), taste disorders, salivary gland dysfunctions, infections, neuropathy and chronic pain, complications of the dentition and periodontium, trismus and loss of elasticity, osteoradionecrosis and osteonecrosis, developmental abnormalities and secondary malignancies. The prominent effects of cancer treatment on the oral mucosa are seen in the early period following treatment and results in oral mucositis. Once mucositis has developed, the oral mucosa is more susceptible to the toxic effects of a second cycle of RT or CT [41]. Patients post allogeneic HSCT may develop oral mucosal GVHD. GVHD is an alloimmune inflammatory process, which results from a donor-origin cellular response against host tissues. GVHD is one of the potential risk factors associated with the development of secondary solid cancers including those presenting in the head and neck area [42].
2. When the oral and pharyngeal mucosa is exposed to radiation, taste receptors are damaged and taste discrimination becomes increasingly compromised. After 3–4

weeks of radiation it is common for patients to complain of an absence of a sense of taste. It will generally take upwards of several months after the end of radiation therapy for taste receptors to recover and become functional, but it may require up to 2 years [43].

3. Long-term salivary gland dysfunction is a common com- plication of cancer treatment, predominantly in RT and in allogeneic HSCT patients. The RT-induced damage to the salivary gland results in a quantitative and qualitative change in saliva. Consequently, there is loss of salivary function, reduction in salivary flow and symptoms of dry mouth. The irradiated volume of salivary gland tissue correlates directly with the severity of oral complications [44]. With cumulative RT dose of 60–70 Gy, more irreversible extensive damage to salivary flow rate is detected. salivary gland impairment is reduced by using IMRT compared to traditional radiotherapy techniques (Rathod et al. 2013). A systematic review concluded that the benefits of IMRT on salivary gland function, xerostomia, and xerostomia-related QOL are most pronounced late (> 6 months) after radio- therapy and there are improvements in xerostomia-related QOL over time [45].
4. Viral, bacterial and fungal infections are common in cancer patients and may manifest years after cancer therapy. Candidal infection is the most prevalent oral fungal infection in cancer patients, either post-RT or post-CT. Herpes Simplex Virus (HSV) reactivation, is common in CT and HSCT patients but rarely occurs during radiation therapy. Bacterial infections are common during immunosuppression, which can persist or recur in patients post chemotherapy or HSCT [46].
5. Post radiation neuropathy (sensory or motor) is well documented following the treatment of head and neck cancers; the interval between treatment and onset ranges from 1 to 10 years, and radiation dosages from 62.5 to 100 Gy [47]. Radiation induced peripheral nerve injury may occur by at least 4 mechanisms: Direct damage to neural tissues by high dose irradiation is one mechanism observed in experimental animal models; Electron microscopy findings are suggestive of axon damage and subsequent nerve fiber loss due to radiation induced hypoxia as a mechanism of late radiation injury to the peripheral nerve. Radiation is also known to suppress proliferation of Schwann cells; and lastly, connective tissue fibrosis has been postulated to mediate neuropathy [48].
6. In the absence of effective preventive regimens, advanced dental caries is observed in patients with dry mouth. This is mostly seen in patients post RT or in patients suffering from GVHD of the salivary glands. This form of dental caries progress rapidly and is typically localized at the cervical aspects of the teeth. The periodontal impairment is manifested in increased probing depth, increased recession on the facial aspects and increased mobility of teeth [49]. This periodontal response to RT is probably due to decreased vascularity and acellularity of the periodontal membrane with rupturing, thickening, and disorientation of Sharpey's fibers and widening of the periodontal space. Trismus may be caused by fibrosis of the muscles of mastication after high-dose RT to the oral cavity or oropharynx. A systematic review of trismus in head and neck oncology showed that radiotherapy (follow-up: 6–12 months), involving the structures of the temporo- mandibular joint and or pterygoid muscles, reduces mouth opening by 18% [50].

7. Osteoradionecrosis (ORN) is a relatively uncommon clinical entity related to hypocellularity, hypovascularity, and ischemia, with a higher incidence after cumulative radiation doses to the bone which exceed 65 Gy. This process may be spontaneous, but it is usually related totrauma such as a tooth extraction and may progress to pathological fracture, infection of surrounding soft tissues,and severe pain. The risk of ORN does not diminish overtime and may even increase [51].
8. Secondary malignancies in the oral tissues have been reported, particularly in Post RT patients. The carcinogenic effect of ionizing radiation has long been recognized. The latent interval between RT and the development of cancer varies from several to many years. Early studies concluded that moderate or high-dose RT did not produce any new squamous cell carcinomas of the oral mucosa (Loprinzi et al. 2004) [52]. A later study showed contrary trends with radiation becoming a risk factor after10 years of follow-up for solid cancers of the oral cavity, pharynx, oesophagus, lung (2.8, 5.9, 3.9, 1.5 times fold than in the healthy population, respectively), and after 1–5 years of follow-up for second primary leukemia (2.5 times fold than in the healthy population) [53].

10.7.1. Lungs

- The lungs are particularly sensitive to RT, and are often the primary dose-limiting structure during thoracic therapy. Radiation injury of the lung is categorized as two distinct phases: acute inflammatory (pneumonitis) and late fibroproliferative. The progression of radiation injury is well established in both mice and humans. In humans, the pneumonitis phase peaks between 2–3 months after radiation exposure. This phase is characterized by a dense inflammatory cell infiltrate, exudation of proteinaceous material, and oedema. The chronic fibroproliferative phase occurs months to years after exposure and is characterized by diffuse interstitial fibrosis, focal scarring, and impaired ventilation [54]. The lung is considered to be a late responding tissue, as the time between exposure and symptomatic injury can last months to years, presumably as a result of innate tissue kinetics. The intercellular conversation is initiated at the moment of irradiation when injury to the cell membrane, DNA, cytoplasmic bodies, and other cell components occurs, resulting in an immediate release of cytokine mRNA [55].
- Coincident with the release of inflammatory cytokines is the development of oxidative stress. Free radical species can participate in a host of cellular signaling events. Indeed, many of the signaling pathways implicated in radiation injury, such as the TGF-b pathway, are sensitive to changes in cellular redox status. The transient nature of ionizing radiation suggests that a mechanism of amplification of ROS/RNS occurs after radiation. Proposed mechanisms include activation of oxidant-generating enzymes, such as NADPH oxidases, mitochondrial leakage, and the respiratory burst from activated inflammatory mediators recruited to the site of injury [56]. In the lung, chronic oxidative stress has been observed using markers for DNA oxidation. oxidative stress can contribute to a number of changes within injured tissue including endothelial cell activation, increased vascular permeability and edema, lipid

peroxidation, inflammation, and fibrosis imbalance between oxidant generating enzymes and antioxidant capacity is a primary cause of hypoperfusion following radiation [57].

- Radiation pneumonitis, typically manifested as shortness of breath, dry cough, and occasionally fever, occurring 1–6 months after treatment. bronchoalveolar lavage (BAL) following unilateral irradiation reveals increased lymphocytes from both the irradiated and unirradiated lung. In patients with symptomatic pneumonitis, physical exam is often normal, although rales or a friction rub can sometimes be appreciated. Radiological studies are often, but not always, abnormal. Thus, pneumonitis is a clinical diagnosis [58]. Radiographic abnormalities without symptoms usually do not warrant intervention. Indeed, asymptomatic patients' frequency has radiologic findings similar to those seen in symptomatic patients. Differentiating radiation pneumonitis from other etiologies (e.g., tumor progression, infection, pulmonary emboli, heart disease) can be challenging [59]. Ideally, one should be reasonably sure that symptoms suggestive of pneumonitis are not due to these other conditions before therapy is initiated. A short course of antibiotics is occasionally useful if there is concern for infection, with a rapid institution of steroids if symptoms do not respond. The culminating event in RT-induced lung injury is replacement of normal lung parenchyma with fibrosis, which is often appreciated on radiographic studies but is usually asymptomatic. In patients treated with high doses of radiation (e.g., >70 Gy), unusual pulmonary complications, such as bronchial stenosis, bronchopleural fistula, and fatal hemoptysis have been reported [60].
- Pulmonary function tests (PFTs) objectively assess multiple pulmonary parameters including lung volumes, the amount and rate of air flow (spirometry), and the ability of the lung to transfer gas at the alveolar level. Diffusing capacity of the lung for carbon monoxide (DLCO) is likely the best parameter to assess lung function after RT, since the ultimate role of the lungs is to facilitate gas exchange. Loss of alveolar surface area and thickening of the intraalveolar septi are the primary causes for reductions in DLCO. Thus, both acute (edema, extravasation of material into the alveoli) and chronic (fibrosis, loss of alveoli) injury can affect DLCO [61].
- Recent data suggest that the volume of lung exposed to relatively low doses of RT (e.g., 5–15 Gy) may be more predictive for pneumonitis than V20–30. This is particularly relevant when IMRT techniques are utilized or when patients with mesothelioma are treated after extrapleural pneumonectomy. Symptomatic bronchial stenosis has been observed with doses > 70 Gy, thus care should be taken when irradiating central structures to high doses [62].
- Several pharmacologic agents have been employed to mitigate the acute and chronic consequences of incidental RT on normal lung tissue (shift the NTCP curve). Amifostine and pentoxifylline have shown the most promising results [63].
- Amifostine (WR-2721; Ethyol, Medimmune Inc, Gaithersburg, MD), is a thio-organic pro-drug which is converted *in vivo* to the active free thiol (WR-1065) by vascular endothelial cell alkaline phosphatase. Amifostine is believed to scavenge harmful free radicals produced by the interaction of ionizing radiation and water molecules [64]. RTOG 9801 Explores the Role of the Radioprotector Amifostine in Locally Advanced Non-Small Cell Lung Cancer. The largest study was performed by

the RTOG (Movsas et al. 2005). The incidence of grade C3 esophagitis, the primary endpoint of the study, was 30% with amifostine versus 34% without ($p = 0.9$). The incidence of grade C3 pulmonary toxicity was lower inpatients receiving amifostine (9 vs. 16%), but this was not statistically significant. This study has been criticized since the drug was given once daily (4 days/week) and the RT was given twice daily (5 days/week), and thus 60% of the RT fractions were delivered without the protector [65].

- Pentoxifylline (Trental, sanofi aventis, Bridgewater, NJ) is an ethyl xanthine derivative with immunomodulating and anti-inflammatory activity. It is primarily prescribed for patients with intermittent claudication secondary to its ability to improve erythrocyte flexibility. pentoxifylline did not mitigate acute decline in lung per-fusion after single fraction RT in rats. However, it did seem to facilitate late recovery in perfusion compared to rats receiving RT alone. In contrast, Stelzer et al. (1996) showed that rats receiving pentoxifylline maintained higher perfusion ratios than irradiated controls during weeks 3–5 [66].
- The traditional treatment for acute pneumonitis is oral steroids, typically prednisone. We recommend oral prednisone (Salinas and Winterbauer 1995), typically 40–60 mg daily for 1–2 weeks, followed by a slow taper (reducing to 10 mg every 1–2 weeks). It must be remembered that there is a differential diagnosis for shortness of breath occurring after RT. This includes tumor progression, drug toxicity, cardiac disease, pulmonary embolus, anemia, and infection. Since steroids can exacerbate an infection, an initial short course of antibiotics may be considered [67].

10.7.2. Esophagus

Clinical RT-induced esophageal injury that has been often divided into two phases: the acute phase, associated with mucosal damage, and the late phase, associated with harm to the muscular wall. There is significant overlap between the two phases, and the strong predictive association between the severity of acute esophagitis and the development of late toxicity. The acute effects of RT on the esophagus are related primarily to damage of the basal epithelial layer, and late effects are associated with RT-induced changes in the submucosa and muscular tissue of the esophageal wall. The basal cell layer may be considered the target for acute RT-induced esophagitis, as this is the region of rapid mitosis and multiplication. Although regeneration of the esophageal mucosal epithelium starts during RT, this period may also include the start of progression toward fibrosis of the esophageal wall. During the subacute period after RT, subepithelial fibrosis may become apparent [68]. The chronic period may be viewed as a continual progression of pathologic changes observed during the subacute period, with increased thickening of the esophageal wall [69].

Table 10.5. LENT SOMA Scoring System of the esophagus

	Grade 1	Grade 2	Grade 3	Grade 4
Subjective				
Dysphagia	Difficulty eating solid foods	Difficulty eating soft foods	Can take liquids only	Totally unable to swallow
Pain	Occasional & minimal	Intermittent & tolerable	Persistent & intense	Refractory & excruciating
Objective				
Weight loss from time of treatment	≥5-10%	>10-20%	>20-30%	>30%
Stricture	>2/3 normal diameter with dilatation	>1/3 – 2/3 normal diameter with dilatation	<1/3 normal diameter	Complete obstruction
Ulceration	Superficial ≤ 1 cm^2	Superficial > 1 cm2	Deep ulcer	Perforation, fistulae
Bleeding (melena or haematemesis)	Occult	Occasional, normal Hb	Intermittent, 10-20% decrease in Hb	Persistent, >20% decrease in Hb
Anaemia		Fatigue	Exhaustion	
Management				
Dysphagia/stricture	Diet modification or antacids	Diet modification and occasional dilatation	Temporary NG tube or regularly dilatation	Parenteral feeding, prosthesis, gastrostomy or permanent NG tube
Weight loss	Diet modification	Nutritional supplement	Tube feeding	Surgical bypass, PEG
Pain/ulceration	Occasional non- narcotic	Regular non- narcotic	Regular narcotic	Surgical interventional
Analytical				
Barium esophagram	Assessment of esophageal lumen, stricture, dilatation			
Endoscopy	Assessment of esophageal lumen, mucosal integrity, ulceration			
CT	Assessment of esophageal wall thickness, lumen, stricture, dilatation			
MRI	Assessment of esophageal wall thickness lumen, stricture, dilatation			
Ultrasonography	Assessment of esophageal wall thickness lumen, stricture, dilatation			
Mobility esophagram	Assessment of motility of bolus and peristalsis			
Electromyogram	Assessment of motility of bolus and peristalsis			

Rates of late esophageal complications after RT have been associated with RT dose, with evidence of a relatively-steep dose–response curve. In their seminal publication of estimated normal tissue dose limits, Rubin and Emami, Lymen, et al. suggested that the doses for whole-esophagus RT that result in a 5 and a 50% rate of stricture or perforation at 5 years are 55 and 68 Gy, respectively, in standard fractionation [70]. Maguire et al. evaluated the associations among incidence of late toxicity with the esophageal volume or surface area exposed to RT doses above 50, 60, and 70 Gy. In their series of NSCLC patients published in 1999, both the volume and the surface area of esophagus receiving>50 Gy (but not >60 or >70 Gy) were significant predictors of late esophageal toxicity [71]. RT plans that delivered 50 Gy or higher to more than 32% of the esophageal volume or surface area resulted in a threefold higher rate of late esophagitis. Lengths >3.2 cm of full-circum-ference irradiated to beyond 50 Gy were associated with a threefold higher risk of late esophagitis [72].

Medical management of acute esophagitis centers uponsupportive care with pain relief and nutritional supple-mentation. Topical anesthetics, opiate analgesics, sucralfate, antacids, prokinetic agents, H2-blockers, proton-pump inhibitors, and antifungal medications are commonly prescribed [73].

Dietary recommendations typically consist of a bland diet of soft foods, with avoidance of spicy, hot or cold foods, as well as tobacco and alcohol. A liquid mixture (''Magic Mouthwash'') commonly used in the radiation oncology clinic is composed of viscous lidocaine (2%), benadryl elixir, saline, and baking soda. This may be used liberally by patients to ease swallowing, particularly around meal time. In general, it is recommended that RT is interrupted after the development of grade 4 esophagitis and is not resumed until esophagitis returns to grade 2 or less. After sufficient time for healing, most cases of acute esophagitis resolve without development of chronic effects [74].

The principal management approach for late esophageal stricture after RT is endoscopy with dilatation. Esophageal dilatation is generally successful at improving patients' symptoms from esophageal stricture. When dilatations are required, the median number of dilatations performed in 2.5 per patient at a median interprocedural interval of 5 months. Dilatation is associated with a small risk of perforation or bleeding, around 0.3%, and this rate may increase with complex strictures [75].

10.7.3. Urinary Bladder

Considering Marks' proposed functional subunit of the bladder, possible targets of radiation-induced damage include the epithelial cell layer, detrusor muscles, nerves, and microvasculature. The bladder responds to radiation injury and other stressors with inflammation, tissue reorganization, and cellular proliferation. Early changes and signs of damage including nuclear irregularity, cellular edema, and increased lysosomes and autophagic vacuoles in intermediate and basal urothelial cells, are seen approximately 3 months after irradiation [76]. By 12 months, there is a dose-dependent increase in cellular proliferation and normal differentiation may be lost in many areas. Radiation injury of the epithelium disrupts the normal tight junctions between urothelial cells and the protective polysaccharide layer, which allows hypertonic urine, toxins, ions, and bacteria to penetrate into the underlying tissue. The resultant damage and inflammation may lead to the onset of early radiation-induced symptoms [77]. Various kind of urinary bladder toxicties and their gradings are enlisted in Table 10.6. Similarly, Endothelial cell edema is observed 3 months after radiation, and endothelial proliferation is identified >6 months after radiation, but does not occur to the same degree as seen in the urothelium. Subsequent late tissue remodelling includes fibroblast proliferation, collagen disposition, and progressive fibrosis, which can lead to decreased bladder compliance, functional restriction of bladder capacity, and bladder contracture [78]. Extensive fibrosis can disrupt/replace the normal musculature. Irreversible, late reduction in bladder compliance occurred at variable time intervals after treatment, and is consistent with clinical contracted bladder syndrome. Early signs of damage, including increase in urinary frequency and decrease in bladder volume, occurred 1–3 weeks after radiation, and typically lasted for less than 1 week. Late toxicity developed 16–40 weeks after fractionated treatment with total doses greater than or equal to 20 Gy, and was typically irreversible [79]. Microscopically, the early, transient damage was not associated with changes in the epithelium or muscle layers of the bladder, but the irreversible late damage was accompanied by epithelial denudation, focal hyperplasia, fibrosis, and ulceration [80]. Late injury is manifested mainly as bladder wall fibrosis, loss of bladder wall compliance and contraction. The existing evidence to date points toward vascular ischemia as the underlying pathophysiology behind these changes, and thus, the vascular endothelial cell has been proposed as the actual target for late radiation-induced bladder injury [81]. endothelial cell injury and remodeling occur months to many years following radiation therapy, while acute epithelial cell injuries do not appear to be correlated with the development of late toxicity. The development of secondary malignancy of the bladder may have a very long latency period with bladder tumors observed as long as 10 years after radiation for ovarian cancer and 20 years after radiation for cervical cancer, which underscores the need for long-term follow-up and a high index of suspicion for secondary malignancy in patients presenting with hematuria after radiation therapy [82]. Most of the data for secondary bladder malignancy after pelvic radiation therapy comes from retrospective series. Duncan et al. observed 8 secondary bladder malignancies in 2,674 patients treated with radiation for cervical cancer, which despite the low total number of cases, represents an incidence rate of 57.6 times that of the general female population [83].

Patient-related risk factors for bladder injury include a history of chronic urinary infections, incontinence, or cystitis. A history of diabetes can exacerbate bladder infections, result in poor wound healing, and increase the likelihood of chronic infections. Patients with portal hypertension may have a high rate of hematuria as do patients medicated with warfarin or other anticoagulation medication [84].

Bladder radiation with respect to dose has been extensively studied and it suggested that it may arise either from whole organ radiation (global injury), such as in treatment to the male or female pelvis, though this is usually to a more limited dose (40–50 Gy), or from higher doses to a small field resulting in focal injury, such as in cone down volumes for bladder cancer (approximately 65 Gy) or prostate cancer (>70 Gy) [85]. Brachytherapy results in significantly higher doses to the bladder than that administered by external beam alone (>75 Gy), but the volumes of bladder exposed to these high doses are much smaller. Marks et al. estimated a clinical complication rate of approx. 5–10% with a whole bladder dose of 50 Gy, and higher complication rates with doses of 50–65 Gy. Irradiation of approximately one-third to half of the bladder volume to a dose of 50–65 Gy resulted in about 5–10% complication rates. Irradiation of smaller portions of the bladder (<20%) to higher doses of 65–75 Gy resulted in late tox- icity in 5–10% of patients [86].

Table 10.6. LENT SOMA scoring system of the urinary bladder

Urinary bladder	Grade 1	Grade 2	Grade 3	Grade 4
Subjective				
Dysuria	Occasional and minimal	Intermittent and tolerable	persistent and intense	Refractory and excruciating
Frequency	3-4 hr intervals	2-3 hr interval	1-2 hr interval	Hourly
Haematuria	Occasional	Intermittent	Persistent with clot	Refractory
Incontinence	<weekly episodes	<daily episodes	$\leq$2 pads/undergarments/day	Refractory
Decreased stream	Occasionally weak	Intermittent	Persistent but incomplete obstruction	Complete obstructions
Objective				
Haematuria	Microscopic, normal haemoglobin	Intermittent macroscopic, <10% decrease in haemoglobin	Persistent macroscopic, 10-20% decrease in haemoglobin	Refractory, >20% decrease in haemoglobin
Endoscopy	Patchy atrophy or telangiectasia without bleeding	Confluent atrophy or telangiectasia with gross bleeding	Ulcerations into muscle	Perforation, fistula
Maximum volume	>300-400 cc	>200-300 cc	>100-200 cc	<100 cc
Residual volume	25cc	>25-100 cc	>100 cc	
Management				
Dysuria	Occasional non- narcotic	Regular non – narcotic	Regular narcotic	Surgical intervention
Frequency	Alkalization	Occasional antispasmodic	Regular narcotic	Surgical interventional
Haematuria/ telangiectasia	Iron therapy	Occasional transfusion or single cauterization	Frequent transfusion or coagulation	Surgical intervention
Incontinence	Occasional use of incontinence pads	Intermittent use of incontinence pads	Regular use of pads or self-catheterization	Permanent catheter
Decreased stream		<once-a-day self- catheterization	Dilation, >once-a day self-catheterization	Permanent catheter, surgical intervention

Table 10.7. LENT SOMA scoring system of the rectum

	Grade 1	Grade 2	Grade 3	Grade 4
Subjective				
Tenesmus	Occasional urgency	Intermittent urgency	Persistent urgency	Refractory
Mucosal loss	Occasional	Intermittent	Persistent	Refractory
Sphincter control	Occasional	Intermittent	Persistent	Refractory
Stool frequency	2-4/day	4-8/day	>8/day	Uncontrolled diarrhea
Pain	Occasional & minimal	Intermittent & tolerable	Persistent & intense	Refractory & excruciating
Objective				
Bleeding	Occult	Occasionally >2/week	Persistent/daily	Gross haemorrhage
Ulceration	Superficial ≥1cm2	Deep ulcer	Perforation, fistulae	
Stricture	>2/3 normal diameter with dilatation	1/3-2/3 normal diameter with dilatation	<1/3 normal diameter	Complete obstruction
Management				
Tenesmus & stool frequency	Occasionally, ≥2 antidiarrheals/week	Regular, >2 antidiarrheals/week	Multiple, >2 antidiarrheals/day	Surgical intervention/ permanent colostomy
Pain	Occasional non- narcotic	Regular non-narcotic	Regular narcotic	Surgical intervention
Bleeding	Stool, softener, iron therapy	Occasional transfusion	Frequent transfusions	Surgical intervention/ permanent colostomy
Ulceration	Diet modification, stool softener	Occasional dilatation	Steroid per enema, hyperbaric oxygen	Surgical intervention/ permanent colostomy
Sphincter control	Occasional use of incontinence pads	Intermittent use of incontinence pads	Persistent use of incontinence pads	Surgical intervention/ permanent colostomy
Analytic				
Barium enema	Assessment of lumen and peristalsis			
Proctoscopy	Assessment of lumen and mucosal surface			
CT	Assessment of wall thickness, sinus, and fistula formation			
MRI	Assessment of wall thickness, sinus, and fistula formation			
Anal manometry	Assessment rectal compliance			
Ultrasound	Assessment of wall thickness, sinus, and fistula formation			

Patients with mild hemorrhagic cystitis can be managed with increased hydration, while persistent bleeding may be medically managed with hyperbaric oxygen, medications such as conjugated estrogens, sodium pentosan polysulfate, or recombinant factor VII. In patients who do not respond to medical management, or with severe hemorrhage resulting in urinary retention, cystoscopy with clot removal, and selective cauterization of bleeding vessels or instillation of alum, silver nitrate or dilute formalin may be helpful. In the relatively rare patients with persistent, recurrent, or severe hemorrhage, more invasive procedures including vesical artery embolization, bladder diversion, or cystectomy and reconstruction may be necessary [87].

Decreased bladder compliance and capacity as a result of fibrosis may eventually cause hydronephrosis and kidney damage, and requires intervention. Initial medical management includes antimuscarinic medications, which may improve bladder compliance via smooth muscle relaxation [88].

10.8. Radiation Induced Rectal Toxicities

Early radiation-induced rectal damage includes mucosal cell loss, acute inflammation in the lamina propria, eosinophilic crypt abscesses, and endothelial swelling in the arterioles which may progress to fibrosis of connective tissue and endarteritis of the arterioles resulting in rectal tissue ischemia, mucosal friability, bleeding, ulcers, strictures, and fistulae. Late rectal toxicity is manifested by a progressive vasculitis leading to thrombosis of small arteries and arterioles resulting in varying degrees of ischemia of the bowel wall [89]. Rectal toxicities along with their gradings are enlisted in Table 10.7.

A four-stage model has been proposed by Sonis to describe the development of radiation-induced mucositis. The four stages are initiation, upregulation, amplification/signalling, and finally ulceration. Although acute rectal toxicity of diarrhoea and frequent stooling can be distressing to a patient while undergoing treatment, it is the late effects of radiation that are most problematic clinically, especially in a patient cured of their cancer [90].

Two of the most important factors in the development of fecal incontinence are connective tissue remodelling of the rectum and diminished neural function of the continence organ. Smooth muscle hypertrophy and myenteric plexus damage may contribute to the reduction in rectal volumes at sensory threshold, constant sensation and maximal tolerance, and in rectal compliance. Chronic radiation proctitis typically occur anywhere from 8 to 13 months after completion of treatment. Bleeding is the most common symptom of chronic radiation proctitis compared to acute radiation proctitis where bleeding is relatively uncommon [91]. Other symptoms of chronic radiation proctitis include mucous discharge, urgency, fecal incontinence, diarrhoea, and pain. Constipation can occur in the presence of a stricture most notably in the sigmoid colon region usually occurring as a result of an intracavitary implant in the treatment of cervical cancer or endometrial cancer. Fibrosis can also be seen following RT [92].

An evidence-based review of the available literature found three-dimensional conformal radiation (3-DCRT) reduced late GI toxicity in patients with prostate cancer, compared to conventional radiation. Intensity modulated radiation therapy appears to further reduce the incidence of radiation-induced late rectal toxicity [93]. Zelefsky et al. reported that IMRT significantly reduced the risk of gastrointestinal toxicity compared to patients treated with 3-D CRT despite the use of higher doses in the IMRT group. More recently, proton beam radiotherapy has been investigated as a means to reduce toxicity in patients receiving radiotherapy for pros- tate cancer. Rectal wall volumes receiving 10–80 Gray Equivalents (GE) were significantly reduced with proton beam therapy compared to IMRT. Endorectal balloons (ERB) have also been found to reduce late rectal mucosal changes detected after 3-D CRT and IMRT [94].

Amifostine, a thiol derivative, acts as a free radical scav- enger with its sulfhydryl compound. Intrarectal amifostine (WR 2721) reduces rectal toxicity in patients undergoing radiotherapy for prostate and gynecologic malignancies. In patients receiving RT for prostate cancer, the addition of 1500 mg of amifostine in a 40-ml aqueous enema solution reduced late rectal toxicity compared to patients who did not receive the amifostine. Sucralfate is a nonabsorbable basic aluminum salt used to treat gastric ulcers and it appears to reduce microvascular injury by stimulating angiogenesis. Since late radiation injury may be mediated by the microvasculature, sucralfate was hypothesized to potentially prevent late radiation change. Misoprostol is a prostaglandin E1 analog that has been used in the treatment and prevention of nonsteroidal anti- inflammatory agent-induced gastric and duodenal ulcers [95].

Management of radiation induced proctitis includes hyperbaric oxygen therapy, laser coagulation, sucralfate and vitamins. Approximately 21 studies evaluating the use of hyperbaric oxygen have been published to date. The atmospheres absolute ranged between 2.0–2.5 with the majority of dives lasting 90 min. Treatment sessions ranged from 3 to 80 with a reported overall improvement of 25–100% [96].

Argon laser therapy has been used to alleviate the symptoms of rectal bleeding in patients suffering from radiation proctitis. Most reports note that patients either improve or have few recurrences of bleeding. The oxidative stress of radiation on the rectum has been thought to play a part in the development of radiation proctitis so it has been hypothesized antioxidants such as vitamins C and E could be used in the treatment of radiation proctitis. Twenty patients with prostate or gynecologic malignancies treated with radiation and experiencing symptoms were given a combination of 400 IU of vitamin E TID and 500 mg of vitamin C TID. A significant reduction in the symptom index for bleeding, diarrhea, and urgency was noted compared prior to treatment. Pain, however was not improved with vitamin treatment [97].

Conclusion

This chapter offered a comprehensive overview of the late effects of radiation therapy on various organs and systems, including the brain, endocrine glands, eyes, ears, lungs, esophagus, urinary bladder, and rectum. It detailed the mechanisms of radiation-induced damage, highlighting how factors such as cumulative dose, fractionation, and individual susceptibility contribute to the risk of chronic toxicity. The text emphasized that late complications, ranging from cognitive decline and hormone deficiencies to fibrosis, necrosis, and secondary malignancies, can significantly impact long-term quality of life for cancer survivors. Management requires multidisciplinary strategies that combine preventive measures, supportive care, medical treatments, and in some cases, surgical interventions. By understanding these delayed effects, clinicians can better balance the benefits of radiation therapy against its long-term risks and tailor treatment plans to improve patient outcomes.

References

[1] Cramer CK, Cummings TL, Andrews RN, Strowd R, Rapp SR, Shaw EG, Chan MD, Lesser GJ. Treatment of radiation-induced cognitive decline in adult brain tumor patients. *Current treatment options in oncology*. 2019 May;20:1-6.

[2] Greene-Schloesser D, Robbins ME, Peiffer AM, Shaw EG, Wheeler KT, Chan MD. Radiation-induced brain injury: a review. *Frontiers in oncology*. 2012 Jul 19;2:73.

[3] DeAngelis LM, Delattre JY, Posner JB. Radiation-induced dementia in patients cured of brain metastases. *Neurology*. 1989 Jun;39(6):789-.

[4] Thomas SR, Khuntia D. Motexafin gadolinium injection for the treatment of brain metastases in patients with non-small cell lung cancer. *International journal of nanomedicine*. 2007 Dec 1;2(1):79-87.

[5] Tohidinezhad F, Di Perri D, Zegers CM, Dijkstra J, Anten M, Dekker A, Van Elmpt W, Eekers DB, Traverso A. Prediction models for radiation-induced neurocognitive decline in adult patients with primary or secondary brain tumors: A systematic review. *Frontiers in psychology*. 2022 Mar 31;13:853472.

[6] MIyatake SI, NoNoguchI N, FuruSe M, Yoritsune E, Miyata T, Kawabata S, Kuroiwa T. Pathophysiology, diagnosis, and treatment of radiation necrosis in the brain. *Neurologia medico-chirurgica*. 2015;55(1):50-9.

[7] Smart D. Radiation toxicity in the central nervous system: mechanisms and strategies for injury reduction. In *Seminars in radiation oncology* 2017 Oct 1 (Vol. 27, No. 4, pp. 332-339). WB Saunders.

[8] Garcia J, Hurwitz HI, Sandler AB, Miles D, Coleman RL, Deurloo R, Chinot OL. Bevacizumab (Avastin®) in cancer treatment: A review of 15 years of clinical experience and future outlook. *Cancer treatment reviews*. 2020 Jun 1;86:102017.

[9] Herman JP, McKlveen JM, Ghosal S, Kopp B, Wulsin A, Makinson R, Scheimann J, Myers B. Regulation of the hypothalamic-pituitary-adrenocortical stress response. *Comprehensive physiology*. 2016;6(2):603.

[10] Lövgren I, Abravan A, Bryce-Atkinson A, Van Herk M. The late effects of cranial irradiation in childhood on the hypothalamic–pituitary axis: a radiotherapist's perspective. *Endocrine Connections*. 2022 Dec 1;11(12).

[11] Merchant TE, Rose SR, Bosley C, Wu S, Xiong X, Lustig RH. Growth hormone secretion after conformal radiation therapy in pediatric patients with localized brain tumors. *Journal of Clinical Oncology*. 2011 Dec 20;29(36):4776-80.

[12] Ayuk J, Sheppard MC. Growth hormone and its disorders. *Postgraduate medical journal*. 2006 Jan;82(963):24-30.

[13] Feldt-Rasmussen U, Klose M. *Adult growth hormone deficiency-clinical management*.

[14] Molitch ME, Clemmons DR, Malozowski S, Merriam GR, Vance ML. Evaluation and treatment of adult growth hormone deficiency: an Endocrine Society clinical practice guideline. *The Journal of Clinical Endocrinology & Metabolism*. 2011 Jun 1;96(6):1587-609.

[15] Gupta V, Lee M. Central hypothyroidism. *Indian journal of endocrinology and metabolism*. 2011 Jul 1;15(Suppl2):S99-106.

[16] Jonklaas J, Bianco AC, Bauer AJ, Burman KD, Cappola AR, Celi FS, Cooper DS, Kim BW, Peeters RP, Rosenthal MS, Sawka AM. Guidelines for the treatment of hypothyroidism: prepared by the american thyroid association task force on thyroid hormone replacement. *Thyroid*. 2014 Dec 1;24(12):1670-751.

[17] Sklar CA, Antal Z, Chemaitilly W, Cohen LE, Follin C, Meacham LR, Murad MH. Hypothalamic–pituitary and growth disorders in survivors of childhood cancer: an Endocrine Society clinical practice guideline. *The Journal of Clinical Endocrinology & Metabolism*. 2018 Aug;103(8):2761-84.

[18] Lin SH, Zhang A, Li LZ, Zhao LC, Wu LX, Fang CT. Isolated adrenocorticotropic hormone deficiency associated with sintilimab therapy in a patient with advanced lung adenocarcinoma: a case report and literature review. *BMC Endocrine Disorders*. 2022 Sep 24;22(1):239.

[19] Roth C, Lakomek M, Schmidberger H, Jarry H. Schädelbestrahlung verursacht vorzeitige Aktivierung des Gonadotropin-Releasinghormon (GnRH)-Pulsgenerators bei Ratten-Ein neuesTiermodell für strahleninduzierte Störungen der Pubertät. *Klinische Pädiatrie*. 2001 Aug;213(04):239-43.

[20] Pekic S, Miljic D, Popovic V. Hypopituitarism following cranial radiotherapy.

[21] Vakilian S, Thébaut J, Ruo R, Marcovitz S, Panet-Raymond V, Shenouda G, Sultanem K, Souhami L. Examination of the dose-effect relationship of radiation-induced hypopituitarism: results of a case-control study. *Advances in Radiation Oncology*. 2021 Jul 1;6(4):100693.

[22] Thapa S, Bhusal K. *Hyperprolactinemia*.[Updated 2021 Jul 26]. StatPearls [Internet]. Treasure Island (FL): StatPearls Publishing; 2021Jan-. Availablefrom: https://www. ncbi. nlm. nih. gov/books/NBK537331. 2023.

[23] Verhelst J, Abs R, Maiter D, Van Den Bruel A, Vandeweghe M, Velkeniers B, Mockel J, Lamberigts G, Petrossians P, Coremans P, Mahler C. Cabergoline in the treatment of hyperprolactinemia: a study in 455 patients. *The Journal of Clinical Endocrinology & Metabolism*. 1999 Jul 1;84(7):2518-22.

[24] Nuzzi R, Trossarello M, Bartoncini S, Marolo P, Franco P, Mantovani C, Ricardi U. Ocular complications after radiation therapy: an observational study. *Clinical Ophthalmology*. 2020 Oct 9:3153-66.

[25] Fang X, Lan G, Lin Y, Xie Z, Zhong Y, Luo S, Xiao X, Luo L, Zhang Y, Li H, Wu H. Inflammation due to ocular surface homeostasis imbalance caused by pterygia: tear lymphotoxin-alpha study and a literature review. *Journal of Ophthalmic Inflammation and Infection*. 2024 Jun 14;14(1):28.

[26] Berry DE, Grewal DS, Mruthyunjaya P. Conjunctival dehiscence and scleral necrosis following iodine-125 plaque brachytherapy for uveal melanoma: a report of 3 cases. *Ocular oncology and pathology*. 2018 Sep 6;4(5):291-6.

[27] Chen X, Badian RA, Hynne H, Amdal CD, Herlofson BB, Utheim ØA, Westgaard KL, Fineide F, Jensen JL, Utheim TP. Alterations in meibomian glands in patients treated with intensity-modulated radiotherapy for head and neck cancer. *Scientific Reports*. 2021 Nov 17;11(1):22419.

[28] Singh AD, Damato B. *Clinical Ophthalmic Oncology Basic Principles and Diagnostic Techniques*.

[29] Ducker L, Rivera RY. Anatomy, Head and Neck: Eye Lacrimal Duct. In *StatPearls* [Internet] 2023 Aug 8. StatPearls Publishing.

[30] Akagunduz OO, Yilmaz SG, Tavlayan E, Baris ME, Afrashi F, Esassolak M. Radiation-induced ocular surface disorders and retinopathy: ocular structures and radiation dose-volume effect. *Cancer Research and Treatment: Official Journal of Korean Cancer Association*. 2022 Apr 1;54(2):417-23.

[31] Nuzzi R, Trossarello M, Bartoncini S, Marolo P, Franco P, Mantovani C, Ricardi U. Ocular complications after radiation therapy: an observational study. *Clinical Ophthalmology*. 2020 Oct 9:3153-66.

[32] Chodick G, Bekiroglu N, Hauptmann M, Alexander BH, Freedman DM, Doody MM, Cheung LC, Simon SL, Weinstock RM, Bouville A, Sigurdson AJ. Risk of cataract after exposure to low doses of ionizing radiation: a 20-year prospective cohort study among US radiologic technologists. *American journal of epidemiology*. 2008 Sep 15;168(6):620-31.

[33] Echegaray JJ, Bechrakis NE, Singh N, Bellerive C, Singh AD. Iodine-125 brachytherapy for uveal melanoma: a systematic review of radiation dose. *Ocular oncology and pathology*. 2017 Sep 5;3(3):193-8.

[34] Chodick G, Sigurdson AJ, Kleinerman RA, Sklar CA, Leisenring W, Mertens AC, Stovall M, Smith SA, Weathers RE, Veiga LH, Robison LL. The risk of cataract among survivors of childhood and adolescent cancer: a report from the childhood cancer survivor study. *Radiation research*. 2016 Apr 1;185(4):366-74.

[35] Sahoo NK, Ranjan R, Tyagi M, Agrawal H, Reddy S. Radiation retinopathy: detection and management strategies. *Clinical ophthalmology*. 2021 Sep 8:3797-809.

[36] Maqueda MA, Romero LZ, Córdoba RM, Soto JM, Torres-Ríos JA, Herrera DB, Camacho AR, Jiménez SM. Effects and assessment of the optic pathway after management with stereotactic radiosurgery for intracranial tumors: a comprehensive literature review. *Cureus*. 2023 Aug;15(8).

[37] Sand M, Sand D, Brors D, Altmeyer P, Mann B, Bechara FG. Cutaneous lesions of the external ear. *Head & face medicine.* 2008 Dec;4:1-3.

[38] Al Aaraj MS, Kelley C. Necrotizing (Malignant) Otitis Externa. In *StatPearls* [Internet] 2023 Oct 29. StatPearls Publishing.

[39] Schilder AG, Chonmaitree T, Cripps AW, Rosenfeld RM, Casselbrant ML, Haggard MP, Venekamp RP. Otitis media. *Nature reviews Disease primers*. 2016 Sep 8;2(1):1-8.

[40] Wang J, Chen YY, Tai A, Chen XL, Huang SM, Yang C, Bao Y, Li NW, Deng XW, Zhao C, Chen M. Sensorineural hearing loss after combined intensity modulated radiation therapy and cisplatin-based chemotherapy for nasopharyngeal carcinoma. *Translational oncology*. 2015 Dec 1;8(6):456-62.

[41] Supportive PD, Board PC. Oral Complications of Chemotherapy and Head/Neck Radiation (PDQ®). In *PDQ Cancer Information Summaries* [Internet] 2016 Dec 16. National Cancer Institute (US).

[42] Fall-Dickson JM, Pavletic SZ, Mays JW, Schubert MM. Oral complications of chronic graft-versus-host disease. *JNCI Monographs*. 2019 Aug 1;2019(53):lgz007.

[43] Asif M, Moore A, Yarom N, Popovtzer A. The effect of radiotherapy on taste sensation in head and neck cancer patients–a prospective study. *Radiation Oncology*. 2020 Dec;15:1-9.

[44] Strojan P, Plavc G, Kokalj M, Mitrovic G, Blatnik O, Lezaic L, Socan A, Bavec A, Tesic N, Hartman K, Svajger U. Post-radiation xerostomia therapy with allogeneic mesenchymal stromal stem cells in patients with head and neck cancer: study protocol for phase I clinical trial. *Radiology and oncology*. 2023 Nov 30;57(4):538-49.

[45] Miah AB, Gulliford SL, Morden J, Newbold KL, Bhide SA, Zaidi SH, Hall E, Harrington KJ, Nutting CM. Recovery of salivary function: contralateral parotid-sparing intensity-modulated radiotherapy versus bilateral superficial lobe parotid-sparing intensity-modulated radiotherapy. *Clinical Oncology*. 2016 Sep 1;28(9):e69-76.

[46] Lalla RV, Latortue MC, Hong CH, Ariyawardana A, D'Amato-Palumbo S, Fischer DJ, Martof A, Nicolatou-Galitis O, Patton LL, Elting LS, Spijkervet FK. A systematic review of oral fungal infections in patients receiving cancer therapy. *Supportive Care in Cancer*. 2010 Aug;18:985-92.

[47] Azzam P, Mroueh M, Francis M, Abou Daher A, Zeidan YH. Radiation-induced neuropathies in head and neck cancer: prevention and treatment modalities. *ecancer medical science*. 2020;14.

[48] Shabeeb D, Musa AE, Keshavarz M, Esmaely F, Hassanzadeh G, Shirazi A, Najafi M. Histopathological and functional evaluation of radiation-induced sciatic nerve damage: melatonin as radioprotector. *Medicina.* 2019 Aug 19;55(8):502.

[49] Gupta N, Pal M, Rawat S, Grewal MS, Garg H, Chauhan D, Ahlawat P, Tandon S, Khurana R, Pahuja AK, Mayank M. Radiation-induced dental caries, prevention and treatment-A systematic review. *National journal of maxillofacial surgery*. 2015 Jul 1;6(2):160-6.

[50] Kassim N, Sirajuddin S, Biswas S, Rafiuddin S, Apine A. Suppl 1: M2: Iatrogenic Damage to the Periodontium Caused by Radiation and Radiotherapy. *The Open Dentistry Journal*. 2015;9:182.

[51] Singh A, Huryn JM, Kronstadt KL, Yom SK, Randazzo JR, Estilo CL. Osteoradionecrosis of the jaw: A mini review. *Frontiers in oral health.* 2022 Jul 28;3:980786.

[52] Dracham CB, Shankar A, Madan R. Radiation induced secondary malignancies: a review article. *Radiation oncology journal*. 2018 Jun;36(2):85.

[53] Hashibe M, Ritz B, Le AD, Li G, Sankaranarayanan R, Zhang ZF. Radiotherapy for oral cancer as a risk factor for second primary cancers. *Cancer letters*. 2005 Apr 8;220(2):185-95.

[54] Arroyo-Hernández M, Maldonado F, Lozano-Ruiz F, Muñoz-Montaño W, Nuñez-Baez M, Arrieta O. Radiation-induced lung injury: current evidence. *BMC pulmonary medicine*. 2021 Dec;21:1-2.

[55] Alberts B, Johnson A, Lewis J, Raff M, Roberts K, Walter P. Pathogens, infection, and innate immunity. *Molecular biology of the cell.* 2008:1485-537.

[56] Chung J, Huda MN, Shin Y, Han S, Akter S, Kang I, Ha J, Choe W, Choi TG, Kim SS. Correlation between oxidative stress and transforming growth factor-beta in cancers. *International Journal of Molecular Sciences*. 2021 Dec 7;22(24):13181.

[57] Bezerra FS, Lanzetti M, Nesi RT, Nagato AC, Silva CP, Kennedy-Feitosa E, Melo AC, Cattani-Cavalieri I, Porto LC, Valenca SS. Oxidative stress and inflammation in acute and chronic lung injuries. *Antioxidants.* 2023 Feb 21;12(3):548.

[58] Jain V, Berman AT. Radiation pneumonitis: old problem, new tricks. *Cancers.* 2018 Jul 3;10(7):222.

[59] Rahi MS, Parekh J, Pednekar P, Parmar G, Abraham S, Nasir S, Subramaniyam R, Jeyashanmugaraja GP, Gunasekaran K. Radiation-induced lung injury—current perspectives and management. *Clinics and Practice*. 2021 Jul 1;11(3):410-29.

[60] Lee MS, Oh JY, Kang CI, Kim ES, Park S, Rhee CK, Jung JY, Jo KW, Heo EY, Park DA, Suh GY. Guideline for antibiotic use in adults with community-acquired pneumonia. *Infection & chemotherapy*. 2018 Jun;50(2):160.

[61] Modi P, Cascella M. *Diffusing capacity of the lungs for carbon monoxide*.

[62] Kristensen CA, Nøttrup TJ, Berthelsen AK, Kjær-Kristoffersen F, Ravn J, Sørensen JB, Engelholm SA. Pulmonary toxicity following IMRT after extrapleural pneumonectomy for malignant pleural mesothelioma. *Radiotherapy and Oncology*. 2009 Jul 1;92(1):96-9.

[63] Komaki R, Lee JS, Milas L, Lee HK, Fossella FV, Herbst RS, Allen PK, Liao Z, Stevens CW, Lu C, Zinner RG. Effects of amifostine on acute toxicity from concurrent chemotherapy and radiotherapy for inoperable non–small-cell lung cancer: report of a randomized comparative trial. *International Journal of Radiation Oncology* Biology* Physics*. 2004 Apr 1;58(5):1369-77.

[64] Alberts DS, Speicher LA, Krutzsch M, Wymer J, Capizzi RL, Conlon J, Barrett A, Aickin M. WR-1065, the active metabolite of amifostine (Ethyol®), does not inhibit the cytotoxic effects of a broad range of standard anticancer drugs against human ovarian and breast cancer cells. *European Journal of Cancer*. 1996 Jan 1;32:S17-20.

[65] Movsas B. Exploring the role of the radioprotector amifostine in locally advanced non-small cell lung cancer: Radiation Therapy Oncology Group trial 98-01. In *Seminars in Radiation Oncology* 2002 Jan 1 (Vol. 12, No. 1, pp. 40-45). WB Saunders.

[66] Annamaraju P, Patel P, Baradhi KM. Pentoxifylline. In *StatPearls* [Internet] 2024 Feb 29. StatPearls Publishing.

[67] Karayama M, Inui N, Inoue Y, Yasui H, Hozumi H, Suzuki Y, Furuhashi K, Fujisawa T, Enomoto N, Asada K, Uto T. Six-week oral prednisolone therapy for immune-related pneumonitis: a single-arm phase II study. *Journal for Immunotherapy of Cancer*. 2023;11(7).

[68] Yang C, Wang J, Yuan S. Chinese clinical practice guidelines for the prevention and treatment of radiation-induced esophagitis. *Precision Radiation Oncology*. 2023 Dec;7(4):225-36.

[69] Desai JP, Moustarah F. Esophageal stricture.

[70] Qiao WB, Zhao YH, Zhao YB, Wang RZ. Clinical and dosimetric factors of radiation-induced esophageal injury: radiation-induced esophageal toxicity. *World journal of gastroenterology*: WJG. 2005 May 5;11(17):2626.

[71] Maguire PD, Sibley GS, Zhou SM, Jamieson TA, Light KL, Antoine PA, Herndon II JE, Anscher MS, Marks LB. Clinical and dosimetric predictors of radiation-induced esophageal toxicity. *International Journal of Radiation Oncology* Biology* Physics*. 1999 Aug 1;45(1):97-103.

[72] Paximadis P, Schipper M, Matuszak M, Feng M, Jolly S, Boike T, Grills I, Kestin L, Movsas B, Griffith K, Gustafson G. Dosimetric predictors for acute esophagitis during radiation therapy for lung cancer: Results of a large statewide observational study. *Practical radiation oncology*. 2018 May 1;8(3):167-73.

[73] Savarino V, Marabotto E, Zentilin P, Demarzo MG, de Bortoli N, Savarino E. Pharmacological management of gastro-esophageal reflux disease: an update of the state-of-the-art. *Drug design, development and therapy*. 2021 Apr 19:1609-21.

[74] Vanhauwaert E, Matthys C, Verdonck L, De Preter V. Low-residue and low-fiber diets in gastrointestinal disease management. *Advances in Nutrition*. 2015 Nov 1;6(6):820-7.

[75] van Boeckel PG, Siersema PD. Refractory esophageal strictures: what to do when dilation fails. *Current treatment options in gastroenterology*. 2015 Mar;13:47-58.

[76] McBride WH, Schaue D. Radiation-induced tissue damage and response. *The Journal of pathology*. 2020 Apr;250(5):647-55.

[77] Jafari NV, Rohn JL. The urothelium: a multi-faceted barrier against a harsh environment. *Mucosal Immunology*. 2022 Nov 1;15(6):1127-42.

[78] Wijerathne H, Langston JC, Yang Q, Sun S, Miyamoto C, Kilpatrick LE, Kiani MF. Mechanisms of radiation-induced endothelium damage: Emerging models and technologies. *Radiotherapy and Oncology*. 2021 May 1;158:21-32.

[79] Kim SJ, Kim J, Na YG, Kim KH. Irreversible bladder remodeling induced by fibrosis. *International Neurourology Journal*. 2021 May;25(Suppl 1):S3.

[80] Bolla SR, Odeluga N, Amraei R, Jetti R. Histology, Bladder.[Updated 2023 Feb 25]. *StatPearls* [Internet]. 2023.

[81] Yang JH, Choi HP, Niu W, Azadzoi KM. Cellular stress and molecular responses in bladder ischemia. *International Journal of Molecular Sciences*. 2021 Nov 1;22(21):11862.

[82] Wijerathne H, Langston JC, Yang Q, Sun S, Miyamoto C, Kilpatrick LE, Kiani MF. Mechanisms of radiation-induced endothelium damage: Emerging models and technologies. *Radiotherapy and Oncology*. 2021 May 1;158:21-32.

[83] Li S, Wei R, Yu G, Liu H, Chen T, Guan X, Wang X, Jiang Z. Risk and prognosis of secondary bladder cancer after radiation therapy for pelvic cancer. *Frontiers in Oncology*. 2022 Aug 24;12:982792.

[84] Bono MJ, Leslie SW, Reygaert WC. *Urinary tract infection.*

[85] Viswanathan AN, Yorke ED, Marks LB, Eifel PJ, Shipley WU. Radiation dose–volume effects of the urinary bladder. *International Journal of Radiation Oncology* Biology* Physics*. 2010 Mar 1;76(3):S116-22.

[86] Xu Z, Yang L, Ma L, Liu Q, Chang AT, Zhou Y, Zhou C, Kong FM, Chen L. Effect of bladder volume on radiation doses to organs at risk and tumor in cervical cancer during imageguided adaptive brachytherapy and treatment outcome analysis. *Molecular and Clinical Oncology*. 2021 Dec 1;15(6):1-8.

[87] Manikandan R, Kumar S, Dorairajan LN. Hemorrhagic cystitis: a challenge to the urologist. *Indian Journal of Urology*. 2010 Apr 1;26(2):159-66.

[88] von Siebenthal M, Akshay A, Besic M, Schneider MP, Hashemi Gheinani A, Burkhard FC, Monastyrskaya K. Molecular characterization of non-neurogenic and neurogenic lower urinary tract dysfunction (LUTD) in SCI-induced and partial bladder outlet obstruction mouse models. *International journal of molecular sciences*. 2023 Jan 26;24(3):2451.

[89] Bansal N, Soni A, Kaur P, Chauhan AK, Kaushal V. Exploring the management of radiation proctitis in current clinical practice. *Journal of clinical and diagnostic research: JCDR*. 2016 Jun;10(6):XE01.

[90] Maria OM, Eliopoulos N, Muanza T. Radiation-induced oral mucositis. *Frontiers in oncology*. 2017 May 22;7:89.

[91] Hayden DM, Weiss EG. Fecal incontinence: etiology, evaluation, and treatment. *Clinics in colon and rectal surgery*. 2011 Mar;24(01):064-70.

[92] Vanneste BG, Van De Voorde L, de Ridder RJ, Van Limbergen EJ, Lambin P, van Lin EN. Chronic radiation proctitis: tricks to prevent and treat. *International journal of colorectal disease*. 2015 Oct;30:1293-303.

[93] Yu T, Zhang Q, Zheng T, Shi H, Liu Y, Feng S, Hao M, Ye L, Wu X, Yang C. The effectiveness of intensity modulated radiation therapy versus three-dimensional radiation therapy in prostate cancer: a meta-analysis of the literatures. *PloS one*. 2016 May 12;11(5):e0154499.

[94] Zelefsky MJ, Levin EJ, Hunt M, Yamada Y, Shippy AM, Jackson A, Amols HI. Incidence of late rectal and urinary toxicities after three-dimensional conformal radiotherapy and intensity-modulated radiotherapy for localized prostate cancer. *International Journal of Radiation Oncology* Biology* Physics*. 2008 Mar 15;70(4):1124-9.

[95] Simone NL, Ménard C, Soule BP, Albert PS, Guion P, Smith S, Godette D, Crouse NS, Sciuto LC, Cooley-Zgela T, Camphausen K. Intrarectal amifostine during external beam radiation therapy for prostate cancer produces significant improvements in Quality of Life measured by EPIC score. *International Journal of Radiation Oncology* Biology* Physics*. 2008 Jan 1;70(1):90-5.

[96] Cooper JS, Hanley ME. *Hyperbaric treatment of radiation proctitis*.

[97] O'Connor JJ. Argon laser treatment of radiation proctitis. *Archives of Surgery*. 1989 Jun 1;124(6):749.

Chapter 11

Radiosensitivity and Resistivity

Mrunal Meshram[1,*], MDS, PhD
Anurag Luharia[2], PhD
Abhinav Puppalwar[3], MD
and Rajesh Amutha[4], MSc

[1]Department of Oral Medicine and Radiology, Datta Meghe Institute of Higher Education and Research, Wardha, India
[2]Department of Radio physics and Radio safety, Datta Meghe Institute of Higher Education and Research, Wardha, India
[3]Department of Radiation Oncology, HCG Hospital, Nagpur, India
[4]Department of Radiotherapy, Rio Bravo Cancer Center, Bakersfield, CA, USA

Abstract

The complex relationship between cell cycle regulators and the development of cancer has been extensively investigated in the field of radiobiology. Oncogenes, which are genes that have the potential to cause cancer, play a crucial role in the progression of cancer. These genes can become activated through various mechanisms, including genetic mutations, gene amplification, and chromosomal rearrangements. Tumor suppressor genes, on the other hand, serve as inhibitory modulators that govern the intricate dynamics of the cellular cycle. The protein p53, commonly referred to as tumor protein p53, plays a critical role as a tumor suppressor by participating in the cellular response to DNA damage. The discovery of oncogenes originated from the investigation of retroviruses, which are RNA tumor viruses that convert their genomes into DNA within animal cells they infect. Experimental animals can be classified into two distinct categories based on the time it takes for tumor formation to occur. Rapid tumor formation can occur within a few days following the injection of acutely transforming retroviruses. Oncogenes can be broadly classified into several types, including growth factors, growth factor receptors, signal transducers, transcription factors, and programmed cell death regulators. These genes have distinct functions and can contribute to the development of cancer in various ways. Radiosensitivity refers to the susceptibility of cells to the effects of radiation. The level of radiosensitivity is higher in cells that divide more frequently and lower in cells that are more specialized or differentiated. Radiation primarily affects

* Corresponidng Author's Email: mrunal.oralmed@dmiher.edu.in

In: Fundamentals of Radiation Biology
Editors: Anurag Luharia, Ashish Uke, Gaurav Mishra et al.
ISBN: 979-8-89530-806-6

actively dividing cells and immature cells. The age-response function in radiobiology focuses on the variations in cell sensitivity during different stages of the cell cycle, specifically in relation to the lethality caused by radiation exposure. The primary cause of sensitivity changes can be attributed to the DNA's role as the main target for cell lethality caused by radiation. Radiosensitizers are substances or agents that sensitize tumor cells to the effects of radiation therapy. The goal of using radiosensitizers is to enhance the efficacy of radiation treatment and improve cancer control while minimizing damage to surrounding healthy tissues. Radioprotectors, on the other hand, are substances or agents that aim to protect normal tissues from the harmful effects of radiation during radiotherapy or radiation exposure.

Keywords: cancer stem cells, DNA repair, oncogenes, radiosensitivity, radioresistance

11.1. Introduction

The concepts of radio resistance and radiosensitivity are fundamental pillars in the captivating realm of radiation biology, governing the intricate dynamics of organismal responses to radiation exposure.

The crux of this concept resides in the interrelationship between oncogenes and radio resistance, wherein genetic elements meticulously modulate cellular reactions to ionizing radiation. Oncogenes, which are genes closely linked to the pathogenesis of cancer, exert a profound influence on the cellular responsiveness to ionizing radiation, thereby engendering a spectrum of radio resistance across diverse cellular lineages. The understanding of these complex systems offers indispensable insights in the development of precision therapies aimed at counteracting cancer and other ailments, while concurrently minimising the potential for radio resistance.

Upon further investigation into the intricate genetic foundations, one discovers the complex relationship of various elements that dictate an organism's innate susceptibility to the effects of radiation exposure. The interplay of diverse genetic elements intricately orchestrates a finely tuned equilibrium between cellular damage and repair processes, thereby ultimately delineating an individual's inherent radiosensitivity. The acquisition of this knowledge presents a myriad of opportunities for the development of personalised treatment strategies, the fine-tuning of radiation doses, and the augmentation of patient prognoses.

In the field of cancer research, it is crucial to acknowledge the significant influence of cancer stem cells in determining the inherent sensitivity of tumours to radiation therapy. The presence of these distinct cellular populations within neoplastic masses exerts a profound influence on the holistic reaction to ionizing radiation treatment. Understanding the intricate characteristics of cancer stem cells provides valuable insights into the development of groundbreaking therapeutic approaches that specifically aim to target these cells, thereby enhancing the overall effectiveness of cancer treatment modalities.

To proficiently navigate the intricacies of radiation therapy, one must possess a profound comprehension of the efficacious survival curve pertaining to a multifraction regimen. Fractionation, a technique employed in radiation therapy, entails the administration of multiple smaller doses of radiation over a specific period. This approach strategically enables healthy tissues to undergo a recovery process while simultaneously maximising the eradication of tumour cells. The effective survival curve, a pivotal instrument in the realm of radiobiology, plays a crucial role in the optimisation of treatment protocols. By providing valuable insights, it facilitates the attainment of an optimal equilibrium between tumour control and the preservation of normal tissues.

The manifestation of biological diversity becomes apparent when contrasting the radiation-induced cellular responses between mammalian organisms and microorganisms. The elucidation of this contrast serves to unveil the distinctive sensitivities exhibited by diverse organisms in response to radiation exposure. Furthermore, the meticulous examination of these disparities presents novel opportunities for scientific inquiry, elucidating the underlying principles dictating the varying degrees of susceptibility to radiation within the intricate web of biological existence.

In the context of cellular exploration, it becomes evident that the presence of oxygen plays a pivotal role in modulating the cellular response to radiation across various phases of the cell cycle. The presence of oxygen is of paramount importance in the context of radiation-induced damage, as it exerts a profound influence on the efficacy of treatments, especially those that exploit the oxygenation state of tissues. The intricate interplay between various factors within this relationship exhibits great potential for the optimisation of treatment outcomes across a wide range of clinical scenarios.

Age is indeed a pivotal variable in our inquiry, exerting a significant influence on the tissue's radiobiological response and subsequently impacting treatment efficacy and the manifestation of toxicities. The age-response function, in the context of radiobiology, offers invaluable insights that can be utilised to customise treatment approaches according to the age of patients. This utilisation of age-related data enables the implementation of more precise and efficacious therapeutic interventions.

The elucidation of the fundamental mechanisms governing the age-related response function holds paramount importance in the quest for precision medicine within the realm of radiobiology. The underlying mechanisms elucidated herein serve as the fundamental basis for the formulation of novel therapeutic strategies customised to distinct age cohorts, thereby augmenting the overall effectiveness of treatment interventions.

As we delve into the realm of radiation therapy, it becomes increasingly apparent that the age-response function in radiotherapy holds significant implications that warrant our attention. The optimisation of treatment outcomes, the minimization of complications, and the enhancement of the therapeutic potential of radiation therapy can be achieved by tailoring treatment strategies to account for age-related variations in radiosensitivity. This approach ensures that patients of all age groups receive the most effective and personalised treatment, taking into consideration their unique biological characteristics and response to radiation. By acknowledging the influence of age on radiosensitivity, treatment plans can be tailored to maximise efficacy while minimising the risk of adverse effects, ultimately leading to improved patient outcomes.

A fundamental comprehension of the underlying mechanisms and diverse applications pertaining to these various aspects serves as a crucial foundation for the development of enhanced and safer radiation therapies, thereby catalysing a paradigm shift within the realm of radiobiology.

11.2. Oncogenes and Radioresistance

11.2.1. Cell Cycle Regulators and Cancer

The complex relationship between cell cycle regulators and the development of cancer has been a subject of extensive investigation in the field of radiobiology. The cell cycle, a highly regulated process that governs the progression of cells through various phases, is tightly controlled by Mutations in cell cycle regulators and cancer are characterised by distinct genetic alterations [1]. In the realm of cellular biology, it is widely recognised that the complex mechanism of cancer development is influenced by two distinct categories of cell cycle regulators. These regulators, namely positive regulators, commonly referred to as oncogenes, and negative regulators, more commonly known as tumour suppressors, have been observed to play pivotal roles in the progression of cancer. The former, oncogenes, have the propensity to undergo excessive activation, while the latter, tumour suppressors, may undergo inactivation, thereby contributing to the detailed landscape of cancer development.

Oncogenes arise as a consequence of genetic alterations occurring in proto-oncogenes, which represent their unaltered and physiologically functional counterparts [2]. These mutations can manifest through diverse mechanisms. Certain genetic alterations can induce modifications in the amino acid sequence of a protein, thereby perturbing its structural conformation and confining it to a constitutively active state. Additional mutations can result in gene amplification, thereby inducing an aberrant upregulation of protein synthesis. Furthermore, aberrations in the intricate mechanisms of DNA repair can lead to the amalgamation of a proto-oncogene with a distinct gene, thereby engendering a chimeric protein endowed with unregulated functionality. Numerous proteins implicated in the transmission of growth factor signals are encoded by proto-oncogenes. In the event of a mutation-induced hyperactivity of these proteins, they possess the ability to propagate signals in the absence of growth factors. In the context of pancreatic cancer, it is noteworthy to mention that oncogenic Ras mutations exhibit a high prevalence. These mutations result in the Ras protein being trapped in a constitutively active conformation.

In contrast, tumour suppressors serve as inhibitory modulators that play a crucial role in governing the intricate dynamics of the cellular cycle. When these genes are operating optimally, they effectively inhibit the development of malignant neoplasms. However, genetic alterations can lead to a reduction in their enzymatic activity or complete loss of function, thereby causing disruptions in the intricate regulation of cellular division. The protein p53, commonly referred to as tumour protein p53, plays a critical role as a tumour suppressor by participating in the cellular response to DNA damage [3]. The primary mode of action of this particular agent is observed at the G1 checkpoint, wherein it effectively arrests the progression of the cell cycle upon encountering instances of DNA damage or unfavourable environmental circumstances. Upon encountering DNA damage, the tumour suppressor protein p53 initiates the transcriptional upregulation of a cell-cycle inhibitory molecule, thereby facilitating a temporary arrest in the progression of the cell cycle, which allows for the execution of DNA repair mechanisms. In the event of irreparable damage, the p53 protein initiates the process of apoptosis, a controlled cellular self-destruction mechanism, in order to impede the propagation of compromised genetic material.

Regrettably, a significant proportion of neoplastic cells exhibit the absence, impaired functionality, or diminished activity of the tumour suppressor protein p53. Mutations in the tumour suppressor gene p53 are commonly detected in various malignancies of human origin. It has been observed that neoplastic cells harbouring aberrant p53 exhibit a propensity for accumulating genetic alterations as time progresses. The abrogation or impairment of p53 facilitates the perpetuation of cellular proliferation in the presence of DNA damage, thereby engendering the transmission of genetic alterations to progeny cells. In conjunction with p53 mutations, alternative mechanisms can effectively incapacitate p53 within neoplastic cells, including heightened protein activities that facilitate the reutilization of p53 [4].

In the context of radiobiology, it is imperative to grasp the significance of cell cycle regulators, encompassing both oncogenes and tumour suppressors, with a particular emphasis on oncogenes. This understanding is pivotal in unravelling the multifaceted molecular basis of cancer. Through comprehensive analysis and precise targeting of these regulatory mechanisms, scientific investigators and medical practitioners can formulate strategic interventions within the intricate cellular cycle, thereby potentially mitigating or pre-emptively addressing neoplastic conditions.

11.3. Oncogenes

The discovery of oncogenes originated from the investigation of retroviruses, which are RNA tumour viruses that convert their genomes into DNA within animal cells they infect [5]. Throughout the progression of an infection, the genetic material of retroviruses is integrated into the chromosomes of the cells they infect. The provirus, known as the integrated retroviral DNA, undergoes replication alongside the host's cellular DNA. The process of transcribing the DNA provirus results in the creation of viral offspring that emerge from the host cell membrane to invade neighbouring cells.

Experimental animals can be classified into two distinct categories based on the time it takes for tumour formation to occur. These categories are specifically assigned to retroviruses. Rapid tumour formation can occur within a few days following the injection of acutely transforming retroviruses. The neoplastic phenotype can also be induced in cell cultures by these retroviruses. Long-term exposure to retroviruses with varying levels of oncogenicity can lead to the development of specific tumours in certain strains of laboratory animals. This occurs after a significant period of time, typically spanning several months. While retroviruses with low oncogenic potential are capable of in vitro replication, they do not induce cellular transformation when cultured.

The identification of oncogenes dates back to the 1970s, and since then, extensive studies have significantly contributed to the development of cancer therapies. Mutated genes known as oncogenes play a significant role in the progression of cancer, whereas proto-oncogenes are responsible for regulating cell growth and division in their normal state. Every cell contains a pair of gene copies or alleles. A particular alteration in a single allele result in the conversion of the typical "proto-oncogene" into an active oncogene, which has the ability to contribute to the development of cancer [6]. Minor alterations can cause a proto-oncogene to transform into an oncogene. There exist three primary methods through which this occurrence can take place:

1. A change occurring in the proto-oncogene or its regulatory region can modify the configuration of the protein, resulting in heightened enzyme functionality or the absence of regulation.
2. Higher levels of protein concentration can occur due to an upregulation in protein synthesis, improved mRNA persistence, or the duplication of genes, resulting in an increased amount of protein within the cellular environment.
3. Chromosomal rearrangements may also have an impact. Certain chromosomal rearrangements can relocate the proto-oncogene, resulting in an upregulation of its expression. Some individuals develop fusion proteins that exhibit increased oncogenic potential.

The dominant nature of the oncogene surpasses that of the proto-oncogene, leading to the production of a protein product that is commonly deregulated and/or persistently active. The process of oncogenic conversion is characterised by the acquisition of a new function, whereas the transformation necessitates the loss or inactivation of both alleles. Tumour suppressors, alternatively referred to as recessive oncogenes or anti-oncogenes, are characterised by their inactivation, which signifies a mutation resulting in the loss of their normal function [7]. The collaboration between oncogene activation and tumour suppressor inactivation plays a crucial role in the gradual development of tumorigenesis.

The formation of cancer, driven by oncogenes, encompasses alterations in both oncogenes and tumour suppressor genes. This process necessitates mutations in numerous genes, resulting in atypical cellular activity. The uncontrolled growth of cells is caused by the accumulation of mutations in proto-oncogenes and tumour suppressor genes. In the realm of cell biology, oncogenes play a pivotal role in stimulating cell growth and division. Interestingly, a mere solitary mutation is sufficient to heighten the risk of cancer. On the other hand, tumour suppressor genes operate in a contrasting manner by mending damaged DNA or eradicating irregular cells. To escalate the risk of cancer, mutations must occur in both copies of these genes. The successful management of cancer has been greatly enhanced through the precise targeting of various oncogenes. This approach has resulted in the development of highly effective treatments such as Gleevec, therapies that specifically target HER2, therapies that specifically target EGFR, and numerous other breakthroughs [8].

Genes that promote cancer have an impact on various elements of cellular growth and division, such as factors that stimulate growth, receptors, proteins involved in transmitting signals, factors that regulate gene expression, proteins that control the cell cycle, regulators of programmed cell death, and the ability of cells to resist radiation. There have been several studies published in scientific journals indicating that the introduction of activated oncogenes into cells grown in a laboratory setting can enhance their ability to withstand radiation, as measured by their clonogenic survival rate [9]. The direct involvement of oncogene expression in the induction of radio resistance remains uncertain, and the extent to which oncogenes contribute to radio resistance in human tumours is even more uncertain. On the other hand, it has been observed that the activation of oncogenes leads to an enhanced ability of cells to withstand radiation.

Gaining knowledge about oncogenes and their significance in the progression of cancer is essential in the pursuit of creating successful therapies and precautionary actions against the disease. Current studies show potential for the effectiveness of immunotherapy in specific types of cancer and the continued progress in the area of radiobiology.

11.3.1. Types of Oncogenes

There are numerous functions associated with oncogenes, corresponding to more than 100. However, these functions can be broadly classified into various types that result in the transformation of a regular cell into an independent cancer cell. Some of these oncogenes even have the ability to generate proteins that operate in multiple domains, commonly referred to as oncoproteins.

They are classified broadly into: (1) growth factors, (2) growth factor receptors, (3) signal transducers, (4) transcription factors, and others, including 5) programmed cell death regulators.

- **Growth Factors**

Growth factors are released peptides that serve as external cues to trigger the multiplication of specific cells [10]. In order for cell proliferation to be induced by a growth factor, it is necessary for the target cells to have distinct receptors capable of binding to the growth factor. Upon their liberation, they swiftly attach themselves to the designated receptors located on the exteriors of target cells. The activation of this connection triggers internal communication pathways, resulting in a sequence of chemical occurrences that ultimately support the proliferation and expansion of cells. A wide range of growth factors exist, each serving distinct purposes and affecting specific cells. Examples include PDGF, nerve growth factor, epidermal growth factor, and fibroblast growth factor.

PDGF, a growth factor extensively studied, is known for its ability to promote the growth of fibroblasts [11]. This growth factor is of utmost importance in the process of wound healing. Some other instances consist of the factor of growth in nerves, the factor of growth in the epidermis, and the factor of growth in fibroblasts.

Developmental factors are crucial for the regeneration of tissues, the healing of wounds, the growth of embryos, and the maintenance of tissue balance. Furthermore, cancer research is significantly impacted by these factors, as certain growth factors can function as oncogenes when expressed in an inappropriate manner.

- **Growth Factor Receptors**

On the cell membrane, growth factor receptors—also called receptor tyrosine kinases—are proteins that bind to growth factors [12]. There are three main areas they focus on: the domain that binds to ligands outside the cell, the domain that spans the cell membrane, and the domain responsible for catalysing tyrosine kinase activity inside the cell.

Upon the binding of a growth factor to the extracellular domain of its receptor, the catalytic domain of the intracellular tyrosine kinase is triggered into activation. The process begins with a signalling cascade that transmits signals promoting growth from the surface of the cell to the nucleus, resulting in the splitting of cells. There are two primary categories of growth factor receptors: receptor protein kinases (including tyrosine kinases and serine/threonine kinases) and GTP-binding proteins (both monomeric and heterotrimeric). Some growth factor receptors that can be found are erb B, erb B-2, fms, kit, met, ret, ras, and trk.

The proper regulation of cell growth heavily relies on growth factor receptors, which can play a significant role in the onset of cancer if they undergo mutations or abnormal expression.

- **Signal Transducers**

Signal sensors are proteins that relay mitogenic signals from growth factor receptors on the cell surface to the cell nucleus through a series for complex pathways called the signal transduction cascade. There are two main categories of signal transducers: receptor protein kinases and GTP-binding proteins. Receptor protein kinases can further be divided into tyrosine kinases and serine/threonine kinases. GTP-binding proteins, on the other hand, can be classified as either monomeric or heterotrimeric. Some signal transducers that can be mentioned are receptor protein kinases like fyn, jak, fgr, and tyrosine kinases such as btk, syk, and tec. Furthermore, signal transducers encompass GTP-binding proteins such as H-ras, K-ras, N-ras, gsp, and gip[13].

The process of signal transduction encompasses the sequential phosphorylation of proteins that interact within the cytosol, along with the participation of guanine nucleotide-binding proteins and secondary messengers. Their function in regulating cellular growth is crucial and often linked to the development of cancer when their behaviour becomes uncontrolled.

- **Transcription Factors**

Transcription factors are nuclear proteins that regulate the expression of target genes. Their mechanism involves attaching to particular DNA sequences, typically found before the desired gene, and influencing alterations in gene expression [14].

Transcription regulators serve as the ultimate connection in the process of signal transduction, transforming external signals received via receptors for growth factors into regulated gene expression. Members of multigene families have the ability to act as transcription factors and possess similar DNA-binding domains such as zinc fingers. Some of the transcription factors that function as proto-oncogenes are erb A, ets, fos, jun, myb, and c-myc.

Cell proliferation is heavily influenced by transcription factors, which are frequently implicated in the onset of cancer when their function is disrupted by chromosomal translocations or genetic mutations.

- **Programmed Cell Death Regulators**

The maintenance of a delicate equilibrium between cell proliferation and cell death serves as essential for normal embryogenesis and organ development in normal tissues. This is achieved through programmed cell death, which plays a vital role in these processes. Apoptosis is a unique type of programmed cell death that is characterised by specific morphological alterations, including membrane blebbing, nuclear condensation, and fragmentation of DNA into nucleosome-sized pieces [15]. Apoptosis can be induced in mature tissues by external factors such as steroids and radiation.

Cancer development and resistance to cancer treatments can be attributed to both uncontrolled cell proliferation and the inability to undergo programmed cell death. bcl-2 is an important proto-oncogene that plays a role in the regulation of programmed cell death. The activation of this gene prevents programmed cell death in lymphoid cells, which classifies it as an oncogene. The protein encoded by the bcl-2 gene is present in different cellular structures, and although its precise mechanism of action is not fully understood, it is still partially unknown. It is believed to have antioxidant properties that help protect cell membranes from lipid peroxidation. bcl-2 has the ability to interact with various proteins, including bax, that are involved in the regulation of programmed cell death [16]. Although bcl-2 is a well-known gene associated with apoptosis and its role in neoplasia, there may be other proto-oncogenes that affect programmed cell death in cancer that have not yet been discovered. The different types of oncogenes are compiled in Table 11.1.

Table 11.1. Types of oncogenes and their examples

Type of Oncogene	Description	Location	Example
Growth Factors	Peptides triggering cell proliferation	Extracellular	PDGF (Platelet-derived growth factor)
Growth Factor Receptors	Proteins binding growth factors on cell membrane	Cell membrane	EGFR (Epidermal growth factor receptor)
Signal Transducers	Proteins relaying signals from receptors to the nucleus	Cytoplasm and cell membrane	Ras (Rat sarcoma)
Transcription Factors	Nuclear proteins regulating gene expression	Nucleus	Myc (Myc proto-oncogene)
Programmed Cell Death	Genes involved in apoptosis regulation	Mitochondrial membrane, ER, nucleus	Bcl-2 (B-cell lymphoma-2)

11.4. Tumour-Suppressive Genes and Blockage of Carcinogenesis

Within a typical cell, in addition to oncogenes, there exist genes known as tumour-suppressive genes. The tumour suppressive genes are compiled in table 11.2. These genes hold significant influence over the cell's regular growth and differentiation processes, effectively impeding the progression of cancer. Tumour-suppressor genes encompass a vast array of members that share a common trait: in some way or another, each of these genes safeguards the organism against the development of neoplasms. For a cancer cell to continue growing and surviving, it is necessary for both copies of a tumour-suppressor gene to be rendered inactive. Cancer is caused by the presence of mutations in tumour-suppressor genes, which result in their lack of function or inactivation. There are numerous genes that act as tumour suppressors and are believed to be located throughout the human genome. These genes are involved in the development of different Forms of neoplasia in humans. Retinoblastoma 1 protein (RB1) and p53 are two well-known tumour-suppressor genes. The p53 gene produces a protein called p53, which functions as a tetramer [17].

Table 11.2. Examples of tumour suppressive genes

Tumour suppressor genes			
Gene	Chromosome	Location	Function
Rb	13	Nucleus	Cell cycle
p53	17	Nucleus	DNA repair, apoptosis
INK4A	9	Nucleus	Cell cycle/p53 function
Bcl2	18	Mitochondria	Apoptosis
nm23	17	Mitochondria	Metastasis
BRCA2	17	Nucleus	DNA repair
APC	5	Cytskeleton	Cell-cell recognition

11.5. DNA Repair Genes

Besides oncogenes and tumour suppressor genes, there exists another category of genes that contribute to cancer known as DNA mending genes [18]. During the process of cellular division, the replication of DNA is essential for the generation of new cells. The procedure at hand is quite complex and on certain occasions, it leads to errors within the DNA. If there is a malfunction in any of these genes responsible for DNA repair, it can result in an accumulation of additional errors within the cell. Certain genetic variations have the potential to influence neighbouring genes, potentially resulting in uncontrolled cellular growth.

Similar to various forms of genetic alterations, modifications in DNA repair genes can be either passed down from a progenitor or acquired over the course of an individual's existence. The BRCA1 and BRCA2 genes are among the major DNA repair genes examples and others are mentioned in Table 11.3 [19].

Table 11.3. Examples of DNA repair genes

Gene Symbol	Gene name	Function	Repair Pathway
CHK2	Checkpoint kinase 2	Serine threonine kinase	Cell cycle and apoptotic regulation in response to DNA damage
EXO1	Exonuclease 1	5' to 3'exonuclease	Homologous recombination; mismatch repair
FANCC	Fanconi anemia Complementation group C	Component of Fanconi repair system core complex	DNA cross link repair
MSH6	MutS homolog 6	Mismatch repair	Mismatch repair
NEIL1	Endonucleas VIII like 1	DNA glycosylase and apurinic/ apyrimidinic lyase	Base excision repair
NUDTI	Nudix hydrolase 1	Hydrolyzes oxidised purine nucleoside triphosphates	Modulation of nucleotide pools
POLB	DNA polymerase beta	DNA polymerase (catalytic subunit)	Base excision repair
POLE	DNA polymerase epsilon	DNA polymerase (catalytic subunit)	Nucleotide excision repair and mismatch repair
POLM	DNA polymerase mu	DNA polymerase (catalytic subunit)	Gap filling during non-homologus end-joining

11.6. The Clonal Theory of Oncogenesis

In accordance with the clonal hypothesis of oncogenesis, neoplasms originate from a solitary cell [20]. However, the tumours' clonal lineage does not imply that a malignant growth arises solely from a solitary genetic mutation. Mutated genes frequently collaborate to induce the development of cancerous cells. For instance, Myc and Ras represent a pair of frequently activated oncogenes in the development of tumours, which have the ability to work in tandem efficiently to produce cancer. In collaboration and in isolation, they direct numerous characteristics of cancer, such as growth, cell death, and the ability to regenerate.

11.7. Programmed Cell Death (Apoptosis)

Eukaryotic cells can undergo two different types of death: Necrosis and apoptosis, also known as programmed cell death [21]. Cellular damage, such as ischemia or physical and chemical injury, can lead to the development of necrosis. During necrosis, alterations happen within the protoplasm leading to an elevation in cell size, demise of the cell, and ultimately the breakdown of DNA due to the discharge of lysosomal enzymes. On the other hand, apoptosis is a regular event in the development of healthy tissues, involving alterations in the nucleus such as nuclear fragmentation. During the process of apoptosis, cell death occurs after DNA fragmentation caused by an internal endonuclease. It seems that the inability of the cell to repair significant DNA damage, rather than the DNA fragmentation itself, is what ultimately leads to cell death in apoptosis.

Considering that apoptosis is the predominant type of cellular death, it is apparent that the suppression of apoptosis plays an essential part in the progression of cancer. The relationship between apoptosis and cancer is closely tied to the roles played by oncogenes, tumour suppressor genes, and DNA repair genes. Apoptosis, when it functions correctly, serves a crucial role in preserving the well-being of cells and inhibiting the survival and growth of cells that possess significant genetic abnormalities. Disruption or failure of programmed cell death, known as apoptosis, can contribute to the emergence and advancement of cancer [22]. This occurs when irregular cells manage to escape the natural process of cell death, enabling them to persist and proliferate without restraint.

11.8. Radio Resistivity

Radio resistance refers to the inherent ability of organisms to mitigate, repair, and eliminate the deleterious effects of ionizing radiation on molecular, cellular, and tissue structures [23]. The efficacy of this trait exhibits significant variation across diverse organisms.

The complex interaction between oncogenes and radio resistance stems from the profound impact of oncogenes on the cellular response to radiation therapy. Oncogenes exert a profound influence on the intricate process of cancer initiation and progression when subjected to mutational events or exhibit heightened expression levels. These alterations precipitate augmented cellular proliferation and enhanced cell viability, thereby contributing to the pathogenesis of cancer. In the realm of oncology, radiation therapy is a widely employed modality for the management of cancer. This therapeutic approach harnesses the potential of high-energy radiation to inflict substantial damage upon malignant cells, ultimately leading to their demise or impairment. Its primary aim is to perturb the DNA of cancer cells, thereby hindering their proliferative capacity and inducing cellular demise. Nevertheless, it is noteworthy that specific oncogenes have the potential to exert an influence on the phenomenon of radio resistance, thereby diminishing the sensitivity of cancer cells or endowing them with resistance against the therapeutic impacts of radiation. Consequently, the emergence of resistance mechanisms can potentially compromise the efficacy of therapeutic interventions, thereby enabling cancerous cells to persist and proliferate unabated in the face of radiation exposure.

Multiple mechanisms are known to contribute to the phenomenon of radio resistance in cancer cells, with certain oncogenes exerting an influential role in this process:

- *DNA Repair*
  Oncogenes have been observed to exhibit the capability of augmenting DNA repair pathways within malignant cells, thereby facilitating the proficient mending of radiation-induced genetic lesions [24]. This phenomenon significantly augments their viability and recuperative capacity following exposure to ionizing radiation.
- *Cellular Cycle Regulation*
  Oncogenes have the potential to perturb the intricate network of cell cycle checkpoints, thereby inducing dysregulated cellular proliferation [25]. Radiation therapy exhibits its maximum efficacy when cancerous cells are undergoing active division, as it capitalises on the vulnerability of dividing cells. However, the impact of radiation is significantly diminished in the presence of cell cycle dysregulation, which disrupts the orderly progression of cell division.
- *Anti-apoptotic signalling*
  Certain oncogenes facilitate the activation of anti-apoptotic signalling pathways, thereby impeding the initiation of programmed cell death (apoptosis) in cancer cells upon exposure to radiation.
- *Hypoxia*
  Tumour cells harbouring active oncogenes have the ability to establish a microenvironment characterised by reduced oxygen levels (hypoxia) [26]. This hypoxic condition confers a protective advantage to cancer cells, rendering them more resistant to the deleterious effects of radiation.

11.8.1. Induced Radio Resistance

Exposure to low levels of ionizing radiation has been found to cause radio resistance in different types of organisms. These include yeast, bacteria, protozoa, algae, plants, insects, as well as mammalian and human cells grown in a laboratory setting. This phenomenon refers to various cellular radioprotection mechanisms that help safeguard cells from the harmful effects of radiation [27]. These mechanisms include changes in protein levels, enhanced gene expression, DNA repair, and other related processes.

Radiation exposure has been found to trigger a self-repair mechanism in organisms, as demonstrated by various studies. During the Goiania accident, a man named Devoir Alves Ferreira was exposed to a significant amount of radiation but managed to survive. Surprisingly, his wife, who received a slightly lower dose of radiation, unfortunately did not survive. The variation in results could be explained by the way Ferreira's dose was divided into smaller fractions and delivered over time. This approach allowed his body's natural repair mechanisms to have more chances to recover. On the other hand, his wife received a continuous dose without any breaks, which hindered her body's ability to repair the radiation damage.

Likewise, several experiments have demonstrated a significant finding: the survival of cells exposed to radiation decreases as the radiation dose increases. This relationship between radiation dose and cell survival has been extensively studied and confirmed through various experiments. In the field of radiobiology, an interesting phenomenon has been noted. When a group of cells is exposed to radiation, followed by a period of rest for recovery, and then subjected to radiation once more, the effectiveness of the radiation in inducing cell death is diminished. The human body is made up of different types of cells, and if a vital organ loses even a single tissue, it can result in death. In radiobiology, short-term radiation deaths can occur due to the detrimental effects on two vital tissues: the bone marrow and the intestinal wall. The bone marrow is responsible for producing blood cells, while the intestinal wall supports digestion. The loss of cells in these tissues can lead to severe consequences and ultimately result in fatalities.

11.8.2. Factors Affecting Radiosensitivity

Radiosensitivity refers to how a tumour responds to radiation treatment. It can be evaluated based on the degree of tumour regression, the speed of response, and how long the response lasts. Radiosensitivity is influenced by various factors [28]. Some major factors affecting the response of cells in radiation therapy include the following:

1. *Ability to repair damage*: Some cells have better mechanisms to repair radiation-induced damage than others. Cells with efficient repair systems are more likely to recover from radiation exposure.
2. *Hypoxia:* Oxygen plays a crucial role in the effectiveness of radiation therapy. Cells in well-oxygenated areas are more susceptible to radiation damage compared to cells in hypoxic (low oxygen) regions [29].
3. *Cell cycle*: Cells go through different phases of the cell cycle, including resting (G0), growth (G1), DNA synthesis (S), and division (M) phases. Cells in the actively dividing phases (G1 The size of the initial tumour can affect the success of tumour eradication.

It is important to distinguish between radiosensitivity and radio curability. While they may sound similar, they have distinct meanings in the field of radiology. Radiation therapy can effectively treat tumours that are relatively resistant to radiation and can be reached with high doses of localised radiation. However, tumours that are sensitive to radiation and have spread extensively throughout the body can only be managed locally, rather than cured.

Squamous cell carcinoma of the cervix is a type of tumour that is relatively resistant to radiation. However, it is still highly curable due to its location and the fact that the surrounding normal tissues are also relatively resistant to radiation.

According to Bergonie and Tribondeau's Law (1906), tissues are more sensitive to radiation if they meet the following criteria:

1. The cells in the tissues are undifferentiated.
2. The tissues have a higher capacity for proliferation.
3. The cells in the tissues divide at a faster rate.

11.8.3. Physical Factors Affecting Radiosensitivity

Physical factors can influence the sensitivity of tissues to radiation. These factors include:

1. *Linear Energy Transfer*
   LET, also known as Linear Energy Transfer, is a term used to describe the speed at which ionizing radiation transfers energy to soft tissue [30]. The tissue weight factor is a crucial parameter in radiation protection as it aids in evaluating the radiation quality and its effects on various tissues. The kiloelectron volts per micrometre is the designated unit of measurement used to express energy transfer in soft tissue. The biological effects of ionizing radiation can be attributed to its potential to cause harm, which becomes more pronounced as the Linear Energy Transfer (LET) of the radiation rises. The approximate value of the Linear Energy Transfer (LET) for diagnostic x-rays is around 3 kiloelectron volts per micrometre (keV/μm).
2. *Relative Biologic Effectiveness*
   Relative Biologic Effectiveness (RBE) is a commonly used term in the field of radiology that refers to the comparative strength of various forms of ionizing radiation in inducing biological harm [31]. The efficiency of a specific form of radiation is evaluated by comparing it to a standard. The potential for radiation to cause biological harm increases as the Linear Energy Transfer (LET) of the radiation increases. The phenomenon is described using the quantification of relative biologic effects (RBE). The Relative Biological Effectiveness (RBE) of diagnostic x-ray is 1, indicating its level of biological impact.
   Radiations that have a lower linear energy transfer (LET) demonstrate a relative biological effectiveness (RBE) value that is below 1. Radiations with a higher Linear Energy Transfer (LET) will demonstrate a Relative Biological Effectiveness (RBE) that is greater than 1. The relative biological effectiveness (RBE) increases as the linear energy transfer (LET) increases. Nevertheless, after reaching its peak, the level gradually declines as a result of excessive force.
3. *Fractionation & Protraction*
   - *Fractionation:* Dose is delivered with some interval and fraction but at a same dose rate.
   - *Protraction:* The delivery of the dose is continuous, but it is administered at a reduced rate.

- The effect of a dose of radiation is diminished if it is administered over a lengthy period of time as opposed to all at once. If the dose is administered slowly rather than rapidly, the dose's effects will be diminished. If the duration of irradiation is prolonged, a greater dosage is required to achieve the same result. Dose protraction and fractionation result in a diminished effect, allowing intracellular repair and tissue recovery time [32].
- If we administer an exposure of 600 rads at a rate of 300 rads/minute, the effects will be less severe than if we administer the same dose at a rate of 600 rads/minute. The term for this is protraction.
- If 600 rads were administered at a rate of 150 rad per day over four days, the effects would be less severe than if 600 rads were administered in a single day. The term for this is fractionation.

11.8.4. Biologic Factors Affecting Radiosensitivity

Several biologic factors influence the degree of radiosensitivity in different tissues. They are:

- **Oxygen Effect**

In the context of radiation, tissues that have oxygen or are in an aerobic condition are more susceptible than tissues that lack oxygen or are in a low-oxygen state. The Oxygen Enhancement Ratio (OER) is a quantitative measure employed to describe tissue characteristics [33].

The effectiveness of diagnostic x-ray in enhancing oxygen relies on the full oxygenation process. The biological effectiveness of radiation is determined by its dependence on Linear Energy Transfer (LET). The maximum value of around 3 is observed for low LET (Linear Energy Transfer) radiation. Conversely, the OER decreases to 1 for high LET radiation, whereas it remains high for low LET radiation like X-rays and gamma rays. As the linear energy transfer (LET) of radiation increases, there is a corresponding decrease in the oxygen enhancement ratio (OER).

- **Age**

Age plays a significant role in determining the susceptibility of biological structures to radiation. It is crucial to acknowledge that the human body experiences different phases of growth, including the prenatal stage. It is widely acknowledged that the human body is highly susceptible to external influences during this period. As individuals grow older, their sensitivity generally diminishes. As people get older, they often become more sensitive.

- **Recovery**

Interphase death can occur when the radiation dose is sufficiently high to eliminate the cell before it undergoes its next division. When the dosage administered is lower than the lethal limit, there is a chance for cells to recover from the harm caused. Some types of cells possess a higher ability to regenerate and heal. Recovery at the whole-body level is supported by the replenishment of remaining cells and the repair that occurs within the cells themselves. Exposure to an appropriate amount of radiation can cause a decrease in size of a tissue or organ. Atrophy refers to a condition where a specific organ or tissue experiences shrinkage or degeneration [34]. Atrophy is a medical condition that is defined by the degeneration and elimination of cells, leading to their eventual disposal as waste.

Chemical substances have the ability to modify the manner in which our bodies react to radiation. Radiosensitizers refer to substances that enhance the efficacy of radiation therapy by rendering cancer cells more vulnerable to the detrimental impacts of radiation. Radioprotectors, in contrast, are substances that aid in minimising the detrimental impacts of radiation on healthy tissues, thus safeguarding them against harm [35].

- **Cell cycle selectors**

  - Actinomycin-D
  - Hydroxyurea
  - Methotrexate
  - 5-flurouracil

These compounds exhibit higher toxicity towards cells in the S-phase, making them effective anti-metabolites. Cells that have been treated with these medications and are in an asynchronous population will exhibit increased radiosensitivity. The reason for this is that the cells that remain alive after being treated with drugs are more inclined to be in the radio-sensitive phases of the cell cycle, such as G1, M, or G2.

Halogenated pyrimidines are considered true sensitizers, unlike other agents. Example, BUdR, or bromodeoxyuridine, is a substance that can be used to replace thymidine in DNA [36]. This replacement prevents a cell from being able to undergo sub-lethal repair.

- **Hyperthermia**

Hyperthermia is a therapeutic approach that capitalises on the differential sensitivity of tumour cells to heat-induced harm in comparison to healthy cells [37]. Thermal stress, specifically exposure to a temperature of 43 degrees Celsius for a duration of 30 to 60 minutes, increases the susceptibility of cells to radiation-induced injury compared to cells that have not been heated. Dose-modifying factors ranging from 2 to 10 have been documented.

11.8.5. Genetic Factors Affecting Radiosensitivity

Genetic factors play a role in determining how sensitive an individual is to radiation-induced damage. These factors can either increase or decrease sensitivity. Genetic factors primarily impact three crucial processes in radiology: DNA repair, antioxidant defence mechanisms, and cell cycle regulation.

- **DNA Repair**

Exposure to ionizing radiation leads to DNA damage in cells. DNA repair mechanisms play a crucial role in repairing damage and preserving the integrity of genetic material. Radiosensitivity can be influenced by genetic variations or polymorphisms in genes related to DNA repair pathways. Genetic variations in genes involved in DNA repair, such as base excision repair, nucleotide excision repair, and double-strand break repair, can impact how efficiently DNA is repaired. This, in turn, can influence how an individual respond to radiation exposure.

- **Antioxidant Defence Mechanisms**

Ionizing radiation has the ability to produce reactive oxygen species (ROS) in cells, which can cause oxidative stress and damage to the cells. Antioxidant enzymes are essential in safeguarding cells against oxidative damage caused by reactive oxygen species (ROS). Three key antioxidant enzymes are superoxide dismutase, catalase, and glutathione peroxidase [38]. These enzymes work together to neutralise ROS and maintain cellular health. Genetic variations in antioxidant enzyme genes can impact how much they are expressed and how well they function. Variations in individuals can impact their vulnerability to radiation-induced oxidative stress.

- **Cell Cycle Regulation**

The cell cycle is a highly controlled process that governs cell growth, duplication, and splitting. The cell cycle must be carefully regulated to ensure that DNA replication and repair occur accurately. Radiosensitivity can be increased when there are genetic alterations that disrupt cell cycle checkpoints [39]. When cells have damaged DNA, it is important for them to either undergo proper repair or undergo programmed cell death, known as apoptosis. If cells with damaged DNA progress through the cell cycle without these processes, it can lead to the accumulation of DNA damage. This accumulation can make tissues or organs more sensitive to radiation.

11.8.6. Classification of Tissue Radiosensitivity

Two systems are typically used to classify tissue radiosensitivity in terms of (represented as a flowchart in Figure 11.1):

- Population kinetics: Casarett's Classification
- Tissue architecture: Michalowski's Classification

- **Casarett's Classification**

Histologic Observation of Early Cell Death Radiosensitivity refers to the susceptibility of mammalian cells to the effects of radiation [40]. By observing early cell death through histologic examination, we can classify cells based on their radiosensitivity. This classification helps us understand how different types of cells respond to radiation exposure. The parenchymal cells in radiology can be categorised into four main groups. The first group includes supporting structures like connective tissue and endothelial cells of small blood vessels. These structures are considered to have intermediate sensitivity, falling between groups II and III of parenchymal cells. Classified as: Group I, Group II, Group III, Group IV.

- *Group I*
  Highly sensitive - Consists of rapidly dividing and undifferentiated cells - Examples include stem cells, the epidermis of the skin and intestine, and primitive cells involved in spermatogenesis.
- *Group II*
  Cells in this group are relatively sensitive and undergo regular division, while also maturing and differentiating between divisions. - Examples include cells in the hematopoietic series that are in intermediate stages of differentiation, as well as more differentiated spermatogonia and spermatocytes.
- *Group III*
  It consists of postmitotic cells that typically do not undergo mitosis. However, they have the ability to divide under specific circumstances, such as when they experience damage or a significant loss of similar cells. These cells exhibit a relatively higher resistance to such conditions - For example, the liver, pancreas, adrenal glands, and thyroid all contain cells.
- *Group IV:*
  These cells are the most resistant to radiation among fixed postmitotic cells. - They are highly differentiated and seem to have lost their ability to divide - Examples of different types of cells include nerve cells, muscle cells, and granulocytes.

- **Michalowski's Classification**

Tissues can be classified as either hierarchical or flexible. This classification model is designed to predict the progression of radiation toxicity over time. Classified tissues as: Hierarchical (H) type and Flexible (F) Type.

- *H-Type*
  There are three different cell types that can be found in a tissue. - The first type is stem cells, which have the ability to divide uncontrollably. - The second type is functional cells, which are fully developed and cannot divide any further. These cells have a limited lifespan and eventually die. - The third type is intermediate cells, which are partially differentiated and still capable of multiplying. These cells are in the process of completing their differentiation. - Examples of tissues that contain these cell types include hematopoietic bone marrow, intestinal epithelium, and epidermis [41].
- *F-Type*
  There is no rigid hierarchy in F-Type. - Tissues consist of cells that typically do not undergo division under normal circumstances. - However, they can be prompted to

divide in response to tissue damage. - Following tissue damage, all cells, including functional ones, enter the cell cycle. - For example, organs such as the liver, thyroid, and dermis.

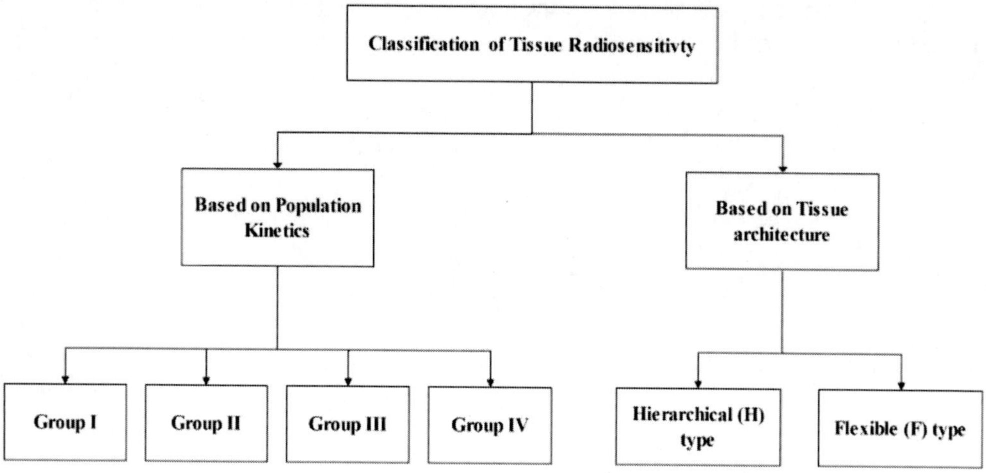

Figure 11.1. Classification of Tissue Radio sensitivity.

11.9. Cell Radiosensitivity

Radiosensitivity has already discussed, refers to the susceptibility of cells to the effects of radiation. It has been observed that the level of radiosensitivity is higher in cells that divide more frequently and lower in cells that are more specialised or differentiated. Radiation primarily affects actively dividing cells and immature cells. Radiosensitive cells refer to cells that are highly responsive to radiation [42]. These cells typically possess certain characteristics: a high rate of division, a high metabolic rate, a non-specialized nature, and good nourishment. Radiation sensitivity varies among different tissues in the body. Some body tissues and their sensitivities are mentioned in Table 11.4.

Table 11.4. Tissues and their relative sensitivities to radiation

High Radiosensitivity
Lymphoid organs, bone marrow, blood, testes, ovaries, intestines
Fairly High Radiosensitivity
Skin and other organs with epithelial cell lining (cornea, oral cavity, oesophagus, rectum, bladder, vagina, uterine cervix, ureters)
Moderate Radiosensitivity
Optic lens, stomach, growing cartilage, fine vasculature, growing bone
Fairly Low Radiosensitivity
Mature cartilage or bones, salivary glands, respiratory organs, kidneys, liver, pancreas, thyroid, adrenal and pituitary glands
Low Radiosensitivity
Muscle, brain, spinal cord

11.9.1. Intrinsic Radiosensitivity and Cancer Stem Cell

It has been widely acknowledged that as cells differentiate, their radiosensitivity alters. Typically, the notion that the more differentiated cancer cells are, the higher their survival rate may seem reasonable, but this is not the case. In actuality, cancer stem cells may be more radiation-resistant than their differentiated counterparts. Due to the potent nature of the free radical scavenger.

However, the greatest impediment to increasing cancer survival rates is the high variability of cancer cells, particularly in locally advanced tumours. Therefore, there is a substantial demand for reliable biomarkers that can aid in stratifying patients for radiation therapy. Stem cells, which have an unlimited capacity for cell division and the ability to differentiate into numerous cell types, play an essential role in the field of cancer stem cells [43]. The origins of cancer stem cells are still a matter of contention, with competing hypotheses proposing either the dysregulation of normal stem cells or the dedifferentiation of terminally differentiated cancer cells. As researchers continue to investigate and comprehend the complex nature of cancer stem cells and their potential implications for cancer treatment and therapies, the mechanisms contributing to the intrinsic radiosensitivity of cancer stem cells cast additional light on this topic.

11.9.2. Mechanisms Contributing to Intrinsic Radiosensitivity of Cancer Stem Cells

Intrinsic radiosensitivity refers to the varying response of tumour cells to radiation therapy. This response is influenced by multiple factors. DNA double-strand breaks (DSBs) are a critical aspect of intrinsic radiosensitivity. Repairing these breaks is crucial as they can cause cell death if left untreated. The distribution of cells in different phases of the cell cycle and their DNA/chromosome content are believed to influence the inherent radiosensitivity of tumour cells. Additionally, it is important to note that radiation can induce apoptosis, particularly in lymphoid tumours. This characteristic plays a role in the varying levels of radiosensitivity observed. In some cases, there have been conflicting findings regarding the relationship between certain parameters and the radiosensitivity of human tumour cells. As a result, the development of a reliable assay that can accurately predict intrinsic radiosensitivity is still being studied.

In radiotherapy, when considering other confounding factors, it is important to note that the radiation dose needed to eliminate a tumour is inversely related to the logarithm of the quantity of cancer stem cells (CSCs). In the field of radiology, it has been observed that Tudors with a lower number of CSCs (Cancer Stem Cells) tend to have higher local control rates [44]. This means that these tumours have a better response to radiotherapy at the same dose compared to tumours with a higher number of CSCs. Experimental and clinical evidence suggests that the number and densities of CSCs (cancer stem cells) in a tumour can affect the effectiveness of local tumour control following radiotherapy. Several studies have demonstrated this correlation. The number of CSCs in a tumour is closely related to the radiation dose required to achieve a permanent cure for 50% of the tumours, known as the tutor control dose 50% (TCD50). This highlights the significant impact of CSCs on the local control of tumours. Radiosensitivity of cancer stem cells (CSCs) and other radiobiological factors can impact the effectiveness of radiation treatment on tumours. This is evident in studies where tumours received the same dose of radiation (TD50), but had different responses in terms of tumour control (TCD50) [45].

Radiosensitivity of tumour cells can vary even within the same histology. In vitro studies have shown this through differences in the survival of colony-forming cells when exposed to 2 Gy of radiation. This variation is measured by the surviving fraction at 2 Gy (SF2) in colony-forming assays. Radiosensitivity varies among different types of tumours and even within the same type of tumour. This has been observed clinically and has been correlated with differences in. The radiosensitivity of clonogenic cells in vitro has shown similar correlations with tumour radio curability in vivo across various tumour type. This emphasises the connection between clonogenicity in the lab and stemness in the body, as well as the significance of the inherent radiosensitivity of cancer stem cells (CSCs) for successful tumour treatment. Preclinical data on established tumour models can offer valuable insights into the biology of cancer stem cells (CSCs). However, in certain cases where detailed gene expressions or interactions between tumours and normal tissues need to be examined, the use of primary xenografts may be necessary.

Tumours can originate from a single type of cell called cancer stem cells (CSCs). If the entire population of CSCs is not completely eliminated, it can lead to treatment failure. Radiation treatment is effective in causing DNA damage in tumour tissue. This is mainly due to its ability to generate reactive oxygen species (ROS) through water metabolism or direct ionisation of DNA molecules. DNA damage can have immediate and lasting effects on cells. These effects can range from temporary or permanent cell arrest to cell death. Surviving cells may also undergo mutagenesis, leading to changes in their genetic makeup. Additionally, DNA damage can cause genomic instability, which can contribute to the development of tumours over time. In cases of DNA damage, cells initiate a response known as the DNA damage response (DDR) [46]. This response involves the activation of mechanisms like DNA repair and checkpoint kinase signalling pathways. These mechanisms play a crucial role in regulating cell cycle progression.

Cancer stem cells (CSCs) have a strong ability to repair DNA damage, which makes them resistant to radiation therapy. This is mainly due to the activation of two important signalling pathways: ATR-Chk1 and ATM-Chk2 [47]. These pathways play a crucial role in the repair of DNA and contribute to the radio resistance of CSCs. Cancer stem cells (CSCs) have effective systems for removing reactive oxygen species (ROS), which helps them maintain lower ROS levels compared to non-CSCs. This ability to scavenge ROS contributes to their resistance against genotoxic stress. Several studies have confirmed this phenomenon. The tumour microenvironment, including the specialised areas where cancer stem cells (CSCs) are found, has a crucial impact on controlling the behaviour of CSCs and their ability to resist radiation treatment. Hypoxic niches shield CSCs from radiation damage and trigger signalling pathways linked to CSC upkeep, including HIF, Notch, WNT, and Hedgehog signalling. Epithelial-mesenchymal transition (EMT) in tumours can lead to radio resistance and the expression of cancer stem cell (CSC) markers, which can impact treatment results. In the field of radiology, it is important to understand that external factors and the way cells interact with each other within the tumour microenvironment can affect the behaviour of cancer stem cells (CSCs) and how they respond to treatment.

Understanding the relationship between CSCs (Cancer Stem Cells) and their sensitivity to radiation, as well as the influence of intrinsic mechanisms and the tumour microenvironment on CSCs' resistance to radiation, is crucial for the development of effective treatment approaches. CSC Radio resistance in Cancer Patients While there are still unanswered questions and ongoing research, it is important to understand the molecular mechanisms behind CSC radio resistance. This knowledge will help in developing targeted therapies and improving treatment outcomes for cancer patients receiving radiation therapy.

CSC radio resistance is a crucial area of study for the development of targeted therapies. It is important to comprehend the molecular mechanisms involved in order to effectively address this issue. Cancer stem cells (CSCs) have developed certain characteristics that make them resistant to radiation therapy. These include changes in DNA repair pathways, an improved ability to respond to DNA damage, and mechanisms to protect against oxidative stress. These factors play a significant role in CSC radio resistance [48]. The tumour microenvironment and tumour repopulation are important factors that can affect treatment outcomes. Mechanisms that contribute to CSC radio resistance can be identified and targeted to enhance the efficacy of radiation therapy in cancer treatment.

However, inconsistent correlations with radiosensitivity of human tumour cells have been reported in this process, and the establishment of a useful assay that predicts intrinsic radiosensitivity is still under investigation.

Certain points that we need to go through when discussing about intrinsic radiosensitivity and cancer stem cells are:

- **Biological Parameters as Biomarkers for Radiation Oncology**

There are a limited number of biological parameters that can serve as potential biomarkers. These include tumour size, hypoxia, and HPV positivity for head and neck squamous cell carcinoma (HNSCC) [49]. Patient stratification is a process that involves categorising patients based on the characteristics of their tumours. The goal is to determine which patients are likely to respond well to radiation therapy and which are not. By doing this, we can improve the effectiveness of cancer treatment and increase the chances of successful outcomes. The approach in radiology is based on the concept of the "5Rs" in radiobiology. These include repair, redistribution, repopulation, reoxygenation, and intrinsic radio resistance.

- **DNA Damage and Repair in Radiotherapy**

Radiotherapy is a crucial treatment for cancer, aiming to cure the disease by damaging the DNA in tumour tissues. The effectiveness of radiotherapy is directly linked to the degree and quality of DNA damage caused. DNA double-strand breaks (DSBs) are a significant type of DNA damage caused by ionizing radiation. When the amount of radiation-induced DNA double-strand breaks (DSBs) is higher than what tumour cells can repair, it can cause the cells to stop dividing, enter a state of senescence, and eventually die. Cellular response to DNA damage is a multifaceted process that encompasses the activation of DNA damage response pathways and DNA repair mechanisms. Radiation-induced DNA damage can give rise to reactive oxygen species (ROS) and reactive nitrogen species (RNS) [50]. These harmful molecules have the potential to cause additional DNA damage, as well as oxidation of proteins and peroxidation of lipids. Ultimately, this can lead to cell senescence and death.

- **CSC Populations and Radioresistance**

Cancer stem cells (CSCs) are a special type of cells that are thought to originate from normal stem cells. These cells possess distinct characteristics that make them resistant to radiation therapy. CSCs (Cancer Stem Cells) are responsible for activating various signalling pathways that contribute to radio resistance. These pathways include epidermal growth factor receptor (EGFR), PI3K/Akt/mTOR, WNT, Notch, and Hedgehog signalling [51]. Exploring molecular pathways as potential therapeutic intervention to overcome CSC radio resistance is currently being explored.

- **Tumour Microenvironment and Radioresistance**

Tumour microenvironment, such as hypoxia and nutrient availability, is important for radiotherapy response [52]. Hypoxia, which refers to low oxygen levels, can lead to resistance against radiotherapy. This resistance occurs because hypoxia reduces the occurrence of DNA double-strand breaks (DSBs), which are caused by the production of free radicals that depend on oxygen. In the context of radiology, it is important to note that hypoxia can have significant effects on tumour metabolism and the maintenance of cancer stem cells (CSCs). This is primarily mediated through the activation of certain pathways, including hypoxia-inducible factor (HIF) signalling, autophagy, and epithelial-mesenchymal transition (EMT).

- **Tumour Recurrences and Repopulation**

Tumour recurrences following radiotherapy can be affected by the regrowth of tumour cells during the course of treatment. Fast-proliferating tumours have the ability to regrow during the intervals between radiotherapy treatments, which can ultimately result in the failure of the therapy. Cancer stem cells (CSCs) possess the remarkable ability to continuously regenerate themselves, which is thought to play a role in the regrowth of tumours. Tumour reoxygenation during treatment has been found to increase the likelihood of symmetric division in cancer stem cells (CSCs), leading to a larger population of CSCs within the tumour.

- **Radiobiological Concept of 5Rs and CSC Tumour Model**

In order to comprehend the impact of radiotherapy on tumour tissues, it is crucial to explore the radiobiological concept known as the "5Rs" within the framework of the cancer stem cell (CSC) tumour model [53]. The concept of repair, redistribution, repopulation, reoxygenation, and intrinsic radio resistance are important factors that affect the response to radiation therapy.

- **Molecular Mechanisms of CSC Radioresistance**

Cancer stem cells (CSCs) have distinct differences in their DNA damage response and repair pathways when compared to non-CSCs. Enhanced activation of ATM, ATR, and their downstream checkpoint kinases (Chk1 and Chk2) is observed [54]. These kinases play a crucial role in regulating the DNA damage response and repair processes. Homologous recombination (HR) is important in cancer stem cell (CSC) radio resistance. On the other hand, non-homologous end joining (NHEJ) is primarily affected by ATM-mediated effects.

- **Reprogramming and Induction of CSCs**

A noteworthy finding is the ability of cancer stem cells (CSCs) to develop resistance to radiotherapy. This resistance can be triggered by genotoxic treatments, which are therapies that damage the DNA of cancer cells. Treatment-induced reprogramming of non-cancer stem cells (CCSCs) into cancer stem cells (CSCs) can occur, which can ultimately contribute to the development of treatment resistance. During the reprogramming process, it is important to note that certain pathways involved in DNA repair may be activated. Additionally, stem cell characteristics may also be induced.

The radiosensitivity of tumour cells is determined by several factors, such as DNA repair capacity, cell cycle distribution, and the likelihood of undergoing apoptosis. There may also be additional unknown factors that can affect intrinsic radiosensitivity [55]. Radiosensitivity is an important factor to consider when it comes to radiation therapy and personalised treatment. It helps in optimising the effectiveness of radiation therapy and developing individualised treatment plans. Additional investigation is required to understand the intricate relationship between these elements and discover dependable biomarkers for accurately forecasting radiosensitivity in various tumour types. Understanding the information provided here will help in better categorising patients and improving the effectiveness of radiation therapy for cancer treatment.

11.10. Effective Cell Survival Curve

Cell culture techniques are crucial for studying the quantitative investigation of cell proliferation and sterilisation. In radiology, the surviving fraction refers to the proportion of cells in an irradiated population that can still divide compared to a unirradiated population. This is determined by plotting the logarithm of the surviving fraction against the radiation dose received, resulting in a survival curve for the cells being studied.

A cell survival curve, as already discussed is a graph that shows the proportion of cells that survive after being exposed to radiation, compared to the proportion of cells that survive without any radiation exposure [56]. Each point on the curve represents a specific radiation dose. Survival data of cellular organisms are typically represented in a logarithmic scale, where the logarithm of the fraction of cells that survive is plotted against the radiation dose administered. The logarithm of the surviving fraction is plotted on the vertical axis, while the dose is represented on the horizontal axis.

Mammalian cell survival curves typically exhibit an exponential reaction to high radiation doses. In the low-dose range, there is a varying width "shoulder" observed [57]. Radiation's impact on cells can be assessed by observing variations in the cell survival curve across various conditions. There are various ways to modify the conditions for optimal results. This can involve utilising diverse radiation modalities, altering the surroundings, adjusting oxygen levels, or administering radiation at specific timings or stages of the cell cycle. Survival curves provide valuable insights into radiation damage, even predating the discovery of DNA's structure.

However, in the realm of radiobiology, when it comes to comparing curves, it becomes advantageous to express them mathematically, utilising theoretical frameworks postulating potential mechanisms underlying the manifestation of lethality. The elucidation of the cellular survival curve's morphology remains a subject of ongoing discourse within the radiobiological community, as does the optimal approach for mathematically modelling such data sets [58].

11.10.1. The Effective Survival Curve: Fractionation

When the dose is given in equal fractions with enough time in between for the body to repair non-lethal damage, the survival curve shows a repeated pattern. The survival curve is formed by combining all the shoulder repetitions. The required dose to achieve a similar decrease in the surviving fraction increases as depicted in Figure 11.2.

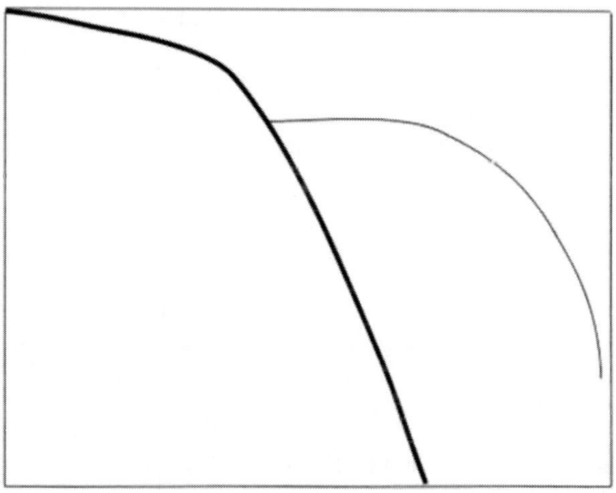

Figure 11.2. The graph on the left depicts a dose/survival curve for a hypothetical group of cells exposed to ionizing radiation. The curve illustrates how the number of cells that survive decreases as the radiation dose increases. The blue line represents cells continuously irradiated without recovery, while the red line represents cells allowed to recover between irradiation sessions. The red line shows better cell survival, indicating the protective effect of fractionation - incorporating rest periods during radiation exposure.

11.11. Cell Survival Curve: Indices

Several indices are derived from the survival curve of cells as shown in Figure 11.3. D1 and D0 are two entities of this type. The initial slope of the survival curve is denoted by D1. D0 represents the ultimate slope of the curve, where it approaches a straight line. D0 also serves as a measure of the relative radiosensitivity of cell populations. D0 is the dose necessary to reduce the proportion of survivors to 37% of the proportion associated with the previous dose. The D0 will vary based on cell type and the local environment in which the cell population is cultured (e.g., oxygen tension; remember that oxygen increases the probability of free radical production). D0 for oxygenated mammalian cells is approximately 1.5 Gy (150 rads). The so-called quasi-threshold dose (Dq) is another component of the parabola [59]. This is also referred to as the sublethal dose.

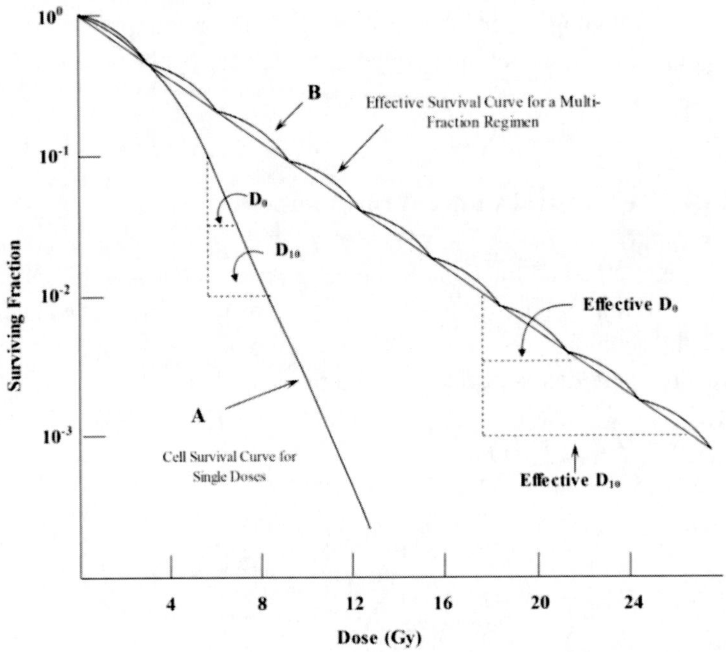

Figure 11.3. A visual representation is provided to showcase the concept of an "effective" survival curve for a multifraction n regimen. When the radiation dose is given in equal fractions with enough time intervals in between for sublethal damage to be repaired, the shoulder of the survival curve is observed multiple times. The dose-survival curve is an exponential function of dose, meaning it follows a straight line from the starting point through a specific point on the survival curve for a daily dose fraction (e.g., 2 Gy). The D10, which represents the dose causing one decade of cell killing, can be calculated using the expression D10 = 2.3 times the Do.

11.11.1. Survival Curve for Mammalian Cells

Survival curves depicting the response of mammalian cells when exposed to low-linear energy transfer (LET) radiation typically exhibit a degree of curvature [60].

11.11.1.1. Region of Cell Survival Curves

The region characterised by a lower rate of cell inactivation per unit dose compared to higher doses is referred to as the initial low dose region, commonly known as the shoulder. Frequently, the region with elevated dosage exhibits a propensity towards a linear trajectory. The parameter D0 can subsequently be employed to characterise the radiosensitivity within this particular region of the curve. The determination of the extrapolation number, denoted as n, involves the process of extending the terminal linear segment of the curve towards the abscissa, as seen in Figure 11.4.

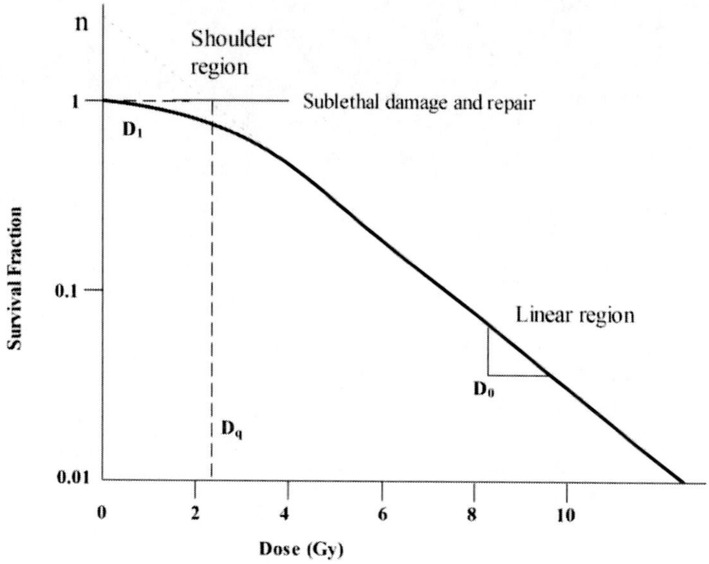

Figure 11.4. Cell survival curve for mammalian cells showing shoulder region and types of damages.

In the context of the dose-response curve, it is observed that within the shoulder region, the cell lethality rate exhibits an upward trend as the administered dose escalates [61].

There are two plausible interpretations in this regard:

- The demise of cells occurs due to the aggregation of events that, on their own, lack the capacity to induce cell death. However, when combined, these events prove fatal for the cell (referred to as target models).
- Lesions, in the context of cellular damage, possess the ability to undergo individual repair processes. However, when the efficiency of enzymatic repair mechanisms decreases in correlation with the number of lesions, the cells reach a state where the lesions become irreparable, ultimately leading to cell death. This phenomenon is governed by repair models that take into account the dose-dependent relationship between the number of lesions and the diminishing efficiency of repair mechanisms.

11.12. Radiosensitivity of Mammalian Cells Compare with Microorganisms

Radiation's effect on living organisms is a complex interaction between the unique characteristics of each different cell and microorganism. Radiosensitivity, which refers to the varying degrees of vulnerability to radiation-induced harm, plays a crucial role in the divergent responses of mammalian cells and microbes (refer Figure 11.5).

The average dose-response relationship for mammalian cells, demonstrates a steep curve. Escherichia coli demonstrates the highest level of resistance among these microorganisms, while yeast exhibits the highest level of resistance. However, Micrococcus radiodurans exhibits the most remarkable resistance, surviving dosages as high as 1,000 Gy without significant cell damage. Compared to the resistance observed in microorganisms such as Escherichia coli, yeast, and Micrococcus radiodurans, the radiosensitivity of mammalian cells is astoundingly high [62].

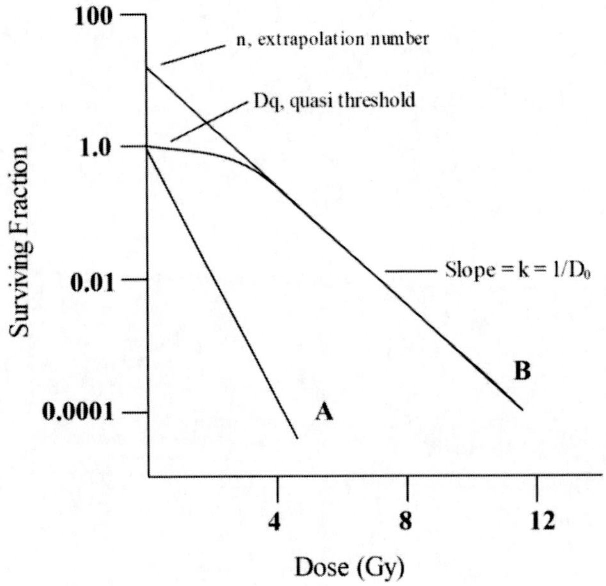

Figure 11.5. Cell survival curves for mammalian cells.

Numerous factors contribute to this wide range of radio sensitivities, with DNA content, DNA repair systems, and the manner of cell death playing the most significant roles. Microorganisms such as E. coli B/r demonstrate the significance of efficient DNA repair systems, whereas mammalian cell susceptibility is primarily determined by DNA content. In addition, the mode of cell death, whether apoptotic or mitotic, also contributes to the differences in radiosensitivity among various organisms.

This observation reveals a number of crucial insights:

- The DNA content is the primary factor influencing this enormous spectrum of radio sensitivities. The high sensitivity of mammalian cells can be attributed to their high DNA content, which creates a larger target for radiation-induced damage.
- Nevertheless, DNA content cannot account for all variation. E. coli and E. coli B/r, for example, have the same DNA content, but their radiosensitivity differs due to B/r's mutant and more efficient DNA repair system. Additionally, the mode of cell death, whether apoptotic or mitotic, influences radiosensitivity in higher organisms.
- Even when objects appear clean, the presence of extremely radioresistant microorganisms necessitates such high concentrations to reduce their population and guarantee sterilisation.

11.13. The Effect of Oxygen at Various Phases of the Cell Cycle

11.13.1. Oxygen and the Cell Cycle

From humans to bacteria, living beings must undergo dramatic changes as they progress through their life cycle. Cells in cell cultures are no different. They too undergo biological changes as they grow and reproduce, giving way to new cells through time. Understanding the cell life cycle and how different conditions, including oxygen, may affect it, is particularly important in modern-day biotechnology [63].

Depending on cell type and location in the body there is a specific physiological amount of oxygen present, and these conditions must be replicated in culture chambers. Cell chambers are often kept at normoxic conditions. Normoxia is the term used to describe oxygen levels between 10–21%. Hypoxic chambers are only now becoming a popular tool in cell culture applications. Hypoxia is a condition of low oxygen tension, typically in the range 1–5% O_2, and is more physiologically relevant for some cell types, such as stem cells.

11.13.2. The Cell Cycle under Normoxic Conditions

There are several important steps for a cell cycle. It must grow, duplicate its genetic material, the DNA, and physically split into two 'daughter' cells. Those daughter cells will follow the same steps, ultimately producing more daughter cells. In eukaryotic cells, those that contain a nucleus, all the steps can be identified by two main phases: Interphase and the mitotic (M) phase. Under normoxic conditions, and if other growing parameters are within a reasonable range for the cells, they will proceed through the cell cycle as intended [64, 65].

11.13.3. Cells under Hypoxic Conditions

While the scientific community is only beginning to understand the role that oxygen plays on the behaviours of cells, it has been discovered that the cellular response to hypoxic conditions of low or no oxygen is governed largely by a group of transcription factors known as hypoxia inducible factors (HIFs). Under hypoxic conditions, this otherwise inactive group of DNA binding proteins accumulate in the cell nucleus, and either activate or deactivate certain cellular responses to mediate the response to hypoxia. Their role varies depending on the cell type as some cells, for example red blood cells, respond better to low oxygen conditions than others [65].

Generally, when the oxygen levels are consistently set too low for the cell, HIFs respond by decreasing metabolic function and inducing cell cycle arrest [66]. As the cells proliferate, they continue to consume oxygen, resulting in an even more hypoxic state. If normal oxygen levels are not returned, eventually, the cells will stop dividing and cell death may occur.

The effects of oxygen on the G1, G2, and S phases of the cell cycle can be significant and can vary depending on the type of cell and the oxygen concentration. In general, low oxygen levels during these phases can have both positive and negative effects on cell growth and proliferation.

I. Positive effects of low oxygen levels on the phases of the cell cycle include:

1. *Increased rate of cell proliferation*: Low oxygen levels can stimulate cell proliferation, as cells respond to the reduced oxygen availability by activating specific pathways that promote cell growth and survival.

2. *Increased resistance to cellular stress*: Low oxygen levels can also increase a cell's resistance to cellular stress, as cells respond to the reduced oxygen availability by activating pathways that protect them from damage.
3. *Maintenance of cell viability*: Oxygen is required for cells to carry out normal metabolic processes, including mitosis, and low oxygen levels can lead to cellular damage and death.
4. *Support of normal cell division*: Adequate oxygen levels are necessary for normal cell division, as cells require oxygen to carry out this process efficiently.

II. Negative effects of low oxygen levels on the phases of the cell cycle include:

1. *Decreased efficiency of cellular metabolism*: Low oxygen levels can decrease the efficiency of cellular metabolism, as cells are less able to generate energy through aerobic respiration.
2. *Increased risk of oxidative stress*: Low oxygen levels can increase the production of reactive oxygen species (ROS), which can cause oxidative stress and damage to cellular components such as DNA, proteins, and lipids.
3. *Impaired cell division*: Low oxygen levels can impair the process of mitosis, the phase of the cell cycle where cells divide into two daughter cells, leading to cell cycle arrest or apoptosis. This can occur because low oxygen levels can inhibit the activity of enzymes involved in cell division and increase the formation of DNA damage.

11.13.4. The Age-Response Function for a Tissue *In Vivo*

The aging process is a complex phenomenon that affects various aspects of an organism's body, including its tissues. As an organism ages, tissues undergo a series of changes and adaptations that can impact their structure, function, and overall health [67].

Certain points to be considered are:

- *Cellular Senescence*
  Cellular senescence is a state in which cells lose their ability to divide and replicate. It is a natural part of the aging process and can occur in various tissues. Senescent cells tend to accumulate over time, leading to tissue dysfunction. These cells secrete inflammatory molecules, growth factors, and enzymes that can have negative effects on surrounding cells and tissues.
- *Telomere Shortening*
  Telomeres are protective caps found at the ends of chromosomes. With each cell division, telomeres gradually shorten. Once they reach a critically short length, cells may undergo senescence or programmed cell death (apoptosis). Telomere shortening is considered a marker of cellular aging and can contribute to tissue deterioration.
- *DNA Damage*
  DNA damage can occur due to various factors, such as oxidative stress, exposure to radiation or toxins, and errors during DNA replication. As an organism ages, the

accumulation of DNA damage increases. If not repaired, this damage can lead to mutations, genomic instability, and impaired cellular function.

- *Decline in Regenerative Capacity*
  Many tissues have the ability to regenerate and repair themselves. This process relies on the presence of stem cells that can differentiate and replenish damaged cells. However, as an organism ages, the regenerative capacity of tissues generally declines. Stem cells become less active, reducing the ability of the tissue to regenerate and heal.
- *Inflammation and Inflammaging*
  Chronic inflammation is a hallmark of aging tissues and is often referred to as "inflammaging." Low-grade, persistent inflammation can be caused by various factors, including cellular senescence, immune dysregulation, and the accumulation of damaged molecules. Inflammaging can disrupt normal tissue homeostasis, impair cellular function, and contribute to age-related diseases [68].
- *Extracellular Matrix Changes*
  The extracellular matrix (ECM) is a complex network of proteins and molecules that provide structural support to tissues. With aging, there are alterations in the composition, structure, and function of the ECM. This can result in tissue stiffness, reduced elasticity, and impaired tissue function. Changes in the ECM contribute to age-related conditions such as osteoporosis and skin aging.
- *Metabolic Alterations*
  Aging tissues undergo metabolic changes that affect their energy production and nutrient utilization. Mitochondrial function, which is responsible for energy production, may decline with age. Alterations in metabolic pathways can also occur, leading to reduced energy production and impaired cellular metabolism.

These age-related changes in tissues can contribute to the development of various age-related diseases and conditions, including neurodegenerative disorders, cardiovascular diseases, osteoporosis, and age-related macular degeneration. It's important to note that the age response of tissues can be influenced by genetic factors, lifestyle choices (such as diet and exercise), exposure to environmental toxins, and overall health status.

11.14. Variation of Sensitivity with Cell Age for High-Linear Energy Transfer Radiations

Radiaton age response is a well-documented phenomenon that has been observed since the 1960s. It pertains to the changes in sensitivity of cultured mammalian cells during different stages of the cell cycle when they are exposed to radiation. The impact of high-LET radiation on cell sensitivity can differ across age groups, influenced by various factors. The comparison of High LET versus that of Low LET can be seen in Figure 11.6.

In the late 1960s and early 1970s, initial studies discovered that high-linear energy transfer (LET) radiations, including fast neutrons, alpha particles, pions, and heavy-ion particle beams, had the potential to reduce the differences in sensitivity between various phases of the cell cycle. This fascinating discovery prompted researchers to investigate the underlying mechanisms that contribute to the variations in radiation response based on age.

Human cells, in contrast to rodent cell lines commonly used in initial research, have longer cell cycle phases. These cells display two distinct peaks of radio resistance to low-LET radiation. One peak occurs during the G1 phase, while the other is observed in the S phase. Recent studies on high-LET radiations have revealed an intriguing finding: these particles are capable of eliminating the X-ray-resistant peak during the early G1 phase, while the resistant peak during the late S phase remains unaffected. This implies that the age-related impact of radio lesions and repair effects may vary depending on the type of radiation exposure.

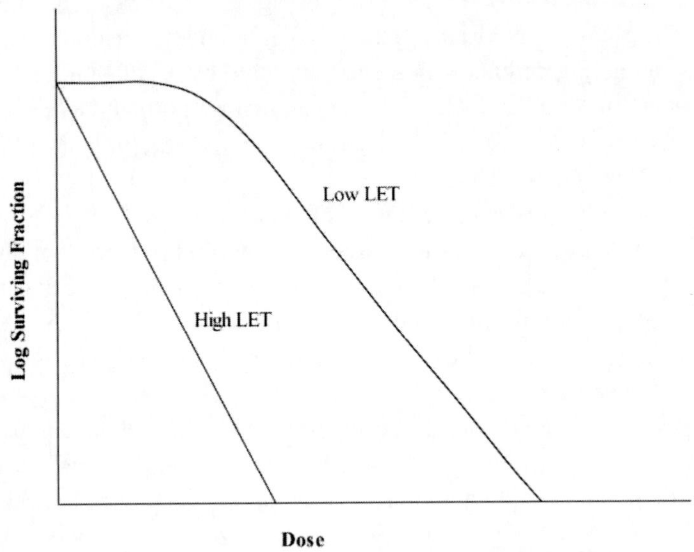

Figure 11.6. Cell survival curves for high-LET particles and low-LET X-rays that are representative. Radiation with a high LET produces steeper curves with little or no shoulder.

As scientists explored the molecular foundation of how radiation affects ageing, initial efforts to attribute this occurrence to a solitary molecular factor or activity, such as DNA synthesis, were found to be insufficient. For example, the provided explanation did not consider the radio resistance that is observed during the G1 phase. To address these limitations, researchers started investigating the functions of intracellular factors that may change depending on the cell cycle stage and impact cell viability.

Glutathione (GSH) is an essential antioxidant molecule found in cells, which plays a significant role in various biological processes [69]. Research has indicated that fluctuations in intracellular non-protein sulfhydryls and GSH concentrations are associated with alterations in the X-ray oxygen enhancement ratio (OER) for cell viability. Nevertheless, the specific processes through which these variations in GSH and other cellular components impact the reaction to radiation are still not completely understood. Nonetheless, it emphasises the significance of comprehending the complex interaction between internal cellular factors and the reaction to radiation at various stages of the cell cycle.

Additionally, studies have shown that intracellular factors such as the levels of glutathione can have an impact on DNA damage, specifically DNA strand breaks. The oxygen concentration seems to play a role in determining the types and amount of base damage caused by radiation. This highlights the importance of the cellular microenvironment in influencing the response to radiation.

Research investigating alterations in radiosensitivity throughout the cell cycle has found a connection between changes in chromatin dispersion and variations in the response to radiation. The similarity in repair kinetics of sublethal and potentially lethal lesions during different phases of the cell cycle may be attributed to the probability of interactions between chromatin. Nevertheless, the precise mechanisms behind the heightened radiosensitivity observed during the G1/S interface phase have yet to be fully elucidated, and continue to be an ongoing focus of research.

The progress made in radiation biology and molecular techniques has opened up new possibilities for understanding the molecular mechanisms that drive the response to radiation-induced ageing. Currently, scientists are dedicated to understanding the functions of particular intracellular factors, DNA repair pathways, and signalling cascades that play a part in the varying levels of sensitivity seen in different phases of the cell cycle. The impact of high-LET radiation on cell sensitivity can differ across age groups due to various factors.

High-LET radiation has the potential to induce various intricate and severe forms of DNA damage in cells. These include double-strand breaks, DNA-protein crosslinks, and clustered lesions. As cells get older, their capacity to fix DNA damage may decrease. The efficiency of DNA repair mechanisms may decline or be compromised, resulting in a decreased ability to repair DNA damage caused by high-LET radiation. As a consequence, there may be a rise in genomic instability and a decline in cell viability.

As cells age, cellular metabolism experiences alterations. Energy metabolism, redox status, and antioxidant defence mechanisms may undergo changes in older cells. The sensitivity to high-LET radiation can be influenced by these modifications. The cellular response to oxidative stress and DNA damage caused by high-LET radiation can be influenced by changes in cellular metabolism. The survival and repair processes of cells can be affected by alterations in energy metabolism and antioxidant defence systems following exposure to high-LET radiation.

The control of the cell cycle is of utmost importance in how cells respond to DNA damage and cellular stress caused by radiation. Changes in cell cycle regulation and checkpoints can be observed in ageing cells. The sensitivity to high-LET radiation can be influenced by these modifications. Cellular survival and prevention of mutations rely heavily on the presence of efficient cell cycle arrest and DNA repair mechanisms [70]. Changes in cell cycle control that occur with age can impact the cell's capacity to effectively address DNA damage caused by high-LET radiation.

As individuals age, there is a possibility for the dysregulation of cellular signalling pathways and apoptotic responses. These alterations can have an impact on the sensitivity to DNA damage and cellular stress caused by high-LET radiation. The ability of ageing cells to initiate programmed cell death in response to severe radiation damage may be compromised due to impaired signalling or resistance to apoptosis. The effect of this can influence the survival of cells and the overall response of tissues to high-LET radiation.

Stem cells are crucial for the regeneration and repair of tissues, as they are present in various tissues and undergo alterations to fulfil this role. As individuals grow older, the regenerative ability of stem cells may diminish. The decrease in tissue response to high-LET radiation could potentially be impacted by this decline. When the function of stem cells is diminished, it can negatively impact the ability of tissues to undergo repair, increasing their vulnerability to damage caused by radiation.

11.14.1. Mechanisms for the Age Response Function

The age-response function in radiobiology focuses on the variations in cell sensitivity during different stages of the cell cycle, specifically in relation to the lethality caused by radiation exposure. Although the precise mechanisms responsible for these variations are not yet fully comprehended, several correlations have been suggested [71].

The primary cause of sensitivity changes can be attributed to the DNA's role as the main target for cell lethality caused by radiation. During the S phase, the DNA content doubles as the genome undergoes replication, and just before mitosis, the chromosome material condenses into discrete entities. These two events occur during periods of minimum and maximum radiosensitivity, respectively. Nevertheless, the precise connection between these alterations in DNA content and sensitivity remains uncertain, and the observed association may not provide a complete explanation for the phenomenon.

Another correlation exists between the levels of naturally occurring sulfhydryl compounds in the cell, which possess strong radioprotective properties. Changes in radiosensitivity are associated with different levels of these compounds during the cell cycle. Although there is some understanding of the relationship between sulfhydryl compounds and sensitivity, the specific mechanisms through which these compounds affect sensitivity are not yet completely comprehended.

The repair mechanisms available for double-strand breaks (DSBs) are influenced by the cell cycle phase. Non-homologous end-joining (NHEJ) is mainly observed during the G phase, specifically when there is an absence of a sister chromatid [72]. In contrast, homologous recombination repair (HRR) is limited to the late S/G2 phase, where it relies on the presence of an intact chromatid as a template for the repair process. The differences in repair mechanisms could potentially play a role in the varying levels of radiation sensitivity observed during different stages of the cell cycle.

To sum up, the age-response function in radiobiology encompasses complex changes in radiation sensitivity as cells advance through their generation cycle. Although there have been suggestions of connections between DNA content and sulfhydryl compounds, the precise mechanisms behind these associations remain unclear. Furthermore, the variations in radiation sensitivity can be attributed to the presence of specific repair mechanisms, such as NHEJ and HRR, which are available at different phases of the cell cycle. Having a comprehensive understanding of these mechanisms is essential in order to enhance the effectiveness of radiation therapy and enhance treatment results for patients across various age ranges. Additional investigation is required to reveal the precise factors contributing to the age-response function and devise specific approaches to improve the efficacy of radiation therapy while mitigating any potential negative consequences.

11.14.2. The Possible Implication of Age Response Function in Radiotherapy

The age response function plays a crucial role in the context of radiotherapy, which is a widely used treatment for cancer patients. Understanding how age influences the response to radiotherapy has important implications for treatment planning, dose fractionation, side effect management, treatment outcomes, and survivorship care. This comprehensive understanding allows healthcare providers to optimize treatment strategies, minimize side effects, and improve overall treatment outcomes for older cancer patients.

Firstly, the age response function helps guide treatment planning decisions. As individuals age, physiological changes occur in their bodies that can impact their response to radiation therapy. For instance, older patients may have reduced tissue tolerance to radiation, increased comorbidities, or compromised organ function. Taking the age response function into account during treatment planning enables healthcare providers to adjust radiation doses and treatment volumes accordingly. By doing so, they can minimize potential side effects and maximize treatment efficacy in older patients.

Secondly, the age response function influences decisions regarding dose fractionation. Dose fractionation involves dividing the total radiation dose into smaller fractions delivered over multiple treatment sessions. The response of normal tissues and tumours to radiation can vary with age. Older patients may exhibit reduced cellular repair mechanisms and increased cellular sensitivity to radiation. By considering the age response function, healthcare providers can optimize treatment outcomes by adjusting the dose fractionation schedule to balance tumour control and normal tissue toxicity.

Moreover, the age response function is crucial for managing side effects associated with radiotherapy. Radiation therapy can cause acute and late side effects, such as fatigue, skin reactions, and damage to surrounding healthy tissues [73]. The age response function provides insights into the likelihood and severity of these side effects based on a patient's age. Older patients may be more susceptible to certain side effects due to age-related changes in tissue resilience and repair mechanisms. By considering the age response function, healthcare providers can implement appropriate strategies to manage and mitigate side effects in older patients, improving their quality of life during and after treatment.

Additionally, the age response function can help predict treatment outcomes in older patients undergoing radiotherapy. Older individuals may have different tumour biology, immune responses, and overall health compared to younger patients. The age response function provides information on the likelihood of tumour response, disease recurrence, and overall survival rates based on age. This knowledge allows clinicians to set realistic treatment goals, discuss prognosis, and tailor treatment strategies for older patients, ultimately improving treatment decision-making and patient care.

Finally, the age response function has implications for survivorship care. As more individuals survive cancer and live longer, survivorship care becomes increasingly important. The age response function informs survivorship care planning for older cancer survivors who have undergone radiotherapy. It helps identify potential long-term effects of radiation treatment based on age, guides screening and surveillance strategies for late effects, and informs supportive care interventions specific to the aging population. By incorporating the age response function into survivorship care, healthcare providers can optimize the long-term health and well-being of older cancer survivors.

11.15. Radiosensitisers and Radioprotectors

11.15.1. Radiosensitizers

Radiosensitizers are substances or agents that sensitize tumour cells to the effects of radiation therapy. The goal of using radiosensitizers is to enhance the efficacy of radiation treatment and improve cancer control while minimizing damage to surrounding healthy tissues [74].

Radiation therapy works by delivering high-energy radiation to the tumour, causing damage to the DNA within the cancer cells. This radiation-induced DNA damage can lead to cell death or impair the tumour's ability to grow and divide. However, some cancer cells may exhibit inherent resistance to radiation or have developed mechanisms to repair the radiation-induced damage, reducing the treatment's effectiveness.

Some of the major functions of Radiosensitizers function are as follows:

- *Enhancing DNA damage*: Radiosensitizers can increase the amount of DNA damage inflicted on cancer cells when combined with radiation therapy. They may create more double-strand breaks or other types of DNA lesions that are difficult for the cancer cells to repair.
- *Inhibiting DNA repai*r: Some radiosensitizers can interfere with the cancer cells' ability to repair radiation-induced DNA damage. By inhibiting specific DNA repair pathways, the cancer cells become more vulnerable to the effects of radiation.
- *Modulating cellular responses*: Radiosensitizers can modify signalling pathways within the cancer cells, leading to changes in their responses to radiation. This can disrupt cell survival mechanisms and promote cell death in the tumour.
- *Targeting hypoxic cells*: Certain radiosensitizers are designed to sensitize cancer cells that exist in areas of low oxygen (hypoxia). These hypoxic cells are often more resistant to radiation, so targeting them can improve overall treatment outcomes.

Radiosensitizers can be chemicals, drugs, or even naturally occurring compounds. Researchers continue to investigate and develop new radiosensitizers to improve the outcomes of radiation therapy for various types of cancer. The use of radiosensitizers is subject to rigorous testing in preclinical studies and clinical trials to ensure their safety and effectiveness before they are incorporated into standard cancer treatment protocols [75].

- **Examples of various radiosensitizers:**

- *Cisplatin*: Cisplatin is a chemotherapy drug that has also been shown to act as a radiosensitizer. It enhances radiation-induced DNA damage in cancer cells and disrupts their repair mechanisms, leading to increased cell death.
- *5-Fluorouracil (5-FU):* 5-FU is another chemotherapy drug that has radio sensitizing properties. It interferes with DNA synthesis and repair processes, making cancer cells more vulnerable to the effects of radiation.
- *Gemcitabine:* Gemcitabine is a chemotherapy drug used in combination with radiation therapy for certain cancers. It inhibits DNA replication and enhances the radiosensitivity of tumour cells.

- *Cetuximab:* Cetuximab is a targeted therapy used in some cases of head and neck cancer and colorectal cancer. It targets the epidermal growth factor receptor (EGFR) and has been shown to sensitize cancer cells to radiation.
- *Veliparib:* Veliparib is a PARP inhibitor, a type of drug that interferes with DNA repair in cancer cells. It has been studied as a radiosensitizer in various types of cancer.
- *Olaparib:* Olaparib is another PARP inhibitor that has shown promise as a radiosensitizer in certain cancers, particularly in those with BRCA mutations.
- *Misonidazole:* Misonidazole is a hypoxic cell radiosensitizer. It is designed to sensitize tumour cells that are deprived of oxygen, which can be common in some solid tumours.
- *Vorinostat:* Vorinostat is a histone deacetylase (HDAC) inhibitor that has been investigated as a radiosensitizer in cancer treatment.

11.15.2. Radioprotectors

Radioprotectors are substances or agents that aim to protect normal tissues from the harmful effects of radiation during radiotherapy or radiation exposure [76, 77]. Unlike radiosensitizers, which enhance the effects of radiation on tumour cells, radioprotectors focus on reducing radiation damage to healthy tissues surrounding the target area. The goal is to minimize side effects and complications associated with radiation therapy while maintaining its effectiveness against the cancerous cells.

Radiation therapy is designed to deliver a focused dose of radiation to the tumour while sparing surrounding healthy tissues as much as possible. However, some healthy tissues, especially those in the proximity of the tumour, may still be exposed to radiation and could experience adverse effects. Radioprotectors work through various mechanisms to mitigate radiation-induced damage to these normal tissues:

Free radical scavenging: Radioprotectors may act as antioxidants, neutralizing harmful free radicals generated by radiation exposure. Free radicals can cause oxidative stress and damage to cells, leading to tissue injury. By scavenging these free radicals, radioprotectors help reduce the potential damage [78].

- **Major functions of radiosensitizers are as follows:**

- *DNA repair enhancement*: Some radioprotectors promote DNA repair mechanisms in healthy cells, enabling them to better recover from radiation-induced damage.
- *Anti-inflammatory properties*: Radiation can trigger an inflammatory response in tissues, which can exacerbate radiation-induced damage. Radioprotectors with anti-inflammatory properties can help reduce inflammation and its harmful effects.
- *Modulation of cell signalling*: Radioprotectors can regulate specific signalling pathways in normal cells, which may enhance their resilience to radiation.
- *Hypoxia protection:* In certain cases, radioprotectors can help protect normal tissues that experience oxygen deprivation (hypoxia) during radiation therapy. This is

particularly useful when dealing with tumours that have areas of low oxygen concentration, as hypoxic cells are generally more resistant to radiation.

Common radioprotectors include certain drugs, chemical compounds, and naturally occurring substances. Researchers continuously study and investigate potential radioprotectors to improve the safety and efficacy of radiation therapy.

It's important to note that while radioprotectors have the potential to reduce radiation-induced damage to healthy tissues, their use must be carefully evaluated through rigorous research and clinical trials to ensure they do not interfere with the intended effects of radiation on cancer cells.

- **Examples for radioprotectors:**

- *Amifostine (Ethyol):* Amifostine is a well-known radioprotector that is commonly used in certain cancer treatments, such as head and neck cancers and ovarian cancer. It acts as a free radical scavenger, helping to protect healthy cells from radiation-induced damage.
- *Cystamine and WR-1065*: Cystamine is a compound that breaks down into the active metabolite WR-1065. WR-1065 is a potent free radical scavenger and has been studied as a radioprotector in various experimental settings [79].
- *Prussian blue:* Prussian blue is an inorganic compound that has been used to protect against certain types of radiation, such as cesium-137 and thallium poisoning. It acts by blocking the absorption of radioactive particles in the body [80].
- *Melatonin:* Melatonin is a hormone produced naturally by the body, often associated with regulating sleep patterns. It has also shown radioprotective properties by acting as an antioxidant and reducing oxidative stress in cells.
- *Vitamin E and other antioxidants:* Antioxidants like vitamin E have been studied for their potential to protect cells from radiation-induced damage by neutralizing free radicals.
- *Aminothio compounds:* Various aminothiol compounds, such as 2-aminothiazole-4-carboxylic acid (ATCA) and 2-(2-aminopropyl) amine-1,3-propanediol (WR-151326), have been investigated as radioprotectors due to their ability to scavenge free radicals and enhance DNA repair.
- *Flavonoids:* Some natural compounds found in fruits and vegetables, like quercetin and rutin, have been studied for their potential radioprotective effects through antioxidant and anti-inflammatory mechanisms.
- *Pentoxifylline:* Pentoxifylline is a drug that has been investigated for its radioprotective properties, mainly by modulating inflammatory responses [81].

The potential applications of radiosensitizers and radioprotectors present promising opportunities for enhancing cancer treatment outcomes and advancing the discipline of radiation oncology. The major differences in the two are compiled in Table 11.5.

Table 11.5. Radiosensitizers vs. radioprotectors

Radiosensitizers	Radioprotectors
Enhance the effects of radiation on tumor cells	Protect normal tissues from radiation-induced damage
Increase DNA damage in cancer cells	Act as antioxidants, scavenging harmful free radicals
Inhibit DNA repair pathways in cancer cells	Promote DNA repair mechanisms in healthy cells
Modulate cellular responses in cancer cells	Regulate cell signaling in normal cells
Target hypoxic cancer cells	Regulate cellular processes in response to radiation
Examples: Cisplatin, 5-Fluorouracil, Caffeine, Oncolytic viruses	Examples: Amifostine, Vitamin E, Melatonin, Dexamethasone, Erythropoietin

Conclusion

This chapter comprehensively explored the concepts of radiosensitivity and radioresistance, describing the complex interplay between oncogenes, tumor suppressor genes, DNA repair pathways, and cancer stem cells in determining cellular responses to radiation. The text detailed how factors such as hypoxia, cell cycle dynamics, genetic variations, and the tumor microenvironment influence radiosensitivity and treatment outcomes. Special attention was given to the mechanisms underlying cancer stem cell radioresistance, including enhanced DNA repair capacity and oxidative stress defense, which pose significant challenges to effective radiotherapy. Understanding these biological, physical, and chemical determinants of radiosensitivity is essential for developing targeted, personalized radiation treatment strategies aimed at improving cancer control while minimizing harm to normal tissues.

References

[1] Collins K, Jacks T, Pavletich NP. The cell cycle and cancer. *Proceedings of the National Academy of Sciences*. 1997 Apr 1;94(7):2776-8.

[2] Kraus MH. Oncogenes. In *Basic science of cancer* 2000 (pp. 41-64). London: Current Medicine Group.

[3] Kastan MB, Onyekwere O, Sidransky D, Vogelstein B, Craig RW. Participation of p53 protein in the cellular response to DNA damage. *Cancer research*. 1991 Dec 1;51(23_Part_1):6304-11.

[4] Brady CA. P53 *Transactivation-Domain Mutant Mice Reveal Context-Specific Differences in P53's Mechanism of Action*. Stanford University; 2011.

[5] Bishop JM. Cellular oncogenes and retroviruses. *Annual review of biochemistry*. 1983 Jul;52(1):301-54.

[6] Anderson MW, Reynolds SH, You M, Maronpot RM. Role of proto-oncogene activation in carcinogenesis. *Environmental health perspectives*. 1992 Nov;98:13-24.

[7] Schmandt R, Mills GB. Genomic components of carcinogenesis. *Clinical chemistry*. 1993 Nov 1;39(11):2375-85.

[8] Hait WN. Targeted cancer therapeutics. *Cancer research*. 2009 Feb 15;69(4):1263-7.

[9] Belli, D. Bettega, P. Calzolari, F. Cera, R. Cherubini, M. Dalla Vecchia, M. Durante, S. Favaretto, G. Gialanella, G. Grossi M. Inactivation of human normal and tumour cells irradiated with low energy protons. *International journal of radiation biology*. 2000 Jan 1;76(6):831-9.

[10] Kim TG, Shin H, Lim DW. Biomimetic scaffolds for tissue engineering. *Advanced Functional Materials*. 2012 Jun 20;22(12):2446-68.

[11] Murakami M, Simons M. Fibroblast growth factor regulation of neovascularization. *Current opinion in hematology*. 2008 May;15(3):215.

[12] Yarden Y, Ullrich A. Growth factor receptor tyrosine kinases. *Annual review of biochemistry*. 1988 Jul;57(1):443-78.

[13] Perugini M. Dissecting signalling contributions of the alpha and beta subunits of the GM-CSF receptor (Doctoral dissertation).

[14] Goffart S, Wiesner RJ. Regulation and co-ordination of nuclear gene expression during mitochondrial biogenesis. *Experimental physiology*. 2003 Jan;88(1):33-40.

[15] Earnshaw WC. Nuclear changes in apoptosis. *Current opinion in cell biology*. 1995 Jan 1;7(3):337-43.

[16] Reed JC, Miyashita T, Takayama S, Wang HG, Sato T, Krajewski S, Aimé-Sempé C, Bodrug S, Kitada S, Hanada M. Bcl-2 family proteins: regulators of cell death involved in the pathogenesis of cancer and resistance to therapy. *Journal of cellular biochemistry*. 1996 Jan 1;60(1):23-32.

[17] McNeish IA, Bell SJ, Lemoine NR. Gene therapy progress and prospects: cancer gene therapy using tumour suppressor genes. *Gene therapy*. 2004 Mar;11(6):497-503.

[18] Minton KW. DNA repair in the extremely radioresistant bacterium Deinococcus radiodurans. *Molecular microbiology*. 1994 Jul;13(1):9-15.

[19] Scully R, Livingston DM. In search of the tumour-suppressor functions of BRCA1 and BRCA2. *Nature*. 2000 Nov 23;408(6811):429-32.

[20] Fialkow PJ. Clonal origin of human tumors. *Annual Review of Medicine*. 1979 Feb;30(1):135-43.

[21] Jorgensen I, Rayamajhi M, Miao EA. Programmed cell death as a defence against infection. *Nature reviews immunology*. 2017 Mar;17(3):151-64.

[22] Bedoui S, Herold MJ, Strasser A. Emerging connectivity of programmed cell death pathways and its physiological implications. *Nature reviews Molecular cell biology*. 2020 Nov;21(11):678-95.

[23] Cortese F, Klokov D, Osipov A, Stefaniak J, Moskalev A, Schastnaya J, Cantor C, Aliper A, Mamoshina P, Ushakov I, Sapetsky A. Vive la radiorésistance!: converging research in radiobiology and biogerontology to enhance human radioresistance for deep space exploration and colonization. *Oncotarget*. 2018 Mar 3;9(18):14692.

[24] Roos WP, Kaina B. DNA damage-induced cell death: from specific DNA lesions to the DNA damage response and apoptosis. *Cancer letters*. 2013 May 28;332(2):237-48.

[25] Chen JS, Faller DV, Spanjaard RA. Short-chain fatty acid inhibitors of histone deacetylases: promising anticancer therapeutics?. *Current cancer drug targets*. 2003 Jun 1;3(3):219-36.

[26] Ruan K, Song G, Ouyang G. Role of hypoxia in the hallmarks of human cancer. *Journal of cellular biochemistry*. 2009 Aug 15;107(6):1053-62.

[27] Bernstein EF, Sullivan FJ, Mitchell JB, Salomon GD, Glatstein E. Biology of chronic radiation effect on tissues and wound healing. *Clinics in plastic surgery*. 1993 Jul 1;20(3):435-53.

[28] Dionysiou, D. D., Stamatakos, G. S., Uzunoglu, N. K., Nikita, K. S. and Marioli, A., 2004. A four-dimensional simulation model of tumour response to radiotherapy *in vivo:* parametric validation considering radiosensitivity, genetic profile and fractionation. *Journal of theoretical biology*, 230(1), pp. 1-20.

[29] Rockwell S, Dobrucki IT, Kim EY, Marrison ST, Vu VT. Hypoxia and radiation therapy: past history, ongoing research, and future promise. *Current molecular medicine*. 2009 May 1;9(4):442-58.

[30] Kraft G, KrÄMer M. Linear energy transfer and track structure. In *Advances in radiation biology* 1993 Jan 1 (Vol. 17, pp. 1-52). Elsevier.

[31] Sørensen BS, Bassler N, Nielsen S, Horsman MR, Grzanka L, Spejlborg H, Swakoń J, Olko P, Overgaard J. Relative biological effectiveness (RBE) and distal edge effects of proton radiation on early damage *in vivo*. *Acta Oncologica*. 2017 Nov 2;56(11):1387-91.

[32] K. SACHS, P. HAHNFELD and DJ BRENNER R. Review the link between low-LET dose-response relations and the underlying kinetics of damage production/repair/misrepair. *International journal of radiation biology*. 1997 Jan 1;72(4):351-74.

[33] Wenzl T, Wilkens JJ. Modelling of the oxygen enhancement ratio for ion beam radiation therapy. *Physics in medicine & biology*. 2011 May 4;56(11):3251.

[34] Bonaldo P, Sandri M. Cellular and molecular mechanisms of muscle atrophy. *Disease models & mechanisms*. 2013 Jan 1;6(1):25-39.

[35] Citrin D, Cotrim AP, Hyodo F, Baum BJ, Krishna MC, Mitchell JB. Radioprotectors and mitigators of radiation-induced normal tissue injury. *The oncologist*. 2010 Apr 1;15(4):360-71.

[36] Mitchell JB, Russo A, Kinsella TJ, Glatstein E. The use of non-hypoxic cell sensitizers in radiobiology and radiotherapy. *International Journal of Radiation Oncology* Biology* Physics*. 1986 Aug 1;12(8):1513-8.

[37] Stewart JR. Prospects for hyperthermia in cancer therapy. *Hyperthermia and oncology*. 2023 Jan 6;1:1-2.

[38] Matés JM, Pérez-Gómez C, De Castro IN. Antioxidant enzymes and human diseases. *Clinical biochemistry*. 1999 Nov 1;32(8):595-603.

[39] Pawlik TM, K. Role of cell cycle Keyomarsi in mediating sensitivity to radiotherapy. *International Journal of Radiation Oncology* Biology* Physics*. 2004 Jul 15;59(4):928-42.

[40] Schwartz JL. Alterations in chromosome structure and variations in the inherent radiation sensitivity of human cells. *Radiation research*. 1998 Apr 1;149(4):319-24.

[41] Marshman E, Booth C, Potten CS. The intestinal epithelial stem cell. *Bioessays*. 2002 Jan;24(1):91-8.

[42] Jeggo P, Lavin MF. Cellular radiosensitivity: how much better do we understand it?. *International journal of radiation biology*. 2009 Dec 1;85(12):1061-81.

[43] Li L, Neaves WB. Normal stem cells and cancer stem cells: the niche matters. *Cancer research*. 2006 May 1;66(9):4553-7.

[44] Huang R, Rofstad EK. Cancer stem cells (CSCs), cervical CSCs and targeted therapies. *Oncotarget*. 2017 May 5;8(21):35351.

[45] Baumann M, Krause M, Thames H, Trott K, Zips D. Cancer stem cells and radiotherapy. *International journal of radiation biology*. 2009 Jan 1;85(5):391-402.

[46] Harper JW, Elledge SJ. The DNA damage response: ten years after. *Molecular cell*. 2007 Dec 14;28(5):739-45.

[47] Hur W, Yoon SK. Molecular pathogenesis of radiation-induced cell toxicity in stem cells. *International journal of molecular sciences*. 2017 Dec 18;18(12):2749.

[48] Schulz A, Meyer F, Dubrovska A, Borgmann K. Cancer stem cells and radioresistance: DNA repair and beyond. *Cancers*. 2019 Jun 21;11(6):862.

[49] Linge, Annett, Fabian Lohaus, Steffen Löck, Alexander Nowak, Volker Gudziol, Chiara Valentini, Cläre von Neubeck et al. "HPV status, cancer stem cell marker expression, hypoxia gene signatures and tumour volume identify good prognosis subgroups in patients with HNSCC after primary radiochemotherapy: A multicentre retrospective study of the German Cancer Consortium Radiation Oncology Group (DKTK-ROG)." *Radiotherapy and Oncology* 121, no. 3 (2016): 364-373.

[50] Wei J, Wang B, Wang H, Meng L, Zhao Q, Li X, Xin Y, Jiang X. Radiation-induced normal tissue damage: oxidative stress and epigenetic mechanisms. *Oxidative medicine and cellular longevity*. 2019 Nov 12;2019.

[51] Ebrahimi M, Nourbakhsh E, Hazara AZ, Mirzaei A, Shafieyari S, Salehi A, Hoseinzadeh M, Payandeh Z, Barati G. PI3K/Akt/mTOR signaling pathway in cancer stem cells.. 2022 Sep 1;237:154010. *Pathology-Research and Practice*

[52] Horsman MR, Vaupel P. Pathophysiological basis for the formation of the tumor microenvironment. *Frontiers in oncology*. 2016 Apr 12;6:66.

[53] Ghaderi N, Jung J, Brüningk SC, Subramanian A, Nassour L, Peacock J. A century of fractionated radiotherapy: How mathematical oncology can break the rules. *International Journal of Molecular Sciences*. 2022 Jan 24;23(3):1316.

[54] Smith J, Tho LM, Xu N, Gillespie DA. The ATM–Chk2 and ATR–Chk1 pathways in DNA damage signaling and cancer. *Advances in cancer research*. 2010 Jan 1;108:73-112.

[55] Pawlik TM, Keyomarsi K. Role of cell cycle in mediating sensitivity to radiotherapy. *International Journal of Radiation Oncology* Biology* Physics*. 2004 Jul 15;59(4):928-42.

[56] Deacon J, Peckham MJ, Steel GG. The radioresponsiveness of human tumours and the initial slope ofthe cell survival curve. *Radiotherapy and Oncology*. 1984 Dec 1;2(4):317-23.

[57] Barendsen GW. Mechanisms of cell reproductive death and shapes of radiation dose-survival curves of mammalian cells. *International journal of radiation biology*. 1990 Jan 1;57(4):885-96.

[58] Aerts AM, Impens NR, Baatout S, Benotmane MA, Camps J, Dabin JM, Derradji H, Grosche B, Horemans N, Jourdain JR, Moreels M. Joint research towards a better radiation protection—highlights of the Fifth MELODI Workshop. *Journal of Radiological Protection*. 2014 Nov 28;34(4):931.

[59] Cox JD, Ang KK. *Radiation oncology E-book: rationale, technique*, results. Elsevier Health Sciences; 2009 Oct 29.
[60] Scholz M. Dose response of biological systems to low-and high-LET radiation. In *Microdosimetric response of physical and biological systems to low-and high-LET radiations* 2006 Jan 1 (pp. 1-73). Elsevier Science.
[61] Timmerman R, Papiez L, McGarry R, Likes L, DesRosiers C, Frost S, Williams M. Extracranial stereotactic radioablation: results of a phase I study in medically inoperable stage I non-small cell lung cancer. *Chest.* 2003 Nov 1;124(5):1946-55.
[62] Dartnell LR, Hunter SJ, Lovell KV, Coates AJ, Ward JM. Low-temperature ionizing radiation resistance of Deinococcus radiodurans and Antarctic Dry Valley bacteria. *Astrobiology.* 2010 Sep 1;10(7):717-32.
[63] Boonstra J, Post JA. Molecular events associated with reactive oxygen species and cell cycle progression in mammalian cells. *Gene.* 2004 Aug 4;337:1-3.
[64] Yoshiba S, Ito D, Nagumo T, Shirota T, Hatori M, Shintani S. Hypoxia induces resistance to 5-fluorouracil in oral cancer cells via G1 phase cell cycle arrest. *Oral oncology.* 2009 Feb 1;45(2):109-15.
[65] Melissa LO, MacDOUGALL JD, Tarnopolsky MA, Cipriano NI, Green HJ. Skeletal muscle adaptations to training under normobaric hypoxic versus normoxic conditions. *Medicine and Science in Sports and Exercise.* 1997 Feb 1;29(2):238-43.
[66] Jeong W, Jung S, Bazer FW, Kim J. Hypoxia-dependent accumulation of hypoxia-inducible factor-1 alpha induces transient cell cycle arrest in porcine trophectoderm cells. *Theriogenology.* 2018 Jul 15;115:9-15.
[67] Wigati KT, Pawiro SA. *Teaching Instructional Design (BRP) Course Radiobiology.*
[68] Guimarães GR, Almeida PP, de Oliveira Santos L, Rodrigues LP, de Carvalho JL, Boroni M. Hallmarks of aging in macrophages: Consequences to skin inflammaging. *Cells.* 2021 May 26;10(6):1323.
[69] Sarıkaya E, Doğan S. Glutathione peroxidase in health and diseases. *Glutathione system and oxidative stress in health and disease.* 2020 Jan 31;49.
[70] Archambault V, Ikui AE, Drapkin BJ, Cross FR. Disruption of mechanisms that prevent rereplication triggers a DNA damage response. *Molecular and cellular biology.* 2005 Aug 1;25(15):6707-21.
[71] Dynlacht JR, Valluri S, Garrett J, Nees J, Caperell-Grant A, DesRosiers C, Bigsby RM. Age and hormonal status as determinants of cataractogenesis induced by ionizing radiation. II. Sparsely ionizing (low-LET) radiation. *Radiation Research.* 2012 Oct 1;178(4):260-5.
[72] Takata M, Sasaki MS, Sonoda E, Morrison C, Hashimoto M, Utsumi H, Yamaguchi-Iwai Y, Shinohara A, Takeda S. Homologous recombination and non-homologous end-joining pathways of DNA double-strand break repair have overlapping roles in the maintenance of chromosomal integrity in vertebrate cells. *The EMBO journal.* 1998 Sep 15;17(18):5497-508.
[73] Mohan G, TP AH, AJ J, KM SD, Narayanasamy A, Vellingiri B. Recent advances in radiotherapy and its associated side effects in cancer—a review. *The Journal of Basic and Applied Zoology.* 2019 Dec;80(1):1-0.
[74] Wang H, Mu X, He H, Zhang XD. Cancer radiosensitizers. *Trends in pharmacological sciences.* 2018 Jan 1;39(1):24-48.
[75] Wardman PJ. Chemical radiosensitizers for use in radiotherapy. *Clinical oncology.* 2007 Aug 1;19(6):397-417.
[76] Nair CK, Parida DK, Nomura T. Radioprotectors in radiotherapy. *Journal of radiation research.* 2001;42(1):21-37.
[77] Purdie JW. A comparative study of the radioprotective effects of cysteamine, WR-2721, and WR-1065 in cultured human cells. *Radiation research.* 1979 Feb 1;77(2):303-11.
[78] Jones JB, Cramer HM, Inch WR, Lampe HB. Radioprotective effect of free radical scavenging enzymes. *The Journal of Otolaryngology.* 1990 Oct 1;19(5):299-306.
[79] Purdie JW. A comparative study of the radioprotective effects of cysteamine, WR-2721, and WR-1065 in cultured human cells. *Radiation research.* 1979 Feb 1;77(2):303-11.

[80] Faruque HA, Choi ES, Kim JH, Kim S, Kim E. *In vivo* removal of radioactive cesium compound using Prussian blue-deposited iron oxide nanoparticles. *Nanomedicine*. 2019 Dec;14(24):3143-58.

[81] Berbée M, Fu Q, Garg S, Kulkarni S, Kumar KS, Hauer-Jensen M. Pentoxifylline enhances the radioprotective properties of γ-tocotrienol: differential effects on the hematopoietic, gastrointestinal and vascular systems. *Radiation research*. 2011 Mar 1;175(3):297-306.

Chapter 12

Hyperthermia and Time-Dose Fractionation in Radiation Therapy

Anurag Luharia[1,*], PhD
Nilesh Ranjan[2], MD
Shweta Dahake[1], MSc
and Anchineyan Pichandi[3], PhD
[1]Department of Radio physics and Radio safety, Datta Meghe Institute of Higher Education and Research, Wardha, India
[2]Department of Radiation Oncology, Health City Hospital, Guwahati, Assam, India
[3]Department of Central Physics, Health Care Global Enterprise Ltd, Banglore, India

Abstract

Hyperthermia, the intentional increase in body temperature, has been used for centuries to treat various diseases, including cancer. Recent studies have shown that hyperthermia can enhance the effects of radiation and chemotherapy in cancer treatment. The cellular effects of heat energy have been found to be comparable to those of radiation, with temperatures between 41° and 45°C exhibiting measurable and time-dependent cytotoxic effects on cells. Hyperthermia has been shown to have distinct additive and synergistic radiosensitizing effects, and several randomized trials have demonstrated its efficacy in conjunction with radiation and chemotherapy for various types of solid tumours. The thermal enhancement ratio (TER) has been quantified for various tissues, and the data exhibit a coherent trend of increasing TER with temperature. Hyperthermia has been found to enhance the activation and function of immune effector cells, and its potential as an adjunct to immunotherapy is being explored. The use of hyperthermia in conjunction with radiation and chemotherapy has been found to improve treatment outcomes in various types of cancer, including cervical cancer, recurrent chest wall breast cancer, and head and neck cancer. The development of non-invasive thermometry technologies, such as magnetic resonance thermal imaging (MRTI), has enabled precise control and measurement of temperature within living tissue. The integration of invasively sampled temperatures with noninvasively measured distributions offers crucial validation for thermal model-based treatment planning. The dose-rate effect, which refers to the impact of radiation dose rate on cell survival, has been found to be significant in both normal

* Corresponding Author's Email: anuragluharia@gmail.com

In: Fundamentals of Radiation Biology
Editors: Anurag Luharia, Ashish Uke, Gaurav Mishra et al.
ISBN: 979-8-89530-806-6

tissues and tumors. The use of low dose-rate radiation has been shown to spare normal tissues while maintaining tumor control.

Keywords: dose-rate effect, hyperthermia, thermal enhancement ratio, thermotolerance, radiosensitization

12.1. Introduction

Radiation therapy is a cornerstone of cancer treatment, with over 50% of cancer patients receiving radiation therapy at some point during their treatment journey. The goal of radiation therapy is to deliver a lethal dose of radiation to cancer cells while minimizing damage to surrounding healthy tissue. To achieve this goal, radiation oncologists and medical physicists use a variety of techniques to optimize radiation delivery, including hyperthermia and time-dose fractionation. Hyperthermia, or heat therapy, is a treatment modality that involves heating cancer cells to temperatures above 40°C to enhance their sensitivity to radiation. This approach is based on the principle that cancer cells are more susceptible to heat-induced damage than normal cells. By combining hyperthermia with radiation therapy, clinicians can increase the effectiveness of radiation treatment while reducing the risk of side effects. Hyperthermia can be applied locally, regionally, or systemically, depending on the location and extent of the tumor. Time-dose fractionation is a critical aspect of radiation therapy that involves dividing the total radiation dose into smaller fractions, or doses, delivered over a specific period. The goal of time-dose fractionation is to balance the need to deliver a sufficient dose of radiation to kill cancer cells with the need to minimize damage to normal tissue. By fractionating the radiation dose, clinicians can take advantage of the differences in radiation sensitivity between cancer cells and normal cells, allowing for more effective treatment with fewer side effects.

12.2. Hyperthermia

The historical background of utilizing medical interventions to regulate body temperature for therapeutic purposes is extensive and captivating. The medical history of several societies worldwide contains ancient records that mention hyperthermia, which refers to the intentional increase in body temperature over the usual range, either in a localized area or throughout the entire body. The cellular effects of heat energy have garnered significant attention from radiation oncologists recently. This interest was first sparked by studies conducted during the 1970s and 1980s. These studies revealed the measurable and time-dependent cytotoxic effects of temperatures within the "heat-shock" range (typically from 41° to 45°C) on cells. These effects were comparable to the consistent and predictable effects of radiation.

Furthermore, it has been observed that hyperthermia within this specific temperature range has distinct additive and synergistic radiosensitizing effects. Several randomized trials have been conducted to investigate the efficacy of hyperthermia in conjunction with radiation and chemotherapy for various types of solid tumors, including deep-seated tumors. These trials have yielded conclusive evidence of substantial clinical advantages. Consequently, at present, certain nations such as the Netherlands and Germany have officially sanctioned and financially supported the integration of hyperthermia into cancer treatment protocols. The current research efforts are focused on optimizing hyperthermia as an adjuvant for various oncologic and non-oncologic disease targets. This is driven by the improved ability to control and measure thermal dose and a better understanding of the biological contribution of hyperthermia in radiochemosensitization. It is currently recognized that the process of heating tumors in their original location, even at temperatures as low as 39° to 42°C, can stimulate various vascular, metabolic, and immunologic factors within the tumor microenvironment. These factors may have an additional impact on enhancing the sensitivity of tumor cells to radiochemotherapy, extending beyond the direct cell death caused by hyperthermia. Furthermore, ongoing research is being conducted to discover additional applications for targeted heat delivery in the field of oncology. One such application involves using thermosensitive liposomes and other nanoparticles to concentrate cytotoxic medications specifically at the tumor site.

- **Early Emphasis on the Direct Cytotoxic Effects of "Heat Shock" Temperatures**

The study, which resulted in the commencement of primary clinical trials in the 1980s and 1990s, aimed to apply localized heat to patients' tumors, raising their temperatures to around 43°C. The primary focus of this research was to investigate the potential of using focused heat energy to induce tumor cell damage, which could enhance or synergize with the antitumor effects of radiation therapy, while avoiding the typical systemic toxicity associated with chemical radiation sensitizers [1]. When cells are subjected to elevated temperatures in an artificial environment, over a prolonged period of time, they undergo a predictable and exponential decline in viability, with the rate of cell death escalating in proportion to the temperature. The cell survival curves for heat exhibit a comparable form to those observed for x-rays, characterized by an initial shoulder followed by an exponential region. However, in the case of heat, the duration of exposure to the elevated temperature serves as a substitute for the absorbed dose of x-rays [2]. The phenomenon becomes more intricate at lower temperatures, as the survival curves exhibit a plateau-like pattern following prolonged exposure to hyperthermia. This observation suggests the potential emergence of "thermotolerance," a state characterized by the acquisition of resistance or tolerance to the heightened temperature. The resemblance observed in the shape of the cell survival curves between heat energy and x-rays can be deceptive. Hence, it is crucial to refrain from making inferences regarding heat only based on the analysis of radiation dose-response curves, as the energy magnitude required for cell inactivation is significantly higher for heat compared to x-rays, by a factor of one thousand [3]. This observation demonstrates the distinct pathways implicated in cellular destruction caused by thermal energy and X-ray radiation. There is evident variation in the susceptibility of cells to cellular damage caused by heat within this particular temperature range. Nevertheless, similar to ionizing radiation, there is a lack of consistent distinction observed between normal and malignant cells when subjected to heat in a controlled laboratory setting.

The survival data of Chinese hamster ovary cells subjected to different levels of hyperthermia, as presented in Figure 12.1 (A), have been graphically represented in Figure 12.1 (B). The y-axis represents the reciprocal of the dose required to achieve a survival fraction of zero (1/D0), while the x-axis represents the reciprocal of the temperature (1/T). The symbol T represents the absolute temperature, while D0 is the reciprocal of the slope of the exponential portion of the survival curve. In other words, D0 refers to the time required at a specific temperature to decrease the fraction of surviving cells to 37% of their initial value.

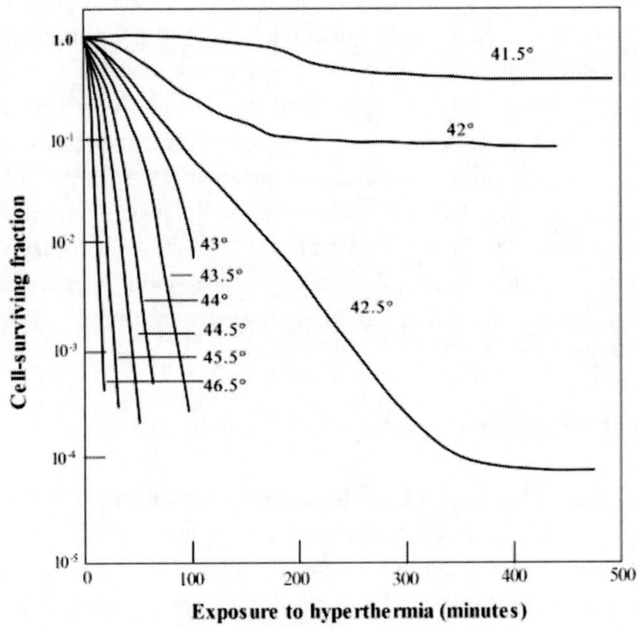

Figure 12.1. (A). Survival curves for mammalian cells in culture (Chinese hamster ovary line) heated at different temperatures for varying lengths of time.

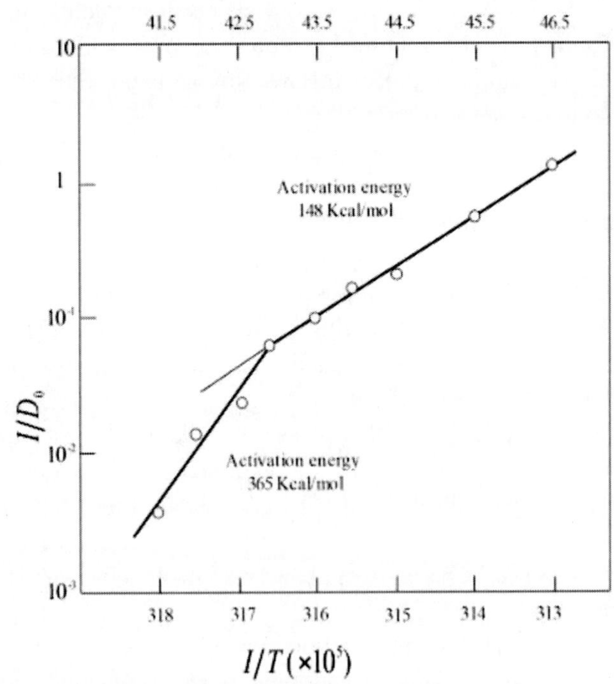

Figure 12.1. (B). An Arrhenius plot for heat inactivation of mammalian cells in culture.

The presentation in question is commonly referred to as an Arrhenius plot, wherein the inclination of the plot provides valuable insights on the activation energy associated with the chemical process responsible for the eradication of cells. The discernible alteration in inclination, a characteristic feature observed in Arrhenius diagrams, transpires at a specific temperature denoted as the "breakpoint" and is around 43°C for human cells [4]. At temperatures exceeding the specified threshold, a rise in temperature by 1°C results in a twofold increase in cell mortality rate. Conversely, below this critical temperature, the rate of cell mortality caused by heat decreases by a factor of 2 to 4 for every decrease of 1° C. The dissimilarity in activation energy observed at temperatures above and below this threshold could potentially indicate distinct mechanisms of cell death, implying alternative targets for cytotoxicity at different temperature ranges. Alternatively, this discrepancy may be attributed to the phenomenon of thermotolerance that occurs inside cells. Significantly, the gradients of Arrhenius plots obtained from numerous *in vitro* and *in vivo* investigations exhibit a remarkable similarity, and this uniformity has rendered the Arrhenius analysis a valuable tool for evaluating thermal dose in clinical hyperthermia applications, maintaining its relevance to the present day.

The hypothesis posits that cellular proteins are the target for heat cell killing within a specific temperature range, based on the similarity between the activation energy for protein denaturation and the activation energy for heat cytotoxicity, as determined using Arrhenius analysis [5]. The heat required for inactivation of cells and the induction of thermal damage is comparable to the energy necessary for protein denaturation, which typically ranges from 130 to 170 kcal/mol. Further evidence supporting the assertion that proteins are the principal focus of thermal cell destruction lies in the significance of heat shock proteins (HSPs) in safeguarding thermotolerant cells against thermal harm. One of the principal roles of Heat Shock Proteins (HSPs) is to facilitate the stabilization and reconstitution of proteins that have undergone denaturation or damage, hence triggering an up regulation in their synthesis [6]. Various cellular components, including as structural chromosomal proteins, nuclear matrix, mitochondria, cytoskeleton, repair enzymes, transport proteins, and other membrane components, have been observed to undergo denaturation in a time-dependent manner when exposed to temperatures ranging from 42° to 45° Enzymes within the respiratory chain have a higher degree of heat sensitivity in comparison to enzymes present in the glycolytic process.

Protein damage is a significant molecular distinction between the cellular damage caused by heat and ionizing radiation. This observation implies that the combination of these two therapies may have an enhanced ability to eliminate tumor cells, perhaps exhibiting an additive effect. Additional distinctions exist between irradiation and heating, implying the potential for cumulative impacts. Cell death occurs during the second or subsequent mitosis following irradiation, unless under exceptional circumstances. Conversely, heat-induced damage manifests early, resulting in cell death by various necrotic or apoptotic processes contingent upon the temperature. Furthermore, the impact of heat extends to both differentiating and dividing cells. Chromosomal abnormalities may arise as a result of exposure to heat if cells are in the S phase of the cell cycle at the time of heating. The delay in x-ray response, which is typically observed due to the time required for stem cells to undergo differentiation and attain functionality, is not present in instances of heat-induced cell death [7].

This is because all cells, regardless of their differentiation status or division activity, are affected by the thermal damage to the tissue. Consequently, if the temperature reaches a sufficiently high level, the tissue will immediately exhibit signs of thermal damage. The DNA repair process exhibits sensitivity to heat, which is potentially one of the underlying mechanisms responsible for heat-induced radiosensitization and chemosensitization. In conclusion, whereas hypoxia has been observed to confer cellular resistance to radiation, its impact on sensitivity to heat remains inconclusive.

12.3. Thermal Enhancement Ratio

The thermal enhancement ratio (TER) is a quantitative measure that compares the dosages of x-rays needed to induce a specific amount of biological damage, with and without the concurrent administration of heat [8]. The tissue equivalent ratio (TER) has been quantified for a range of typical tissues, such as skin, cartilage, and intestinal epithelium. The data exhibit a coherent trend wherein the thermal efficiency ratio (TER) steadily rises as the temperature increases. This trend persists until reaching a threshold of about 2 for a heat treatment (HT) duration of 1 hour at 43°C. Measuring the thermal enhancement ratio (TER) in transplanted malignancies in laboratory animals poses greater challenges due to the predominant influence of the direct cytotoxic action of heat. Heat can potentially manage experimental tumors while minimizing harm to healthy tissues effectively. This is due to the fact that heat-induced cell death is significantly intensified by nutritional deprivation and heightened acidity, which are commonly observed in the inadequately vascularized regions of solid tumors. Therefore, it has been observed that a moderate hyperthermia treatment, which is within the tolerance range of well-vascularized normal tissues, effectively eradicates a significant part of cells in various solid tumors during experimental studies conducted on animals. In the instances when thermal radiosensitization has been examined, the observed thermal enhancement ratio (TER) values are commonly reported as 1.4 at 41°C, 2.7 at 42.5°C, and 4.3 at 43°C, with a duration of 1 hour for heat application. Tumor-specific expression regulators (TERs) have been successfully devised for both canine and human neoplasms, as evidenced by the research conducted by Gillette et al. and Overgaard et al. The aforementioned estimations were derived from retrospective investigations that examined the connections between dosage and its effects, both with and without the presence of hyperthermia. The predicted incidence rate of canine oral squamous cell carcinomas was approximately 1.15 when heat was provided twice a week in conjunction with fractionated radiation. So far, the utilization of hyperthermia resulted in an elevation of the gradient of the TCD50 curve, so ensuring that the dosages necessary to attain a substantial degree of localized tumor control were consistently maintained at levels far lower than those that induced harm to healthy tissues, specifically defined as bone necrosis in this context. The Tumor-to-Extracellular Ratio (TER) has been calculated to be approximately 1.5 for various superficial human tumor types.

12.4. Heat and the Therapeutic Gain Factor

The therapeutic gain factor can be described as the quotient obtained by dividing the tumor-to-normal tissue equivalent ratio (TER) in the tumor by the TER in normal tissues. The use of heat in conjunction with lower doses of X-rays lacks any discernible benefit in the absence of therapeutic advancements compared to the exclusive application of greater X-rays. The therapeutic gain factor issue becomes intricate when considering heat-based treatments, as the temperatures of tumor and normal tissues may not align uniformly [9]. If one asserts that tumor cells are more susceptible to heat damage than normal tissue, it is implicitly assumed that both types of cells are exposed to the same temperature. In real-world scenarios, however, this is not invariably the situation. In the case of a tumor with inadequate vascularization, the application of microwaves as a treatment modality can result in the tumor attaining a greater temperature compared to the surrounding healthy tissue. This discrepancy arises due to the diminished heat dissipation caused by reduced blood flow within the tumor. Furthermore, the outermost layer of the integumentary system can be actively chilled by applying air currents or using a cold-water compress. Under these conditions, the normal tissues can have a considerably lower temperature compared to the tumor. This discrepancy in temperature amplifies the differential response beneficially.

12.5. Factors that Modify Direct Cellular Damage from Hyperthermia

Due to the initial motivation of enhancing protein denaturation and cellular harm caused by direct heat exposure, researchers have dedicated significant efforts to investigating aspects that could alter tumor cells' thermal sensitivity. For instance, the manipulation of the lipid composition of the cell membrane or the application of membrane-active substances, such as alcohols, has been observed to enhance the susceptibility of cells to heat-induced cell death. This increased sensitivity is likely attributed to the disruption of the membrane structure, particularly in relation to the interactions between lipids and proteins. Cells exposed to an acidic pH environment exhibit heightened susceptibility to thermal destruction [10]. The impact of pH history on the pH-dependent cytotoxicity at increased temperatures is evident. Cells have the ability to adapt to alterations in pH levels, hence mitigating the heat sensitivity typically observed under conditions of low pH. Cells that lack essential nutrients have a heightened sensitivity to heat. This phenomenon can be observed in cultured cells, where the sensitivity to heat gradually intensifies as the cells experience a compromised energy source. This can occur by either glucose deprivation or the administration of a medication that disrupts oxidative phosphorylation. The aforementioned findings on pH and nutrient levels, which were derived from experiments conducted on cultured cells under controlled circumstances, have prompted the hypothesis that tumor cells, which are situated far from blood capillaries and hence experience nutritional deprivation and acidic pH, may exhibit heightened susceptibility to heat. Due to the prevailing environmental conditions, it is probable that these cells are currently in a state of cell cycle arrest and potentially experiencing hypoxia as well. It may be hypothesized that heat and x-rays exhibit a complementary effect in this particular scenario. This is due to the observation that cells that are more resilient to X-rays, as they are not actively dividing and are deprived of oxygen due to their distance from a blood vessel, tend to have an increased susceptibility to heat [11]. Another contributing factor that enhances the complementary interaction between hyperthermia and radiation is the presence of poorly developed vasculature and potential hypoxia in certain tumor regions. These regions tend to have elevated temperatures due to reduced cooling effects caused by limited blood flow.

12.6. Thermotolerance

Examining the evolving perception of the significance of "thermotolerance" in hyperthermia provides a valuable illustration of the progressive development of our comprehension regarding the radiosensitizing impacts of hyperthermia during the last two to three decades [12]. Thermotolerance, also known as induced thermal resistance, is typically characterized as acquiring a temporary and non-heritable resistance to future heat exposure following an initial high-temperature treatment. The results obtained from in vitro clonogenic experiments of thermal cytotoxicity indicate that while an initial heat treatment significantly reduces cell viability, repeated daily treatments show a relatively limited effectiveness in inducing cell death. The onset of thermotolerance can manifest within a few hours following the initial treatment and may persist for up to a week before gradually diminishing. This observation implies that the issue of thermotolerance becomes clinically relevant when heat is paired with fractionated irradiation. Consequently, the majority of clinical trials were structured in a manner that aimed to mitigate thermotolerance by incorporating many days of interval between hyperthermia portions. Nevertheless, it has become evident that in real-life localized tumors, the augmentation of blood flow and subsequent improvement in oxygen supply resulting from heating can substantially enhance the effectiveness of radiotherapy on tumors to a greater extent than any reduction in thermal killing caused by the development of thermotolerance. Moreover, the phenomenon of heat-induced radiosensitization does not exhibit thermotolerance. Therefore, despite the historical significance of concerns about thermotolerance in the scheduling of hyperthermia for patients, it is now evident that under the typical heating conditions employed in clinical settings, the induction of thermotolerance is unlikely to occur to a significant extent. Recent trials that are now being developed aim to incorporate more frequent applications of heating, which is anticipated to lead to enhanced clinical benefits.

Another area of research that has had significant development in the knowledge of radiation sensitization by hyperthermia is the study of Heat Shock Proteins (HSPs). The phenomenon of increased expression levels of proteins with specific molecular weights or families with exposure of cells to heat has been well-documented over an extended period of time[13]. Previous studies have demonstrated a correlation between the emergence of heat shock proteins (HSPs) and the acquisition of thermotolerance, while the decline of thermotolerance aligns with eliminating these HSPs. Subsequent molecular investigations that selectively manipulated the expression of specific heat shock proteins (HSPs) have provided compelling evidence of their substantial protective influence against potentially fatal heat exposures. It has long been recognized that families of heat shock proteins (HSPs) are widely distributed throughout evolution and present in all organisms. Likewise, thermotolerance can be observed as a conserved evolutionary response, as evidenced by the upregulation of specific genes in response to exposure to various stressors. Nevertheless, despite the initial association of HSPs with thermotolerance, it is now well acknowledged that these proteins fulfill crucial activities in several macromolecular processes both in normal physiological settings and during periods of stress. Currently, a substantial body of research is investigating the production of heat shock proteins (HSPs) through hyperthermia treatments, mostly due to their potential involvement in enhancing immune responses against tumors.

12.7. Immunologic Effects of Hyperthermia

One of the emerging areas of study in the field of thermal medicine pertains to investigating the potential impact of thermal stimulation on the antitumor immune response [14]. This research aims to determine whether such stimulation can lead to enhanced local control or long-term survival outcomes for patients undergoing hyperthermia treatments. The medical origins of hyperthermic oncology are historically associated with some of the earliest endeavors to utilize immunotherapy in cancer treatment. It has been reported that cancer patients who received injections of infectious agents, specifically Coley toxins, in an effort to treat tumors and subsequently experienced the most elevated fevers, may have also exhibited the longest survival periods. While hyperthermia and fever exhibit significant distinctions, they both entail an elevation in body temperature, a phenomenon that has been extensively linked to enhanced survival rates after infection across several animals. One potential consideration is that clinical hyperthermia might activate thermally sensitive sites within the immune system that have developed over an extensive period of time to react to fever. One intriguing prospect is that strategically administered HTs could potentially function as an adjunct, aiding in the mitigation of certain tumor evasion strategies employed by malignancies to elude immune detection and eradication. Despite the need for further research, existing evidence suggests the plausibility of this hypothesis. This evidence includes the observation of increased immunogenicity and expression of heat shock proteins (HSP) following heat application to tumor cells. Additionally, heat has been found to enhance the activation and function of immune effector cells, as well as improve vascular perfusion and facilitate the delivery or movement of immune effector cells to tumors. The current objective of the study in this rapidly expanding field is to determine the specific function of heat shock proteins (HSPs) in facilitating heightened T lymphocyte responses under thermal stress. Additionally, researchers aim to develop heating procedures that optimize the utilization of thermally controlled immune effector pathways. While the majority of hyperthermia applications have been focused on attaining temperatures of 42° to 45°C, or above, typical body temperatures during fever seldom surpass 40°C and typically range between 38° and 39°C [15]. Multiple studies have provided evidence indicating that immune system cells exhibit a higher degree of sensitivity to rising temperatures compared to other types of cells.

Nevertheless, it is important to consider that thermal ablation procedures can still result in the formation of thermal gradients at the tumor's boundaries and surrounding healthy tissue, where the rise in temperature may be relatively slight. Moreover, it is anticipated that there will be extensive areas of healthy tissue that receive heated blood from the heated tumor region. These distant draining tissues and blood cells may remain at a slightly elevated temperature for significant durations, which is sufficient to induce various immunological effects.

12.8. Phase III Clinical Trials Testing Benefit of Hyperthermia for Enhancing Radiation Therapy

12.8.1. Carcinoma of the Cervix

One phase III trial conducted by a Dutch group played a significant role in establishing hyperthermia as a standard treatment for certain cancers in certain regions of Europe. This trial compared the efficacy of radiation therapy alone to the combination of radiation therapy and hyperthermia in patients with locally advanced pelvic tumors, including cervical carcinoma, bladder tumors, and rectal tumors [16]. The study involved a randomized sample of 361 patients. In this research, HT was administered on a weekly basis for a total of five treatment sessions. It is noteworthy that while several individuals previously believed that hyperthermia would exclusively benefit superficial tumors, the used heating technology in this study yielded satisfactory deep heating, demonstrating its efficacy in heating pelvic cancers. While there were observed enhancements in the treatment outcomes for all forms of tumors, the majority of the advantages seemed to be concentrated among patients diagnosed with cervical cancer. The rate of complete response (CR) following the combination of radiation therapy (RT) and hyperthermia (HT) was found to be 83%, whereas the rate of complete response after RT alone was 57%. The three-year survival rate for patients with cervical cancer who received radiation therapy alone was 27%, while those who received a combination of radiation therapy and hyperthermia had a three-year survival rate of 51% ($p < 0.003$). Significantly, there is continued evidence of substantial survival benefits in patients who had hyperthermia, as indicated by more recent long-term follow-up studies conducted between 2008 and 2009 [17]. Nevertheless, once the trial had commenced, it became evident that the inclusion of cisplatin in conjunction with radiation therapy yielded superior outcomes compared to radiation therapy alone in the context of cervical cancer treatment. Consequently, by the conclusion of the trial, the control group's therapeutic approach could be deemed suboptimal and subject to criticism. Therefore, a phase III clinical research has been launched to compare the efficacy of cisplatin treatment (CT) in combination with radiation therapy (RT) and hyperthermia (HT) to the combination of CT and RT [18]. It is noteworthy to mention that recent research conducted by Frankena et al. demonstrates that hyperthermia can provide survival advantages to patients who are unable to undergo chemoradiation. Furthermore, the inclusion of just one hyperthermia treatment can enhance the likelihood of achieving a complete response.

12.8.2. Recurrent Chest Wall Breast Cancer

The management and treatment of recurrent breast cancer in the chest wall pose a considerable challenge for both patients and healthcare providers. Nevertheless, within this particular context, it is evident that hyperthermia plays a substantial role in providing advantageous outcomes. Consequently, initiating additional clinical trials to further investigate and validate these benefits is imperative. A total of five distinct phase III studies were conducted, ultimately amalgamated into an international joint study. In this study, participants were randomly assigned to two groups: one receiving radiation therapy (RT) alone and the other receiving a combination of radiation therapy (RT) and hyperthermia (HT). The results demonstrated a statistically significant enhancement in the complete response (CR) rate among patients who received the combined treatment of RT and HT, as compared to those who received RT alone. It is worth mentioning that the most significant impact was noticed in patients who had lesions in places that had previously undergone radiation therapy, so restricting their capacity to receive the most effective subsequent irradiation. In relation to this trial, findings from a retrospective evaluation conducted across seven institutions regarding the management of chest wall recurrence were reported at the 2006 meeting of the American Society for Therapeutic Radiology and Oncology [19].

12.8.3. Superficial Malignancies

Jones et al. conducted a significant prospective randomized trial at a single institution, focusing on the use of radiation and hyperthermia for the treatment of various superficial tumors, primarily recurrent chest wall breast tumors. The study specifically included patients who were eligible for local radiation therapy for superficial lesions with a thickness of less than 3 cm. In this research, the researchers decided to ascertain a tumor's thermal susceptibility before randomization initially. This was achieved by administering a test hyperthermia treatment and assessing the tumor's ability to reach a predetermined temperature before to the actual experiment. Subsequently, all patients whose tumors were determined to be susceptible to thermal treatment were randomly assigned to two groups: one receiving radiation therapy alone without extra thermal intervention, and the other receiving a combination of radiation therapy and hyperthermia. The hyperthermia/radiation group's response rate was 66%, which is much higher than the radiation-alone group, where the response rate was just 42%. Once again, it is worth noting that patients previously exposed to radiation saw the most significant advantage. Specifically, they exhibited a response rate of 68.2% when subjected to a combination of hyperthermia and radiation, whereas the response rate was only 23.5% for patients who received radiation treatment alone [20]. This study was the initial investigation to exploit the concept that in order for hyperthermia to function as a radiation sensitizer, it is imperative that the tumor is susceptible to heating. Furthermore, this study will undoubtedly contribute to the establishment of the necessity for enhanced pre-treatment identification of patients who are most likely to derive advantages from hyperthermia in the future. Furthermore, as previously mentioned, this study presents compelling evidence that despite the intended purpose of heating to achieve a minimum tumor temperature of 43°C, the resulting CEM 43°C T90 is considerably lower. This finding implies that mild hyperthermia can exert substantial radiosensitizing effects, which may not be attributed to thermal cytotoxicity.

Thrall et al. conducted a significant canine trial, referred to as the second phase III trial, which has been completed. This trial prospectively assessed the heat-ability of tumors prior to randomization. The study focused on pet dogs that had spontaneous soft tissue sarcomas. The data obtained from this trial further validate the advantages of tumor heat-ability in terms of clinical benefits.

12.8.4. Head and Neck Cancer

The addition of hyperthermia to radiotherapy has been shown to greatly enhance the response of head and neck malignancies [21]. According to research conducted by Valdagni et al., patients in stage III who had a combination of radiotherapy (RT) and hormone therapy (HT) achieved a complete response (CR) rate of 58%, which was significantly higher compared to the 20% CR rate observed in the group receiving only radiotherapy. Similarly, it was shown that patients diagnosed with stage IV illness attained a complete response (CR) rate of 38%, but those who received radiation therapy (RT) alone had a CR rate of 7%. In spite of the challenges associated with heating tumors in the head and neck area, this study examined both the main site and neck nodes. In a separate study conducted by the aforementioned research team, the focus was solely on the treatment of metastatic cervical lymph nodes in patients diagnosed with advanced local regional squamous cell carcinoma. The results indicated that the complete response (CR) rate for combined radiotherapy (RT) and hyperthermia (HT) was 83%, whereas the CR rate for radiation treatment alone was 41%. Surprisingly, the 5-year survival rate was 0% for patients who had radiation therapy alone, but it was 53% for those who received both radiation therapy and hyperthermia.

Hyperthermia may benefit brain malignancies, specifically glioblastoma multiforme [22]. The research team led by Sneed et al. from the University of California in San Francisco assessed the efficacy of combining interstitial hyperthermia with brachytherapy radiation in treating individuals diagnosed with glioblastoma multiforme. The study enrolled patients whose tumors were suitable for implantation in brachytherapy after undergoing external beam radiation and chemotherapy. These patients were randomly assigned to receive either brachytherapy alone or a combination of brachytherapy plus hyperthermia. Remarkably, in the context of this swiftly advancing form of cancer, patients who had hyperthermia treatment exhibited notable enhancements in both tumor progression time and 2-year survival rates, as compared to those who just received brachytherapy [23]. Specifically, the group that received hyperthermia shown a 31% survival rate, whereas the group treated with brachytherapy alone exhibited a 15% survival rate. Nevertheless, there was a marginal increase in toxicity observed among patients who underwent hyperthermia treatment, highlighting the significance of addressing this issue in order to expand the use of hyperthermia therapy to the brain.

12.9. Isolated Limb Perfusion, Limb Infusion, and Hyperthermic Intraperitoneal Chemotherapy

Mild hyperthermia is becoming recognized as a valuable component in significant surgical techniques involving chemotherapy, such as isolated limb perfusion (ILP), isolated limb infusion (ILI), and intraperitoneal chemotherapy [24].

Intra-arterial limb perfusion (ILP) is a therapeutic approach designed to prevent the need for limb amputation in cases where there are large tumors or multiple small tumors (such as in the case of melanoma metastases) by delivering drugs directly to the affected region. This method allows for drug concentrations that are 15 to 25 times higher than those achieved through systemic administration, thereby minimizing systemic side effects while maximizing the exposure of tumors to potent drug concentrations. The achievement of ILP often involves clamping and cannulation of significant blood arteries, connecting an oxygenated extracorporeal circuit, ligating collateral vessels, and using a tourniquet. Melphalan, also known as L-phenylalanine mustard, has emerged as the prevailing pharmaceutical agent employed in this particular medical procedure. Nevertheless, it has been observed that the inclusion of tumor necrosis factor-alpha (TNF-α) plays a crucial role in achieving clinical effectiveness. This is primarily due to its capacity to augment the drug uptake by tumor vasculature. Consequently, the utilization of TNF-α has contributed to the approval of this therapeutic approach in Europe. The ILP procedure additionally includes the application of mild hyperthermia, often ranging from 39° to 40°C. This addition has been found to have a beneficial effect on vascular function and the transportation of drugs into big tumors.

Nevertheless, if the temperature exceeds 41°C, it is seen that there is a heightened occurrence of local toxicity, hence constraining the advantages associated with isolated limb perfusion (ILP). Mild hyperthermia is also utilized in a surgical modification of isolated limb perfusion (ILP) known as isolated limb infusion (ILI)[25]. This treatment is simpler since it does not necessitate the insertion of arterial and venous catheters through the surgical incision, hence reducing the associated morbidity.

Mild hyperthermia is becoming recognized as a valuable component in significant surgical techniques involving chemotherapy, such as isolated limb perfusion (ILP), isolated limb infusion (ILI), and intraperitoneal chemotherapy.

Intra-arterial limb perfusion (ILP) is a therapeutic approach designed to prevent the need for limb amputation in cases where there are large tumors or multiple small tumors (such as in the case of melanoma metastases) by delivering drugs directly to the affected region. This method allows for drug concentrations that are 15 to 25 times higher than those achieved through systemic administration, thereby minimizing systemic side effects while maximizing the exposure of tumors to potent drug concentrations. The achievement of ILP often involves the clamping and cannulation of significant blood arteries, the connection of an oxygenated extracorporeal circuit, the ligation of collateral vessels, and the use of a tourniquet. Melphalan, also known as L-phenylalanine mustard, has emerged as the prevailing pharmaceutical agent employed in this particular medical procedure [26]. Nevertheless, it has been observed that the inclusion of tumor necrosis factor-alpha (TNF-α) plays a crucial role in achieving clinical effectiveness. This is primarily due to its capacity to augment the drug uptake by tumor vasculature.

Consequently, the utilization of TNF-α has contributed to the approval of this therapeutic approach in Europe. The ILP procedure additionally includes the application of mild hyperthermia, often ranging from 39° to 40° C. This addition has been found to have a beneficial effect on vascular function and the transportation of drugs into big tumors. Nevertheless, in the event that the temperature exceeds 41° C, it is seen that there is a heightened occurrence of local toxicity, hence constraining the advantages associated with isolated limb perfusion (ILP). Mild hyperthermia is also utilized in a surgical modification of isolated limb perfusion (ILP) known as isolated limb infusion (ILI). This treatment is simpler since it does not necessitate the insertion of arterial and venous catheters through the surgical incision, hence reducing the associated morbidity [27].

12.10. Hyperthermic Intraperitoneal Chemotherapy

A significant number of patients have a heightened susceptibility to the development of abdominal tumors due to the presence of residual disease at a microscopic level subsequent to surgical intervention. Additionally, some patients exhibit tumors that affect the ovaries or abdominal organs, including the pancreas, while others harbor cancerous cells within the ascites fluid [28]. In these instances, the utilization of intraoperative chemotherapy is being integrated with hyperthermia through the process of heating the chemotherapy solution before introducing it into the abdominal cavity. This allows the organs within the cavity to be exposed to the heated solution, typically at a temperature of around 40°C, for varying durations. It is widely believed that heat has the potential to enhance the efficacy of chemotherapy through its ability to decrease the resistance of tumor cells. A number of recent clinical trials have shown enhanced survival rates and overall improvements in quality of life when hyperthermic intraperitoneal chemotherapy is employed, as compared to conventional chemotherapy. Nevertheless, further research is required to elucidate the precise advantages of hyperthermia in this particular context.

- **Systemic or Whole-Body Applications**

Furthermore, Bull et al. have conducted phase I and phase II clinical studies that explore the viability and safety of employing mild temperature whole body treatments, with temperatures ranging from 39° to 40° C, in conjunction with chemotherapy [29]. These investigations complement the existing research on deep regional or part-body hyperthermia studies. Further research and experimentation are required to advance the progress of systemic heat therapies. However, it is probable that the mechanisms behind the impact of whole body and part-body hyperthermia procedures on the effectiveness of chemotherapy exhibit similarities. Moreover, the comprehensive or systemic approach offers the potential benefit of treating extensively spread cancers in patients with metastasis, using the same hormone therapy.

- **Major methods of tumor heating**

The majority of initial laboratory investigations that contributed to the development of clinical implementations of local hyperthermia involved the utilization of *in vitro* cell cultures, typically subjected to elevated temperatures through the application of hot-water baths. Undoubtedly, the most straightforward and dependable method for heating cells in a petri dish or for heating a tumor cultivated in the limb of a rodent involves submerging the target in a water bath that is regulated by a thermostat [30]. The aforementioned methodology has been often employed in preclinical investigations of hyperthermia for approximately 30 years. Water temperature management can be achieved with a high degree of precision, allowing for adjustments within a narrow range. Additionally, the measurement of water temperature has no significant challenges. Nevertheless, in this rudimentary scenario of rodent tumor heating, it is plausible that the temperature of the tumor may not align with that of the skin (or water bath). This discrepancy arises due to the continuous circulation of cooler blood from non-heated areas of the body, which drains and replenishes the heated tumor.

Furthermore, it is common practice to administer anesthesia to rodents in water-bath experiments. However, this practice can have a substantial impact on the study of neurovascular regulation in response to tissue heating. Anesthesia during these experiments can lead to aberrant temperature gradients due to significant heat loss. Due to the mice's significant surface-to-volume ratio, their core temperature can be readily and rapidly manipulated. Consequently, Repasky and colleagues have devised a practical approach involving warm air incubators to induce systemic alterations in the temperature of mice with tumors. The present procedure does not necessitate the administration of anesthesia and leads to a prompt elevation in core body temperature, which is expected to elicit supplementary thermoregulatory vascular responses. A recent study conducted by Bull and colleagues employed a technique to simulate systemic heating, wherein sedated rats were predominantly submerged in warm water. The determination of an "optimal" heating procedure for rodent tumors to closely replicate the conditions that may arise in patients should take into consideration the specific research topic at hand and the characteristics of the tumor or heating technique under investigation. Due to inherent disparities in thermoregulatory mechanisms between rodents and humans, it is probable that no rodent model can fully replicate human hyperthermia treatments. Consequently, the clinical studies conducted on larger canine models by Thrall et al. hold particular significance. Contrary to the comparatively straightforward scenario of heating cultured cells or rodents with tumors, the development of equipment that can effectively heat patients' tumors without causing harm to the surrounding healthy tissues has demanded substantial engineering endeavors. These efforts persistently progress in the present era.

In order to create localized hyperthermia in human malignancies using microwaves, RF-induced currents, or ultrasound, several significant technological challenges have needed to be addressed. When considering microwaves, it is possible to achieve effective localization at shallow depths. However, as the tumor depth increases, even with a lower frequency to facilitate deeper penetration, the localization becomes significantly less accurate. Additionally, the effectiveness of therapy is limited by surface heating. The utilization of ultrasound may result in aberrations of the heating pattern when bone or air cavities are present. However, in soft tissues, particularly with the use of ultrasound in focused arrays, sufficient penetration and uniform temperature distributions can be attained [31]. In practical application, superficial tumors such as recurrent chest wall nodules can be effectively treated using microwaves or plane wave ultrasound. Theoretically, it should be feasible to apply focused ultrasound, regional microwave devices, or interstitial techniques to heat deep-seated tumors located below the diaphragm.

Regardless of the specific scenario, the issue of heating methods presents a multifaceted challenge. Nevertheless, notable advancements have been achieved through the astute utilization of targeted arrays. An illustration of this concept is the utilization of multi-phased arrays, which enables the attainment of temperature homogeneity throughout the entire field, including its peripheri [32]. The complexity depicted in the image suggests that a singular, straightforward solution to the intricate array of challenges is improbable. Currently, this field is experiencing significant activity, and the subsequent overview of existing heating systems is expected to undergo revisions in the near future due to emerging advancements. Due to spatial constraints, the present review is restricted to devices now employed in clinical settings or those with the potential for imminent commercial availability. There has been a significant proliferation of various systems that have been invented and subjected to testing throughout the past three decades. However, only a limited number of these systems have been successfully manufactured and made available in the commercial market. This can be attributed, at least in part, to the classification of hyperthermia devices by the U.S. Food and Drug Administration.

12.11. Clinical Thermometry

12.11.1. Invasive Thermometry Methods

For a significant period of time, the exclusive approach to treatment monitoring, control, and thermal dose computation during clinical hyperthermia involved the use of invasive sensors to detect temperatures directly. In order to ensure accurate and precise temperature measurements, it is important for sensors to possess the capability to measure temperatures with an accuracy and precision of around 0.1° C when immersed in a water bath, and approximately 0.2° C when operating within powerful electromagnetic (EM) or ultrasonic fields *in vivo* [33]. There exist three fundamental categories of intrusive thermometers, namely: (1) electrically conducting thermometers, (2) minimally conducting thermometers, and (3) nonconducting (optical) sensors. Thermistors and thermocouple sensors equipped with metallic leads are illustrative of the first category, which are deemed unsuitable for electromagnetic hyperthermia. One often employed sensor with limited conductivity is the high-resistivity thermistor, which features carbon-impregnated plastic leads. The utilization of high-resistivity materials enables precise measurements to be conducted in environments with high levels of electromagnetic interference. Nonconducting optical sensors employ materials located at the end of an optical fiber, where the optical properties of these materials are established as a recognized function of temperature. The utilization of the second and third types of sensors is prevalent in the field of electromagnetic hyperthermia.

Temperature measurements may be subject to inaccuracies due to the direct heating of either the sensor or the catheter in which the sensor is located. The elimination of such mistakes in electromagnetic (EM) systems has been achieved through the implementation of high-resistive thermistors and optical sensors [34]. In the context of ultrasonic hyperthermia, it is important to acknowledge the potential occurrence of artifacts with varying degrees. These artifacts may arise due to the absorption of acoustic waves by the catheter or sensor-coating material and the generation of frictional (viscous) heating in the sensors. Furthermore, the measurement accuracy can be influenced by thermal conduction heat transfer occurring along metallic leads. Typically, using thin needle thermocouple sensors and monitoring temperature fluctuations during brief intervals of ultrasonic power can effectively mitigate the occurrence of ultrasound artifacts. An adequate quantity of thermometry sensors is crucial to ensure precise assessment of the effectiveness of hyperthermia treatment and the computation of the thermal dosage administered. Typically, a higher number of monitored locations during treatment leads to improved evaluation and estimation of thermal dose. In order to achieve this objective, a combination of multisensor probes, thermal mapping methodologies, and quality assurance procedures have been implemented. In addition, sophisticated heating systems require comprehensive thermometry to efficiently utilize temperature feedback for power regulation.

Nevertheless, it is crucial to acknowledge the clinical fact that the utilization of invasive catheters is both restricted and logistically challenging [35]. In order to enhance the delivery, monitoring, control, assessment, and quality of hyperthermia, it is imperative to have a more comprehensive understanding of the temperature distribution within the human body during treatment. This has spurred a significant amount of study in noninvasive thermometry technologies.

12.11.2. Progress Toward Clinically Achievable Non-invasive Thermometry

One of the primary objectives in the field of hyperthermia research is the attainment of precise control and measurement of temperature within living tissue in patients. Specifically, there is a significant demand for a noninvasive technology capable of offering comprehensive temperature distributions during the course of treatment. Numerous noninvasive methods for measuring thermal properties are currently being studied. These include infrared thermography, thermal monitoring sheet fiber optic arrays (limited to surface distributions), electrical impedance tomography, microwave tomography, microwave radiometry, ultrasonic temperature estimation techniques, and Magnetic Resonance Thermal Imaging (MRTI) [36]. Proton resonance frequency shift (PRFS)-based magnetic resonance temperature imaging (MRTI) has emerged as the most promising method thus far for monitoring comprehensive three-dimensional tissue temperature distributions during thermal therapy. The aforementioned technique has been effectively employed in the monitoring of temperatures during thermal therapy utilizing both electromagnetic and ultrasonic heating methodologies. The utilization of Proton Resonance Frequency Shift (PRFS) in Magnetic Resonance Temperature Imaging (MRTI) has exhibited a precision of approximately 1 degree Celsius per cubic centimeter of tissue in the acquisition of numerous slices, with a minimum frequency of once per minute. The utilization of this noninvasive technology enables precise assessment of the volumetric temperature distribution, facilitating the targeted delivery of heat to the tumor. Furthermore, the utilization of magnetic resonance imaging (MRI) for treatment monitoring offers valuable information for the development of treatment strategies, the regulation of treatment administration, and the evaluation of tissue damage both during and after treatment. This data has the potential to predict the clinical response to treatment. The integration of invasively sampled temperatures with noninvasively measured distributions offers crucial validation for thermal model-based treatment planning, which has the potential to enhance the administration of appropriate thermal doses. The enhanced characterization of tissue temperature made available by Magnetic Resonance Temperature Imaging (MRTI) is expected to significantly improve the interpretation of forthcoming clinical trials involving hyperthermia [37].

12.12. Thermal Ablation Applications in Thermal Medicine

The primary objective of topic is to examine the utilization of hyperthermia treatments in conjunction with radiation and chemotherapy applications. However, it is worth noting that thermal tumor ablation is emerging as a prominent clinically employed method of hyperthermia. This technique involves subjecting tumors (such as those found in the liver, kidney, lung, bone, adrenal gland, or prostate) to brief periods of high temperature ranging from 50°C to 100°C, with the intention of thermally "ablate" the nodules. At a temperature of 50°C, the process of cell death requires a short duration of time, but at temperatures exceeding 60°C, the same process occurs within a significantly shorter timeframe. Furthermore, ongoing clinical trials are currently investigating the combination of thermal ablation with conventional hyperthermia techniques to enhance medication delivery. This is achieved by utilizing thermosensitive liposomes at the periphery of ablated tumors. Ablative heating is generated through the utilization of needle-type radiofrequency (RF) or microwave applicators, which have a diameter of 1.5 mm. These applicators are injected into the tumor with the assistance of imaging guidance, such as computed tomography (CT) or ultrasound. The surrounding tissue is then heated by the RF electric current or microwaves emitted by the applicator. The expansion of the tissue coagulation zone occurs due to the thermal conduction of heat from the vicinity of the applicator, where it is hot, into the surrounding tissue [38]. The cessation of blood flow occurs within the coagulation zone, resulting in less perfusion effects when compared to moderate hyperthermia. The size of the final coagulation zones varies between 3 to 5 cm in diameter, depending on the specific device being used. Tumor ablation procedures can be conducted with minimal invasiveness by interventional radiologists or as part of surgical interventions, such as laparoscopy or open surgery. The long-term outcomes of primary and metastatic liver cancer demonstrate encouraging results, with comparable survival rates to those achieved through surgical intervention when appropriate patient selection is employed. An advantage of ablation, in comparison to other therapeutic approaches like chemotherapy and radiation, is its potential for recurrent application, even in cases of tumor recurrence. This is due to the fact that cancer cells do not exhibit resistance to thermal ablation.

Currently, thermal ablation is typically not utilized in conjunction with other therapies, like as chemotherapy, in clinical settings. However, there is ongoing and rigorous preclinical research aimed at exploring the possibilities of combining ablation with chemotherapy and radiation, in order to maximize their potential. Furthermore, the acknowledgement of the presence of an inflammatory tissue rim, which has been subjected to lower temperatures, at the periphery of an ablated zone has sparked interest in utilizing the immune responses triggered by inflammation to facilitate sustained protection against the recurrence of tumors. As previously stated, ongoing clinical trials are currently investigating the use of thermosensitive liposomes. These liposomes are specifically engineered to release their contents in the outer regions of the ablation zone, where temperatures can potentially decrease to as low as 41° to 42°C. This temperature range serves as a trigger for the liposomes to release the encapsulated drug.

12.13. The Dose-Rate Effect

The utilization of multifraction regimens in conventional radiation therapy can be primarily attributed to radiobiologic investigations conducted in France throughout the 1920s and 1930s [39]. The study revealed that subjecting a ram's testes to a single dose of radiation resulted in significant scrotal skin damage, making sterilization unfeasible. However, when the radiation was administered in smaller daily fractions over several weeks, sterilization could be achieved without causing unacceptable harm to the skin. The hypothesis was put forward that the testes may serve as a representative model for studying tumor growth, while the skin of the scrotum was identified as a normal tissue with a limited tolerance for radiation exposure. Although the reasoning employed in the argument may contain flaws, the ultimate conclusion reached is indeed valid. In the majority of situations, the fractionation of the radiation dose has been observed to yield superior tumor control compared to administering a single high dose, while maintaining a similar degree of normal tissue harm.

The dose rates employed in most radiobiological investigations on cellular and tissue samples typically fall within the range of 1-5 Gy min^{-1}, which aligns with the average dose rates commonly utilized in external beam radiation for clinical purposes. The duration of exposure required to achieve a dose of 2 Gy should not exceed a few minutes. During this brief duration, the initial chemical reactions induced by radiation, specifically the formation of free radicals, can occur. However, the exposure periods are typically insufficient for the repair of DNA damage or for significant progression of other biological processes. As the dose rate decreases, the duration required to administer a specific radiation dose increases [40]. Consequently, this extended exposure period allows for various biological processes to occur during irradiation, potentially altering the measured radiation response. The four R's of radiation, namely recovery (or repair), redistribution in the cell cycle, repopulation (proliferation), and reoxygenation, have been utilized to define these processes.

The extent to which each process has an influence is contingent upon its velocity, hence determining the range of dose rates. The process of intracellular repair has the highest rate among these processes, with a half-time of approximately 1 hour. Consequently, when the period of exposure is around 1 hour, a significant amount of repair will occur. Based on the calculations conducted, it has been determined that the repair process conducted at this particular pace will result in alterations to the radiation effects within the dose-rate range of approximately 1 Gy min^{-1} to around 0.1 cGy min^{-1}. Changes in dose rate can lead to minor impacts on tolerance, even within the range of clinical external beam dose rates. On the other hand, the process of repopulation is considerably more gradual. The doubling durations for repopulation in human tumors (or normal tissues) are constrained to a minimum of 1 day, with a potentially extensive range spanning from a few days to several weeks [41]. Hence, it is only when the exposure period surpasses around 24 hours that substantial repopulation will occur within a solitary instance of radiation exposure. The influence of repopulation on cellular response, whether in tumors or normal tissues, is observed within a narrower range of dose rates, typically below 2 cGy min^{-1}, and is contingent upon the cell growth rate. The modification in response throughout an intermediate range of dose rates, as well as the impact of reoxygenation in tumors, can be attributed to redistribution, specifically in terms of cell-cycle progression.

12.13.1. The Effect of Dose Rate on Cell Survival

As the radiation dose rate is reduced within the range of 1 Gy min^{-1} to 1 cGy min^{-1}, the impact per unit dose diminishes, resulting in a progressive transition from curved cell-survival curves found at high dose rates to straighter curves. The relationship between dose rate with cell survival is shown in Figure 12.2.

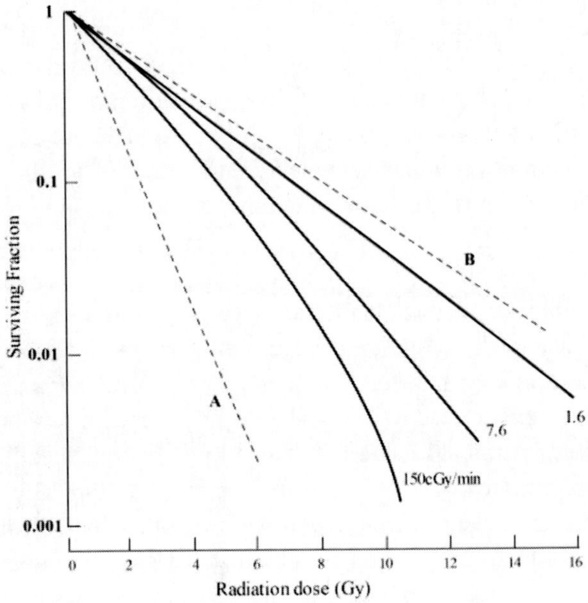

Figure 12.2. Effect of dose rate on cell survival with respect to radiation dose.

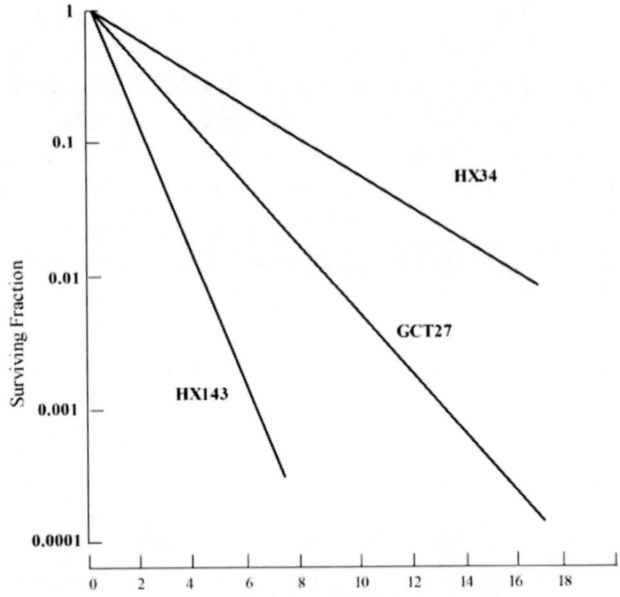

Figure 12.3. Cell survival curves for different human cancer cell lines.

The survival curve exhibits a noticeable curvature when exposed to a dose rate of 150 cGy min^{-1}, but at a dose rate of 1.6 cGy min^{-1}, it appears nearly linear on the semi-log plot and appears to extend the initial slope of the high-dose-rate (HDR) curve [42]. The degree of sparing resulting from the drop-in dose rate can be quantified by examining the radiation doses that yield a consistent survival fraction, such as 0.01. Specifically, these values are 7.7 Gy at a dose rate of 150 cGy min^{-1} and 12.8 Gy at a dose rate of 1.6 cGy min^{-1}.

The dose-recovery factor (DRF) is defined as the ratio of the doses, specifically 12.8 divided by 7.7, resulting in a value of 1.6. The data presented in Figure have been subjected to a simultaneous fitting process using Curtis' lethal, potentially lethal (LPL) model. This particular model is known for its utility in characterizing the dose-rate impact. This enables the estimation of the cellular recovery half-time (0.16 hours) and also provides predictions for cell survival in the absence of repair (line A) or with complete repair (line B). Figure 1 displays three further instances of low dose rate (LDR) survival curves seen in human tumor cell lines, thus demonstrating the almost linear nature of these survival curves.

The Figure 12.3 displays cell-survival curves for four specific human cancer cell lines, depicting two different dosage rates (150 and 1.6 cGy min^{-1}) as shown in Figure 12.4 (A) and Figure 12.4 (B). The presented datasets exemplify the dose-rate impact and demonstrate the spectrum of radiosensitivities observed in human tumor cells [43]. Within the context of high-dose rate (HDR) radiation therapy, a spectrum spanning around three units of radiation dosage corresponds to a survival rate of 0.01. This specific dose is commonly referred to as the D0.01. In the context of Low dose rate radiation (LDRs), it can be observed that the curves diverge and after that assume a linear or near-linear trajectory. Specifically, the range of D0.01 values is around 7. This observation highlights a significant attribute of low dose rate (LDR) irradiation, namely its superior ability compared to high dose rate (HDR) irradiation, to differentiate between cell lines with varying levels of radiosensitivity.

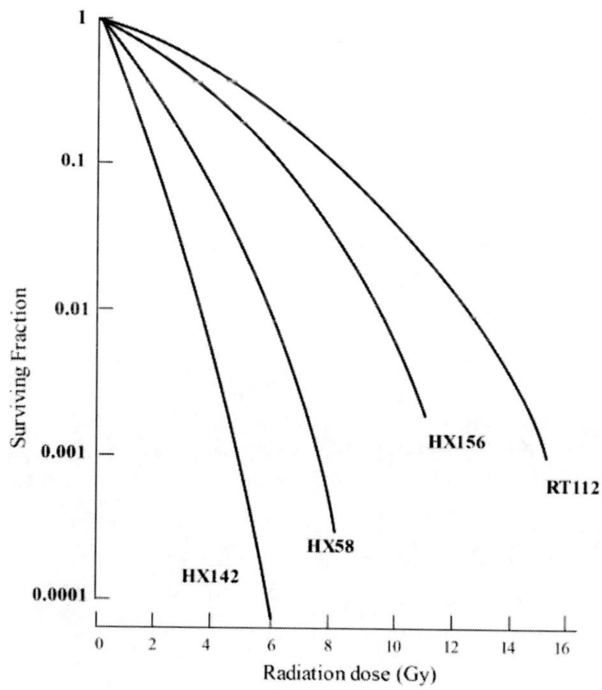

Figure 12.4. (A). Cell survival curves in with a dose rate of 150 cGy min^{-1}.

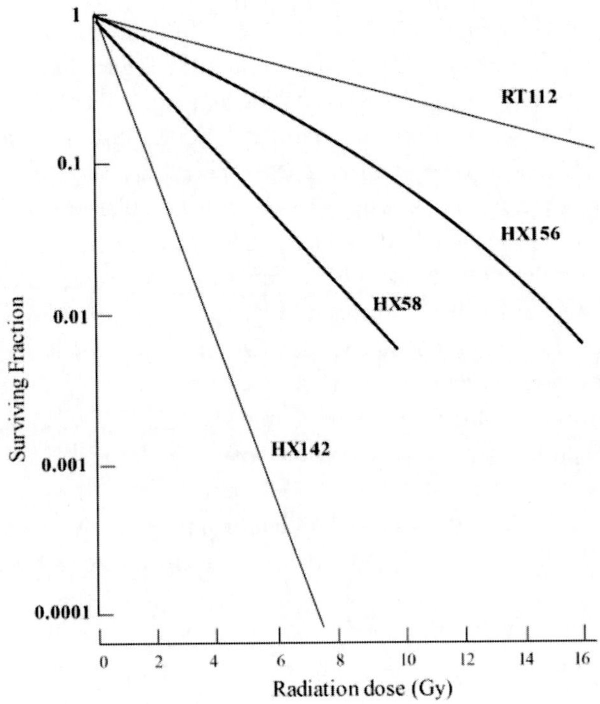

Figure 12.4. (B). Cell survival curves in with a dose rate of 1.6 cGy min.$^{-1}$.

12.13.2. Dose-Rate Effect in Normal Tissues

Significant preservation of most normal tissues is observed when the dosage rate is decreased. The thorax of awake mice was irradiated with 60Co γ rays, and subsequent damage to the lung was assessed by a breathing-rate assay. The radiation dosage required to induce early pneumonitis in 50% of the mice, also known as the ED50, was found to be 13.3 Gy when administered at a rate of 100 cGy min^{-1}. However, this dose jumped to 34.2 Gy when the lowest dose rate of 2 cGy min^{-1} was used, resulting in a dose rate factor (DRF) of 2.6. It should be noted that other researchers have also achieved a comparable level of sparing with the use of fractionated high-dose-rate (HDR) irradiation, employing a dosage of 2 Gy each fraction.

Furthermore, an even greater level of sparing has been observed when the dosage is reduced to 1 Gy per fragment. It is important to note that the curve exhibits a rapid increase even at a dose rate of 2 cGy min^{-1}. Due to the challenges associated with immobilizing the mice for extended durations, achieving dose rates lower than 2 cGy min^{-1} in the conducted tests was not feasible.

The comparison between a single exposure to low dose rate (LDR) radiation at a rate of 2 cGy per minute and fractionated high dose rate (HDR) irradiation at a dose of 2 Gy per fraction enables a significant conclusion to be inferred. If the fractions are administered daily, the total duration required to deliver an ED50 dose of 34 Gy is 17 days. A single LDR treatment yields an equivalent outcome within 28 hours [44]. Therefore, continuous exposure to low-dose radiation (LDR) is considered the most effective method for facilitating optimal tissue repair within a minimal timeframe. Reducing cell proliferation has the benefit of mitigating harm to tumor cells. However, this poses a drawback for the tolerance of early responding normal tissues that heavily rely on proliferation for (intra) cellular healing.

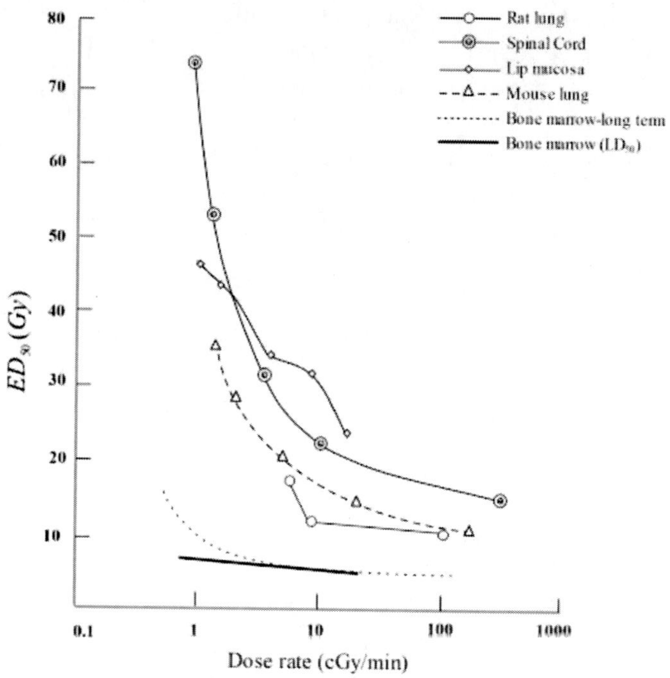

Figure 12.5. Dose-rate effect on normal tissues in rodent.

The above Figure 12.5 shows some examples of other studies of the dose-rate effect on normal tissues in rodents: lip mucosa, lung, spinal cord, and bone marrow. When comparing two typical late-responding tissues (lung and spinal cord) with an early-responding tissue (lip mucosa in the mouse), the patterns of recovery are similar, with the largest sparing in the spinal cord [45]. This is to be expected for the central nervous system as this tissue shows the largest increase in tolerance when decreasing the fraction size (low α/β value). For early-responding epithelial tissues like the lip mucosa, the dose-rate effect is less pronounced, but for overall times longer than 1–2 days, proliferation adds to a rapid increase in tolerance, in contrast to late-responding tissues.

The two bone-marrow endpoints, lethality due to bone-marrow syndrome and long-term repopulation of hemopoietic stem cells, show only a minimal recovery for dose rates as low as 1 cGy min^{-1}. This is predominantly due to the high sensitivity of the bone marrow, as a LD50 dose in the range of 6–9 Gy is even at 1 cGy min^{-1} delivered in a total time of only 10–15 hours. It is of interest to note that a slow proliferating haemopoietic stem cell population showed a significant recovery when lowering the dose rate to approximately 0.5 cGy min^{-1}, in agreement with a low α/β value.

12.14. Effect of Cell Proliferation

The effect of proliferation at very low dose rates is graphically illustrated in above Figure 12.6. These calculations are made for a hypothetical cell population with an α/β value of 3.7 Gy and a repair half-time of 0.85 hours. Cell proliferation is assumed to occur with the doubling times shown in the figure, and no account has been taken of radiation effects on the rate of proliferation (if this occurred, it would reduce the effect of proliferation at the higher dose rates) [46]. For these parameter values, there is no effect of proliferation at dose rates above 1 cGy min^{-1} but as the dose rate is lowered to 0.1 cGy min^{-1} the isoeffective dose rises steeply. The implication for brachytherapy is that above 1 cGy min^{-1} repopulation effects can be ignored, but below this dose rate, they will be substantial, both in tumors and in early responding normal tissues.

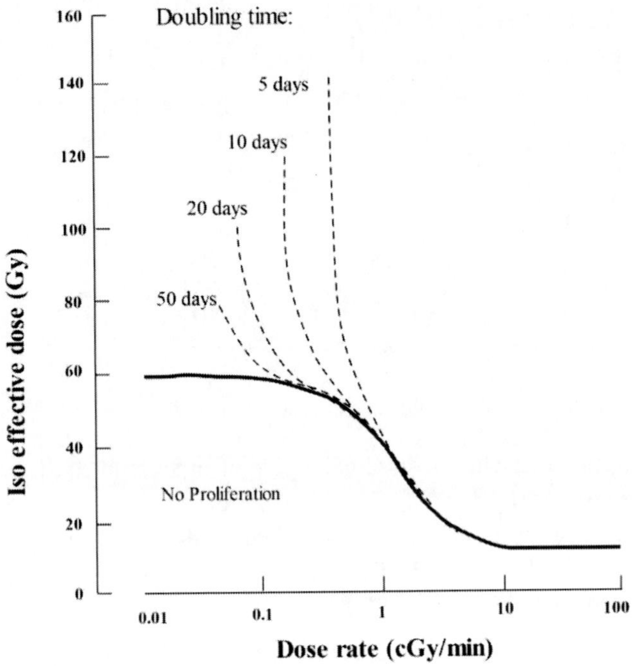

Figure 12.6. Effect of very low dose rate on cellular proliferation.

12.14.1. The Inverse Dose Rate Effect

While it is often observed that cellular sensitivity declines as the dose rate drops in clinical practice, there have been instances where exceptions to this norm have been seen. In previous investigations conducted by Mitchell and Bedford on the phenomenon of cell death in mammalian cell lines, a minor reversal was sometimes observed [47]. This reversal was attributed to a reduced dosage rate, which facilitated the progression of cells through various phases of the cell cycle, ultimately leading to increased vulnerability and subsequent harm. Further elucidation of the mechanism underlying the inverse dose-rate effect has been achieved by recent experimental investigations pertaining to the phenomenon known as "low-dose hyper radiosensitivity" (HRS), initially discovered by Joiner et al. In cellular models exhibiting a prominent hypersensitive response (HRS) at doses lower than 0.4 Gy, a contrary effect to the typical protection reported at low dosage rates (LDRs) might be detected at dose rates below 1.5 cGy min^{-1} [48].

12.14.2. IMRT and Dose Rate

Intensity-modulated radiation treatment (IMRT) is widely recognized as a highly precise method of delivering external beam radiotherapy. It is generally acknowledged as the optimal approach for achieving dose escalation inside the target volume using conventional photons, while minimizing radiation exposure to the adjacent normal tissues. The attainment of better precision was initially accomplished through the utilization of a more intricate technological approach, involving a substantial quantity of distinct segments. Consequently, the administration of the whole dose fraction sometimes necessitated lengthier delivery periods exceeding 30 minutes. Therefore, a portion of the increased dosage may undergo biological loss through repair mechanisms during the course of treatment. Several researchers have examined this question using *in vitro* cell culture techniques. A series of studies and a comprehensive literature study determined that, as a general trend, the efficacy of cell eradication may experience a reduction of up to 20% when treatment durations range from 20 to 30 minutes [49]. The findings indicated that the observed decline in efficacy did not manifest when cells were exposed to high linear energy transfer d(48.5) + Be neutrons as opposed to megavoltage X-rays, hence corroborating DNA repair as the underlying process. One notable observation is that the aforementioned figures exhibit variations among different cell lines, with their values being more influenced by the pace of repair rather than the α/β value [50]. This finding aligns with the predictions made by the LPL and partial repair models. To date, there have been no published signs of a diminished efficacy of intensity-modulated radiation therapy (IMRT) treatments [51]. It is important to acknowledge that the success of therapy is not only decided by the inherent susceptibility of tumor cells. A noteworthy aspect in this regard pertains to an experimental investigation examining the correlation between radiosensitivity *in vitro* and cancer response *in vivo* within the same cell line. The study revealed that the diminished efficacy resulting from less cell destruction was counterbalanced *in vivo* by prompt reoxygenation.

In contrast to the initial applications of intensity-modulated radiation treatment (IMRT), volumetric modulated arc therapy (VMAT) has emerged as an IMRT technology that enables the administration of dose fractions within a considerably shorter timeframe, often less than 10 minutes [52]. Numerous treatment facilities currently use flattening-filter-free (FFF) beams, which have the potential to yield increased average dosage rates and hence enable expedited treatment administration. The advent of speedier treatment delivery has raised inquiries on the potential impact of increased dose rates, namely the instantaneous dose rate during beam pulses, on treatment efficacy in comparison to average dose rates below 5 Gy min^{-1}. In a research investigation involving two human cell lines that were exposed to radiation in a controlled laboratory setting using a clinical linear accelerator, it was shown that there was no discernible alteration in the observed outcomes up to an average dose rate of 30 Gy per minute, which is equivalent to an instantaneous dosage rate of 338 Gy per second. This lack of change was observed for doses up to 10 Gy. Nevertheless, a thorough examination of the existing body of literature reveals that elevated X-ray and electron dose rates, reaching approximately 109 Gy s^{-1}, can lead to the depletion of cellular oxygen. This depletion has the potential to induce significant alterations in the radiosensitivity of cells, especially those already experiencing low oxygen tension, typically around 3 mm Hg or 0.4% [53]. Such conditions are commonly observed in tumorous growths. It is improbable that linear accelerator–based X-ray radiation could attain such high dose rates. However, there is a possibility that high-energy proton or carbon-ion beams could induce localized oxygen depletion, perhaps leading to radioresistance.

12.15. Radiobiological Aspects of Brachytherapy

12.15.1. Variation in Cell Killing Around an Implanted Radioactive Source

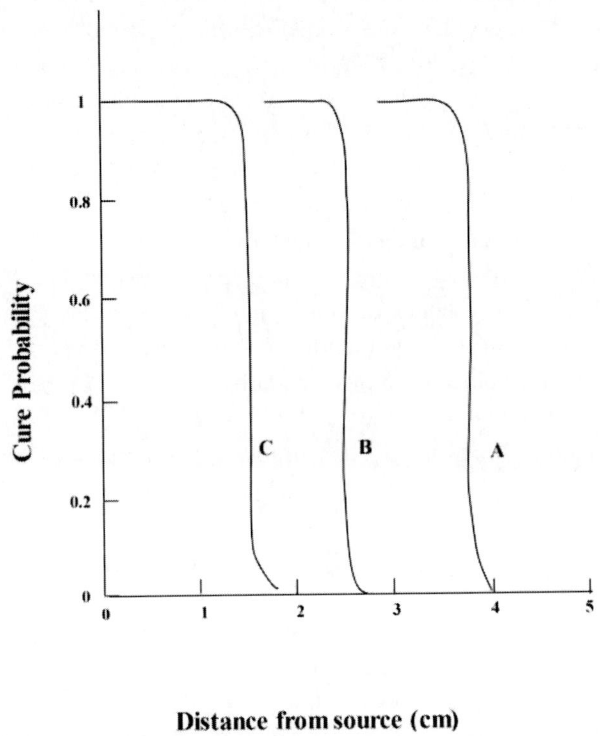

Figure 12.7. Probability of the cell kill with respect to distance from the radioactive source.

The lack of uniformity in the radiation zone surrounding an implanted source has significant implications in the science of radiobiology [54]. As shown in Figure 12.7, In proximity to the radiation source, the dose rate is elevated, resulting in a cell-killing effect that closely aligns with the predictions derived from the acute-radiation survival curve. As the distance from the source increases, two notable alterations occur: firstly, the cells exhibit reduced sensitivity to lower dose rates, and secondly, the accumulated dose within a specific period of implantation diminishes as well. These two variables contribute to a significant and swift decline in cellular mortality as the distance from the source increases. In tissues, whether they are tumor or normal, in close proximity to the radiation source, the extent of cellular destruction will be sufficiently elevated to result in the eradication of cells exhibiting a wide range of radiosensitivity. At greater distances, the impact will be sufficiently minimal that even the most susceptible cells to radiation will be able to endure [55]. Within the spectrum of these two extremes exists a crucial region characterized by the occurrence of differential cell death. According to the findings of Steel et al. it can be inferred that cells with varying levels of radiosensitivity exhibit a distinct transition from a high to low local cure probability, resembling a cliff-like pattern. This transition occurs within a radial radius of a few millimeters, as depicted in the accompanying Figure. The proximity of the cliff to the source is contingent upon the radiosensitivity of the cells during low dose rate (LDR) exposure, with radioresistant cells being situated closer and radiosensitive cells being positioned farther away.

12.16. Pulsed Brachytherapy

The advent of computer-controlled high-dose-rate (HDR) afterloading devices has facilitated the administration of interstitial or intracavitary radiation through a sequence of pulses, known as pulsed-dose-rate (PDR) therapy [56]. The intervals between pulses offer enhanced flexibility for patients, heightened safety for nursing personnel, and technical benefits, such as the ability to make adjustments for the degradation of the radioactive source, so minimizing any impact on the efficacy of the treatment.

Transitioning from continuous exposure to therapy with intervals presents a radiobiological drawback. This phenomenon occurs due to the greater dosage rate inside each pulse, limiting the potential for healing radiation-induced damage. The tissue repair process that occurs at a sluggish pace will consequently face some disadvantages, leading to a diminished therapeutic index. This discrepancy in repair rates between rapidly regenerating tumor tissues and the comparatively slower healing of normal tissues will result in a loss of balance [57]. Brenner and Hall (3) analyzed the magnitude of this phenomenon and determined that, for a range of pulse intervals of 60 minutes or less, the radiobiological deficit may be deemed an acceptable compromise in light of the enhanced dosimetric localization achieved in the target volume. Subsequently, extensive theoretical discourse has been conducted regarding the principles governing the safe administration of pulsed brachytherapy. The group of Pettersen in Oslo has conducted comprehensive laboratory investigations comparing photodynamic therapy (PDR) with continuous low-dose radiation (CLDR) using *in vitro* cell models. The researchers concluded that PDR exhibited a higher magnitude of impact in certain cell lines than what was initially anticipated. The inverse dose-rate effect does not provide an adequate explanation for this phenomenon. The observed inverse dose-rate impact was consistent across cell lines, regardless of whether they were exposed to continuous low dose-rate (CLDR) or pulsed dose-rate (PDR) conditions [58].

Previous research has conducted theoretical investigations to analyze the impact of repair half-times on both normal and tumor tissues. These studies have also explored the presence of various components with distinct half-times within each tissue . Conducting brachytherapy research on laboratory animals presents technical challenges, mostly due to the inherent size disparities between rats and humans. Nonetheless, comprehensive investigations have been conducted to examine the effects of brachytherapy on the spinal cord of rats.

The utilization of clinical pulsed brachytherapy technology, which enables the sequential movement of a solitary high-intensity source throughout the treatment field, has become prevalent in contemporary medical practice [59]. These systems offer a significant level of control. However, it is imperative to exercise caution when applying the procedure, as there may be consequences in terms of treatment quality if pulse sizes are very big or if the period between pulses exceeds 1 hour. The implementation of high dose rate (HDR) post loading systems may provide a potential inclination to reduce the overall treatment duration. As previously mentioned, this inclination could result in heightened early reactions to radiotherapy and an augmented resistance of tumors to radiation due to insufficient reoxygenation. A comparative clinical trial was conducted at the Princess Margaret Hospital in Toronto, Canada, to evaluate the effectiveness of CLDR and PDR in the treatment of cervical cancer. There was no statistically significant difference detected in terms of survival or late toxicity. Consequently, the authors concluded that PDR (pulsed dose rate) offers the advantage of improved dosage adjustment. The utilization of PDR (Pulse Dose Rate) in conjunction with IMRT (Intensity-Modulated Radiation Therapy) has the potential to offer optimal possibilities for dose escalation, since it enables the delivery of high doses inside the intended target volume [60].

Conclusion

This chapter comprehensively discussed the role of hyperthermia as a radiosensitizer in cancer therapy and its integration with time-dose fractionation strategies. The mechanisms by which heat induces cytotoxicity, enhances radiation effects, and potentially stimulates immune responses were explored in detail, along with the technological advances that enable precise tumor heating. Clinical evidence from randomized trials was presented, demonstrating significant improvements in treatment outcomes for various malignancies when hyperthermia is combined with radiotherapy or chemotherapy. The text also reviewed the effects of dose rate on cell survival and normal tissue sparing, emphasizing the importance of optimizing treatment parameters to balance efficacy and toxicity. As non-invasive thermometry and innovative heating methods evolve, hyperthermia is poised to become an increasingly valuable adjunct in the multidisciplinary management of cancer.

References

[1] Bergs JW, Wacker MG, Hehlgans S, Piiper A, Multhoff G, Roedel C, Roedel F. The role of recent nanotechnology in enhancing the efficacy of radiation therapy. Biochimica et Biophysica Acta (BBA)-*Reviews on Cancer*. 2015 Aug 1;1856(1):130-43.

[2] Bartzsch S, Oelfke U. Line focus x-ray tubes—a new concept to produce high brilliance x-rays. *Physics in Medicine & Biology*. 2017 Oct 27;62(22):8600.

[3] DiCarlo AL, Perez Horta Z, Rios CI, Satyamitra MM, Taliaferro LP, Cassatt DR. Study logistics that can impact medical countermeasure efficacy testing in mouse models of radiation injury. *International journal of radiation biology*. 2021 Dec 3;97(sup1):S151-67.

[4] Bhowmick S. *Supraphysiological thermal therapy in the treatment of prostate cancer: linking thermal history to cellular and tissue level injury mechanisms*. University of Minnesota; 2000.

[5] Lang BJ, Guerrero ME, Prince TL, Okusha Y, Bonorino C, Calderwood SK. The functions and regulation of heat shock proteins; key orchestrators of proteostasis and the heat shock response. *Archives of toxicology*. 2021 Jun;95(6):1943-70.

[6] Parsell DA, Lindquist S. The function of heat-shock proteins in stress tolerance: degradation and reactivation of damaged proteins. *Annual review of genetics*. 1993 Dec;27(1):437-96.

[7] Field SB, Bleehen NM. Hyperthermia in the treatment of cancer. *Cancer treatment reviews*. 1979 Jun 1;6(2):63-94.

[8] Myers R, Robinson JE, Field SB. The relationship between heating time and temperature for inhibition of growth in baby rat cartilage by combined hyperthermia and X-rays. *International Journal of Radiation Biology and Related Studies in Physics, Chemistry and Medicine*. 1980 Jan 1;38(4):373-82.

[9] Petryk AA. *Magnetic nanoparticle hyperthermia as an adjuvant cancer therapy with chemotherapy*. Dartmouth College; 2013.

[10] Nam J, Won N, Jin H, Chung H, Kim S. pH-induced aggregation of gold nanoparticles for photothermal cancer therapy. Journal of the American Chemical Society. 2009 Sep 30;131(38):13639-45.

[11] Denekamp J. Vascular attack as a therapeutic strategy for cancer. *Cancer and Metastasis Reviews*. 1990 Nov;9:267-82.

[12] Arruebo M, Vilaboa N, Sáez-Gutierrez B, Lambea J, Tres A, Valladares M, González-Fernández Á. Assessment of the evolution of cancer treatment therapies. *Cancers*. 2011 Aug 12;3(3):3279-330.

[13] Neuer A, Spandorfer SD, Giraldo P, Dieterle S, Rosenwaks Z, Witkin SS. The role of heat shock proteins in reproduction. *Human reproduction update*. 2000 Mar 1;6(2):149-59.

[14] Curley CT, Sheybani ND, Bullock TN, Price RJ. Focused ultrasound immunotherapy for central nervous system pathologies: challenges and opportunities. *Theranostics*. 2017;7(15):3608.

[15] Hildebrandt B, Wust P, Ahlers O, Dieing A, Sreenivasa G, Kerner T, Felix R, Riess H. The cellular and molecular basis of hyperthermia. *Critical reviews in oncology/hematology*. 2002 Jul 1;43(1):33-56.

[16] Franckena M, Stalpers LJ, Koper PC, Wiggenraad RG, Hoogenraad WJ, van Dijk JD, Wárlám-Rodenhuis CC, Jobsen JJ, van Rhoon GC, van der Zee J. Long-term improvement in treatment outcome after radiotherapy and hyperthermia in locoregionally advanced cervix cancer: an update of the Dutch Deep Hyperthermia Trial. *International Journal of Radiation Oncology* Biology* Physics*. 2008 Mar 15;70(4):1176-82.

[17] Peetsold MG, Heij HA, Kneepkens CM, Nagelkerke AF, Huisman J, Gemke RJ. The long-term follow-up of patients with a congenital diaphragmatic hernia: a broad spectrum of morbidity. *Pediatric surgery international*. 2009 Jan;25:1-7.

[18] Verma V, Simone II CB. Combining Cytotoxic Chemotherapy and Radiation Therapy. *Precision Radiation Oncology*. 2018 May 24.

[19] Howard MA, Polo K, Pusic AL, Cordeiro PG, Hidalgo DA, Mehrara B, Disa JJ. Breast cancer local recurrence after mastectomy and TRAM flap reconstruction: incidence and treatment options. *Plastic and reconstructive surgery*. 2006 Apr 15;117(5):1381-6.

[20] Kok HP, Cressman EN, Ceelen W, Brace CL, Ivkov R, Grüll H, Ter Haar G, Wust P, Crezee J. Heating technology for malignant tumors: A review. *International Journal of Hyperthermia*. 2020 Jan 1;37(1):711-41.

[21] Horsman MR, Overgaard J. Hyperthermia: a potent enhancer of radiotherapy. *Clinical oncology*. 2007 Aug 1;19(6):418-26.

[22] Pinel S, Thomas N, Boura C, Barberi-Heyob M. Approaches to physical stimulation of metallic nanoparticles for glioblastoma treatment. *Advanced Drug Delivery Reviews*. 2019 Jan 1;138:344-57.

[23] Datta NR, Ordóñez SG, Gaipl US, Paulides MM, Crezee H, Gellermann J, Marder D, Puric E, Bodis S. Local hyperthermia combined with radiotherapy and-/or chemotherapy: Recent advances and promises for the future. *Cancer treatment reviews*. 2015 Nov 1;41(9):742-53.

[24] Habib MR, Morris DL. Local and Regional Hyperthermia. Induction Chemotherapy: Integrated Treatment Programs for Locally *Advanced Cancers*. 2011:51-8.

[25] Kroon HM, Moncrieff M, Kam PC, Thompson JF. Outcomes following isolated limb infusion for melanoma. A 14-year experience. *Annals of surgical oncology*. 2008 Nov;15:3003-13.

[26] Grubbs EG, Abdel-Wahab O, Cheng TY, Abdel-Wahab Z, Peterson B, Pruitt SK, Colvin OM, Friedman HS, Tyler DS. In-transit melanoma: the role of alkylating-agent resistance in regional therapy. *Journal of the American College of Surgeons*. 2004 Sep 1;199(3):419-27.

[27] Soens MA, Birnbach DJ, Ranasinghe JS, van Zundert A. Obstetric anesthesia for the obese and morbidly obese patient: an ounce of prevention is worth more than a pound of treatment. *Acta anaesthesiologica scandinavica*. 2008 Jan;52(1):6-19.

[28] Bankert RB, Balu-Iyer SV, Odunsi K, Shultz LD, Kelleher Jr RJ, Barnas JL, Simpson-Abelson M, Parsons R, Yokota SJ. Humanized mouse model of ovarian cancer recapitulates patient solid tumor progression, ascites formation, and metastasis. *PloS one*. 2011 Sep 15;6(9):e24420.

[29] Issels RD. Hyperthermia adds to chemotherapy. *European journal of cancer*. 2008 Nov 1;44(17):2546-54.

[30] Yadav PR. *Cell culture*. Discovery Publishing House; 2005.

[31] Hynynen K, Jones RM. Image-guided ultrasound phased arrays are a disruptive technology for non-invasive therapy. *Physics in Medicine & Biology*. 2016 Aug 5;61(17):R206.

[32] Pribat D, Plais F, Legagneux P, Reita C. Thin films for large area electronics. In *Science and technology of thin films* 1995 (pp. 293-359).

[33] Cetas TC. Temperature measurement. In *Heat Transfer in Medicine and Biology: Analysis and Applications*. Volume 2 1985 (pp. 373-392). Boston, MA: Springer US.

[34] Satapathy A, Mahimkar K, Mondal S, Pathaare Y, Kandasubramanian B. Attenuation of electromagnetic waves in polymeric terahertz imbibers. *Journal of Materials Science: Materials in Electronics*. 2023 Feb;34(6):516.

[35] Sipsas NV, Kontoyiannis DP. Invasive fungal infections in patients with cancer in the Intensive Care Unit. *International journal of antimicrobial agents*. 2012 Jun 1;39(6):464-71.

[36] Brüser C, Antink CH, Wartzek T, Walter M, Leonhardt S. Ambient and unobtrusive cardiorespiratory monitoring techniques. *IEEE reviews in biomedical engineering*. 2015 Mar 18;8:30-43.

[37] Grüll H, Langereis S. Hyperthermia-triggered drug delivery from temperature-sensitive liposomes using MRI-guided high intensity focused ultrasound. *Journal of Controlled Release*. 2012 Jul 20;161(2):317-27.

[38] Lopresto V, Strigari L, Farina L, Minosse S, Pinto R, D'Alessio D, Cassano B, Cavagnaro M. CT-based investigation of the contraction of ex vivo tissue undergoing microwave thermal ablation. *Physics in Medicine & Biology*. 2018 Mar 7;63(5):055019.

[39] Hall EJ. 2 Review of essential and topical radiobiology. In *Radiobiological Modelling in Radiation* Oncology 2007 Oct 1 (pp. 12-34). The British Institute of Radiology.

[40] McCollough CH, Primak AN, Braun N, Kofler J, Yu L, Christner J. Strategies for reducing radiation dose in CT. *Radiologic Clinics*. 2009 Jan 1;47(1):27-40.

[41] Fowler JF. Optimum overall times II: Extended modelling for head and neck radiotherapy. *Clinical oncology*. 2008 Mar 1;20(2):113-26.

[42] van der Kogel AJ, Joiner MC. *The dose-rate effect. InBasic clinical radiobiology* 2018 Aug 28 (pp. 143-151). CRC Press.

[43] Wang JZ, Guerrero M, Li XA. How low is the α/β ratio for prostate cancer?. *International Journal of Radiation Oncology* Biology* Physics*. 2003 Jan 1;55(1):194-203.

[44] Iqbal F, Shabbir MI. Genetic analysis with pyrosequencing using loop pipetting and a light-dependent resistor. *Analytical Methods*. 2021;13(42):5035-47.

[45] Gregoire V, Grau C, Haustermans K, Muren LP, Stewart F. Principles of radiotherapy. *UICC Manual of Clinical Oncology*. 2015 Aug 14:108-23.

[46] Tracqui P, Cruywagen GC, Woodward DE, Bartoo GT, Murray JD, Alvord Jr EC. A mathematical model of glioma growth: the effect of chemotherapy on spatio-temporal growth. *Cell proliferation*. 1995 Jan;28(1):17-31.

[47] Mitchell JB, Bedford JS, Bailey SM. Observations of the first postirradiation division of HeLa cells following continuous or fractionated exposure to γ rays. *Radiation Research*. 1979 Oct 1;80(1):186-97.

[48] Fernandez-Palomo C, Seymour C, Mothersill C. Inter-relationship between low-dose hyper-radiosensitivity and radiation-induced bystander effects in the human T98G glioma and the epithelial HaCaT cell line. *Radiation research*. 2016 Feb 1;185(2):124-33.

[49] Emery P, Fleischmann R, Filipowicz-Sosnowska A, Schechtman J, Szczepanski L, Kavanaugh A, Racewicz AJ, van Vollenhoven RF, Li NF, Agarwal S, Hessey EW. The efficacy and safety of rituximab in patients with active rheumatoid arthritis despite methotrexate treatment: results of a phase IIB randomized, double-blind, placebo-controlled, dose-ranging trial. *Arthritis & Rheumatism: Official Journal of the American College of Rheumatology*. 2006 May;54(5):1390-400.

[50] Unkel S, Belka C, Lauber K. On the analysis of clonogenic survival data: Statistical alternatives to the linear-quadratic model. *Radiation oncology*. 2016 Dec;11(1):1-1.

[51] Du T, Xiao J, Qiu Z, Wu K. The effectiveness of intensity-modulated radiation therapy versus 2D-RT for the treatment of nasopharyngeal carcinoma: A systematic review and meta-analysis. *PloS one*. 2019 Jul 10;14(7):e0219611.

[52] Pacelli R, Caroprese M, Palma G, Oliviero C, Clemente S, Cella L, Conson M. Technological evolution of radiation treatment: Implications for clinical applications. In *Seminars in oncology* 2019 Jun 1 (Vol. 46, No. 3, pp. 193-201). WB Saunders.

[53] Wilson P, Jones B, Yokoi T, Hill M, Vojnovic B. Revisiting the ultra-high dose rate effect: implications for charged particle radiotherapy using protons and light ions. *The British journal of radiology*. 2012 Oct;85(1018):e933-9.

[54] DiCarlo AL, Perez Horta Z, Rios CI, Satyamitra MM, Taliaferro LP, Cassatt DR. Study logistics that can impact medical countermeasure efficacy testing in mouse models of radiation injury. *International journal of radiation biology*. 2021 Dec 3;97(sup1):S151-67.

[55] Mettler Jr FA, Voelz GL. Major radiation exposure—what to expect and how to respond. *New England Journal of Medicine*. 2002 May 16;346(20):1554-61.

[56] Gao XZ, Hou ZX, Guo Z, Liu JX, Chen XQ. Energy management strategy for solar-powered high-altitude long-endurance aircraft. *Energy conversion and management*. 2013 Jun 1;70:20-30.

[57] Butterfield TA, Best TM, Merrick MA. The dual roles of neutrophils and macrophages in inflammation: a critical balance between tissue damage and repair. *Journal of athletic training*. 2006 Oct;41(4):457.

[58] Furre, M. Koritzinsky, Dr. Olsen, Eo Pettersen T. Inverse dose-rate effect due to pre-mitotic accumulation during continuous low dose-rate irradiation of cervix carcinoma cells. *International journal of radiation biology*. 1999 Jan 1;75(6):699-707.

[59] Kennedy JE, ter Haar GR, Cranston D. High intensity focused ultrasound: surgery of the future?. *The British journal of radiology*. 2003 Sep;76(909):590-9.

[60] Tanderup K, Georg D, Pötter R, Kirisits C, Grau C, Lindegaard JC. Adaptive management of cervical cancer radiotherapy. In *Seminars in radiation oncology* 2010 Apr 1 (Vol. 20, No. 2, pp. 121-129). WB Saunders.

Chapter 13

Radiation Safety

Anurag Luharia[1,*], PhD
Mary Joan[2], PhD
Rajesh Amutha[3], MSc
and Nilavarasu Shanmugam[4], MSc

[1]Department of Radio physics and Radio safety, Datta Meghe Institute of Higher Education and Research, Wardha, India
[2]Department of Radiation Oncology, Christian Medical College and Hospital, Ludhiana, India
[3]Department of Radiotherapy, Rio Bravo Cancer Center, Bakersfield, CA, USA
[4]Department of Radiotherapy, All India Institute of Medical Sciences, Nagpur, India

Abstract

Radiation safety is a critical concern in various settings, including occupational, public, and medical exposure. The International Commission on Radiological Protection (ICRP) provides guidelines to ensure the safe use of radiation and nuclear technology. The ICRP's recommendations focus on preventing tissue reactions and limiting the risk of stochastic effects, such as cancer and heritable effects, to a reasonable level. The Commission's guidelines are based on three fundamental principles: justification, optimization, and limitation. Justification involves ensuring that the benefits of a radiation exposure outweigh the risks, while optimization requires minimizing harm to individuals and society. Limitation involves setting individual dose restrictions to prevent excessive exposure. Effective radiation safety requires a comprehensive approach that includes risk assessment, dose monitoring, and optimization of protection. The ICRP's recommendations provide a framework for radiation safety professionals to ensure the safe use of radiation and nuclear technology.

Keywords: ALARA principle, occupational exposure, dose limits, ICRP guidelines, radiation protection

* Corresponding Author's Email: auragluharia@gmail.com

In: Fundamentals of Radiation Biology
Editors: Anurag Luharia, Ashish Uke, Gaurav Mishra et al.
ISBN: 979-8-89530-806-6

13.1. Introduction

Radiological protection limits how much ionizing radiation people are exposed to so that tissue reactions do not happen and the chance of random effects is in a safer range. Dosimetric quantities were made by the International Commission on Radiation Units and Measurements (ICRU) and the International Commission on Radiological Protection (ICRP) to help examine how much radiation a person has been exposed to. The ICRP's basic protection numbers are based on measurements of how much energy is given to the organs and tissues of the body. With these numbers, it is possible to measure the amount of exposure to ionizing radiation that comes from both outside radiation sources and radionuclides taken in. The estimated doses can then be compared to the proposed limits for people exposed at work and the general public.

13.2. International Commission on Radiological Protection

The second International Congress of Radiology founded ICRP in 1928 to address medical concerns about ionizing radiation. International X-ray and Radium Protection Committee (IXRPC) was the first name. It became the International Commission on Radiological Protection [1]. The goal was to better account for radiation usage outside medicine, hence the generalised name.

Since 1977, ICRP has published its recommendations in the shape of a scientific journal. The series of publications is called Annals of the ICRP, now published by SAGE UK. The work is based on critical scientific evaluation and documented data [2]. The designing of scientific recommendations at various national and international levels is shown in Figure 13.1.

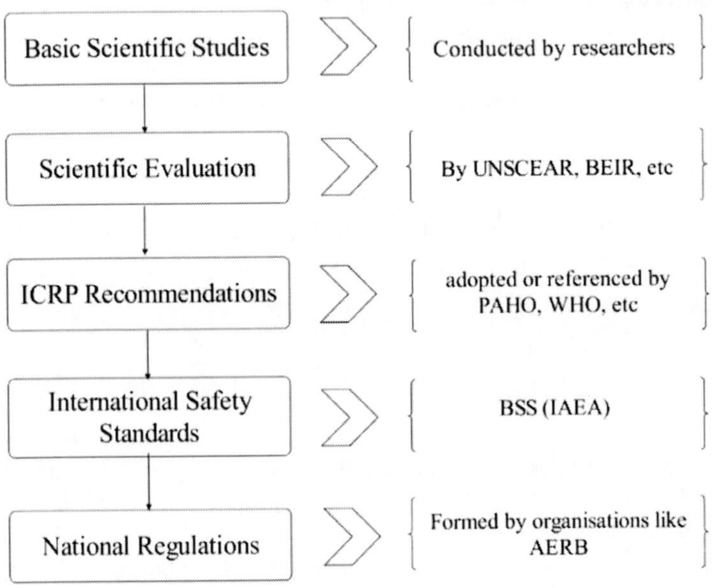

Figure 13.1. Flow of framing the regulations at national and international level.

13.3. The National Council on Radiation Protection and Measurements (NCRP)

The National Council on Radiation Protection and Measurements (NCRP) in USA was followed alongside the ICRP in 1928. The mission of the National Council on Radiation Protection and Measurements (NCRP) is to develop and disseminate extensively radiation protection and measurement information, guidance, and recommendations that reflect the best available scientific knowledge [3]. The Council is constantly looking for new topics in which the creation and dissemination of NCRP materials might significantly advance the common good.

Since its formation as "The Advisory Committee on X-Ray and Radium Protection" in 1929, NCRP has been an essential aspect of radiation protection and monitoring [4].

13.3.1. Radiation Protection and Radiation Safety

There are two distinct forms of damage caused by ionizing radiation. The first kind of harm occurs when cells in an organ or tissue are eliminated. The second type of consequence results from radiation's effects on cells that are not killed but are altered or modified. The International Commission on Radiological Protection (ICRP) has designated specific labels for each phenomenon. Radiation-induced cell death and subsequent tissue or organ damage have traditionally been called a deterministic effect but are now more commonly referred to as a tissue reaction [5]. While some stem cells in a self-renewing system would die after receiving a low radiation dose, the organ or tissue would still function generally because new cells would quickly replace the dead ones.

Therefore, a tissue reaction requires a certain amount of exposure. There is a 100% possibility of a tissue reaction if the radiation dose is high enough to severely deplete the stem cell compartment, which can happen at any radiation dose. As a result, a tissue reaction's dose-response curve takes the form of a threshold sigmoid [6].

A tissue reaction is characterised by the effect being related to damage to numerous cells and becoming more severe with a dose above the threshold. Tissue reactions include things like changes in fertility, death from whole-body radiation exposure, and kidney failure.

The effects caused due to cells, not being totally eliminated, instead undergoing random mutations are called stochastic. Cancer is the most consequential stochastic impact; the others are heritable. The severity of a stochastic impact is not dose-dependent, but the likelihood of its occurrence does increase with increasing doses. The effect is likely related to damage to a single or a small number of cells because most malignancies are monoclonal. For radiation protection purposes, it is considered safe to presume that any dose, no matter how tiny, has some likelihood of creating an effect. However, this probability decreases with decreasing dose [7]. Other than the lower dose threshold, for which experimental data is available, no one knows if more thresholds are present and if those doses can show effects. The thresholds set through experimentation are mentioned Table13.1.

Table 13.1. Dose Thresholds set for different observed effects due to radiation exposure

Stochastic Effects	Tissue Reactions (Formerly Known as Deterministic Effects)
Occupational exposure should be permitted above the age of 18 years	
The effective dose in any year should not exceed 50 mSv (5 rem).	50 mGy per year for the lens of the eye
The individual worker's lifetime effective dose should not exceed age in years × 10 mSv	500 mSv per year for localized areas of the skin and the hands and feet
Note: These limits apply to the sum of the effective dose from external radiation and the committed effective dose from internal exposures.	Note: The poor sensitivity of the specific tissues implicated to radiation-induced malignancy necessitates these extra restrictions for tissue reactivity.

13.4. Assessment of Radiation Exposure

13.4.1. External Radiation Exposure

Dose assessments from environmental radiation exposure are typically performed through prospective assessments where H*(10) is measured or estimated and appropriate conversion coefficients are applied or through individual monitoring using personal dosimeters worn on the body. Hp (10) and Hp (0.07) are the operating numbers for individual monitoring. Hp (10) offers a practical dose value sufficiently exact for radiological protection purposes at low doses and on the assumption of a uniform whole-body exposure, assuming the personal dosimeter is worn on a body position typical of its exposure [8].

13.4.2. B. Internal Radiation Exposure

The dose assessment system for radioactive intakes relies on radionuclide intake computation, an operational number for dose assessment from internal exposure. Direct and indirect measurements (such as urine or faeces), ambient samples, and biokinetic models can estimate consumption. The Commission recommends dose factors for many radionuclides to calculate the effective dosage after delivery. Public occupational dose coefficients are age-specific and adult-specific.

The half-life and biological retention of radionuclides within the body influence the time they radiate the tissues. As a result, their doses to bodily tissues may only become apparent for a short time short time after consumption. Committed dose quantities have been defined as regulating radionuclide exposures and the buildup of radiation dosage over time. The predicted total dose delivery from a radionuclide that has been included is known as the "committed dose," and it is expected to be delivered within a specific time frame [9].

The Commission's recommendation that the year of intake be allocated to the committed dose to determine compliance with dose restrictions remains unchanged. The Commission has arbitrarily set the commitment term at 50 years because it believes this is a reasonable approximation of a young person's expected working life. Hence, the committed dose is typically assessed over 50 years after ingestion for workers. Public dose estimates using the committed effective dose from radionuclide ingestion are also performed. Adults'

Assessments must be planned on a commitment period of at least 50 years. Dose assessment for newborns and children is performed up to age 70.

The reference dose coefficient is used with the worker's intake to determine the effective dose from occupational exposure to radionuclides. For some radionuclides (Sv, Bq), the dosage coefficients are computed using predetermined biokinetic and dosimetric models. Radionuclides can enter the body in various chemical forms, and their entry, distribution, and retention within the blood are all modelled [10]. Calculating the percentage of energy emitted from a source region S absorbed in a target region T using the computational male and female phantoms for several different sources is also possible. The majority of radiation protection activities may be completed with these approximations.

13.4.3. Occupational Exposure

Workers' background radiation dosimeter's output is Hp (10). This figure estimates the effective dose under uniform whole-body exposure. Radionuclide intakes are measured by bioassay or other methods to establish committed effective doses for internal exposure. The dose coefficient multiplies the dose received. Occupational radiation exposures and radionuclide intakes are added to produce the Total Effective Dose, E. Calculating the effective dosage from specific radionuclides may require considering the material taken into the body.

Reference Male Reference Female anatomical, physiological, and biokinetic factors (ICRP, 2002) determined dose coefficients. Consider the activity median aerodynamic diameter (AMAD) of the inhaled aerosol and the chemical form of the particulate matter to which the designated radionuclide is connected. A worker's effective dose is the Reference Person's exposure to the same radiation fields and activity levels. The 50-year commitment period estimates dose accumulation during a working life for radionuclides with long physical half-lives and tissue retention [11].

Uncontrolled wound radionuclide uptake has consequences beyond work practice compliance and is excluded. Worker exposure should be curtailed after assessing these instances and providing proper medical care.

In the exceedingly uncommon occurrence of a significant contribution to external exposure to weakly penetrating radiation, the skin dose and the terms for effective dose estimation must be considered. Dose assessment may also include radiation from radon isotopes, especially radon-222, and their decay products (ICRP 1993a).

When personal dosimeters are not used, such as aircrew exposure, H*(10) can be used to estimate effective dosage [12]. The effective dosage is then calculated from radiation field data or the appropriate parameters.

13.4.4. Public Exposure

Estimating effective doses follows the same fundamental principles for the general public and workers. The effective dose received by the public within a year due to external exposure and the effective dosage promised due to radionuclides included within this year are added together to form the yearly effective dose. The dose is often established using effluent and environmental measurements, habit data, and modelling rather than through direct measurement of individual exposures, as is done for occupational exposure, for apparent reasons. Effluent monitoring for existing installations or forecast of effluents from the installation or source over the design period can be used to estimate the component owing to discharges of radioactive effluents [13]. To evaluate doses from external radiation exposure and intakes of radionuclides, scientists use data on concentrations of radionuclides in effluents and the environment in conjunction with radioecological modelling (pathway analysis of environmental transport through air, water, soil, sediments, plants, and animals to humans).

13.5. Medical Exposure of Patients

The equivalent or absorbed dose to irradiated tissues is the crucial parameter for planning patient exposure and risk-benefit assessments. Patients' exposures cannot be accurately quantified using effective dose alone; other factors must be considered. Comparing effective doses across diagnostic procedures, similar technologies and procedures across hospitals, and different technologies for the same medical examination can all be helpful. However, the equivalent or absorbed dose to irradiated tissues is the pertinent quantity for planning patient exposure and risk-benefit analyses [14]. When organs and tissues only receive partial or very heterogeneous exposure, as is the situation especially with x-ray diagnostics, it is very difficult to quantify and interpret effective dose from medical exposure of patients.

13.5.1. Types of Exposure Situations

The Commission intends that its Recommendations apply to all sources of radiation and any and all individuals exposed to radiation in the following three categories of exposure conditions.

The deliberate introduction and operation of sources constitutes a *"planned exposure situation."* Both normal exposures (those that are expected to happen) and prospective exposures (those that are not expected to happen) can arise from planned exposure circumstances [15].

In order to avoid or mitigate potentially disastrous outcomes, quick action is required in emergency exposure circumstances, which might arise during the execution of a planned situation, as a result of malicious activity, or as a result of any other unforeseen circumstance.

Any *pre-existing exposure situation*, such as extended exposure conditions following emergencies, must be considered when making a control decision.

What the Commission has termed 'practices' may be the root of preexisting, unexpected, and deliberate disclosure. Patient medical exposures are examples of planned exposure circumstances but are discussed separately due to their unique qualities. The same precautionary principles that apply to anticipated hazards also apply to the safety of workers amid unexpected or ongoing hazards.

13.5.2. Categories of Exposure and Identification of the Exposed Individuals

The Commission classifies exposures as either "occupational," "public," or "medical," depending on where they occurred. Volunteer study participants and those providing comfort and care are considered sources of exposure. At least three groups of exposed people—workers, the general public, and patients—must be addressed independently. They roughly correlate to those whose exposures fall into one of the three types described in the section before this one. Any person may be vulnerable to exposure in their roles as employees, members of the general public, or patients.

13.5.3. Occupational Exposure

The Commission considers any radiation exposure sustained by an employee during their employment to be occupational exposure. The Commission has taken note of the common understanding that any exposure to a hazardous chemical in the workplace counts as occupational exposure. However, the direct application of this term to radiation would imply that all workers should be subject to a regime of radiological protection due to the widespread nature of radiation. Therefore, the Commission restricts its usage of 'occupational exposures' to those involving radiation exposures sustained during employment due to circumstances that can be legitimately regarded as falling under the purview of the operating management [16]. In occupational safety, it is unnecessary to consider risks associated with exposures that are either excluded or result from exempt activities or sources.

The onus for employees' safety ultimately rests with their company. However, the licensee responsible for the source (if not the same as the employer) also must ensure the safety of workers from radiation exposure. The licensee and the employer should work together by exchanging information and ensuring that workers are provided with adequate radiological protection if their employment involves or may involve a source not under the licensee's control.

13.5.4. Definition of a Worker and Their Safety

The Commission considers anyone working for an employer, permanently or temporarily, to be a worker and have rights and responsibilities in occupational radiological protection. A self-employed person is responsible for being an employer and an employee. Radiation exposure is an occupational hazard for those in specific medical fields.

One of the responsibilities of an employer or licensee is to ensure the safety of employees who are subjected to hazards in the workplace [17]. The Commission's continued recommendation to categorise jobs rather than individuals is intended to facilitate this goal.

They formally designate the workplace regions where sources are located, aiding their management. The Commission uses two types of these classifications: regulated areas and supervised areas. A controlled area is a delineated space that requires, or may require, special precautions and safety measures to ensure that typical exposures are minimised or that contamination is contained under normal working conditions. Workplace conditions are monitored in a supervised location, although additional steps are usually unnecessary. A supervised area typically contains a regulated area. However, this is only sometimes the case.

Workers in "controlled areas" of workplaces should be in the know, have had additional training, and stand out as a distinct unit. These personnel often undergo occupational radiation monitoring and, on rare occasions, additional medical monitoring.

Workers who are nursing or expecting should not be exposed.

The Commission determined in its 1990 Recommendations that there was no need to differentiate between the sexes when regulating workplace exposure. These Recommendations represent the continuation of the Commission's previous stance [18]. Additional precautions for the safety of the embryo/fetus must be taken into account if a female worker has disclosed (i.e., notified her employer) that she is pregnant. The Commission's position is that pregnant women should be afforded the same level of protection at work for their unborn children as the general public. If the mother is exposed before she declares her pregnancy, the Commission believes that the protection it has advocated will effectively apply this policy. Once a company is made aware of a pregnancy, precautions can be taken to ensure the safety of the unborn child. Following a pregnancy declaration, a pregnant worker's working conditions should be adjusted so that the increased dose to the embryo/fetus does not exceed roughly 1 mSv.

Due to the dose limitation placed on the developing embryo and fetus, it is not required that pregnant women refrain from all contact with radiation or radioactive materials or be barred from visiting or working in radiation-controlled locations. However, it does suggest that the company assess the working conditions of pregnant women closely. More specifically, their working conditions should be altered to greatly reduce the likelihood of accidental doses and radioactive intakes during pregnancy. Publications 84 and 88 (ICRP, 2000a, 2001a) offer detailed guidance for employers on how to limit their employees' exposure to harmful substances while they are pregnant. The Commission has also made available data in Publication 95 (ICRP, 2004c) that can be used to estimate the doses received by nursing infants due to maternal intakes [19]. Women who have publicly stated that they are pregnant or nursing should not participate in emergency measures that expose them to potentially harmful levels of radiation, as recommended by the International Commission on Radiological Protection (ICRP) (2005a).

13.5.5. Public Exposure

In contrast to occupational and patient medical exposures, public exposure includes all general public exposures —various types of radiation exposure cause it. Although the proportion of public exposure attributable to natural sources is much more significant, this fact does not justify paying less attention to the much smaller proportion attributable to sources that can be more easily managed. Pregnant workers' exposures to harmful substances are treated as public exposures and subject to the same regulations.

13.6. Definition of Members of the Public and Representative Man

The Commission considers everyone exposed outside of an employment or medical setting to be a member of the public. People are exposed to various hazards from both natural and anthropogenic sources.

In the case of widespread exposure, doses from each source will be spread out among several people. The Commission has adopted the 'critical group' concept to define an individual receiving a dosage typical of the most heavily exposed members of the population for public safety (ICRP, 1977) [20]. The average dose in the correct critical group has been capped. The critical group concept has been widely used for several decades, resulting in a wealth of learned wisdom. Methods for gauging exposure in the general population have also advanced, with probabilistic methods becoming increasingly common. The word "critical" suggests an emergency, which was never the intention of the Commission. Further, the measured dose is to an individual. Therefore, the word "group" may be misleading.

The Commission has shifted its focus from the critical group to the 'Representative Person' for radiological protection of the public. Publication 101 (ICRP, 2006a) from the Commission offers advice on defining the Representative Person and determining dosages for the Representative Person.

Though fictitious, the Representative Person should be based on the average behaviour of a subset of the population that shares the characteristics of the most at-risk members rather than the outlier behaviour of a single member of that subset. This includes the Representative Person's diet, breathing rate, location, and use of local resources.

13.6.1. Medical Exposure of Patients

Diagnostic and therapeutic procedures all expose patients to radiation. Various aspects of medical radiology call for a strategy distinct from that used for radiation protection in other cases of deliberate exposure. This is a calculated risk taken for the patient's good. The biological effects of high-dose radiation, such as cell death, are harnessed for therapeutic purposes in radiotherapy, which is used to treat cancer and other disorders [21]. Therefore, additional direction is needed regarding how these Recommendations apply to the medicinal uses of radiation.

13.6.2. Definition of Patients

The person who goes through a diagnostic, therapeutic, or interventional treatment is called the patient by the Commission. Since the Commission's dose limits and dose limitations could make diagnosing or treating a patient harder, they are not suggested for use with individual patients. So, the focus is on making sure that medical procedures are necessary, security is as good as possible and using diagnostic reference levels for diagnostic procedures.

13.6.3. The Objectives of Radiation Protection

The principles of radiation protection and their implementation are designed around some objectives. These objectives form the crux or central idea around which rules are framed. The two objectives of Radiation Protection are:

1. To prevent clinically significant radiation-induced tissue reactions by adhering to dose limits that are below the apparent or practical dose threshold
2. To limit the risk of stochastic effects (cancer and heritable effects) to a reasonable level about societal needs, values, and benefits gained

13.6.4. Radiation Safety Guiding Principles

With its guidelines from 1993, NCRP designed a radiation protection framework consisting of three essential elements:

1. Justification: the obligation to show that the predicted benefits to society outweigh the overall costs of an activity that exposes people to radiation.

According to the Commission's recommendations, the predicted change in radiation detriment should be explicitly addressed in the decision-making process whenever actions involving an increased or decreased level of radiation exposure or risk of possible exposure are being evaluated. There are a variety of other dangers, costs, and benefits of the activity to consider in addition to those directly related to radiation. In some cases, the harm from radiation will only account for a negligible fraction of the whole. Therefore, justification extends far beyond the realm of radiation safety. Because of this, the Commission only suggests making a positive net benefit a requirement for justification [22]. Authorities in charge of radiological safety do not have to spend time determining which of several options is the best.

- **Justification as a guiding concept**

The principle of justification can be applied in two ways in cases of occupational and public exposure, depending on whether or not the source can be directly controlled. If new activities require radiation protection and time is available to prepare the source, then the first method can be adopted. According to the justification principle, no circumstance involving intentional exposure should be introduced unless it results in a net benefit to the exposed individuals or society that exceeds the radiation damage caused by the intentional exposure. Conclusions about the appropriateness of introducing or maintaining specific planned situations involving exposure to ionizing radiation are crucial. New evidence or advances in technology may necessitate reevaluating the rationale.

The second strategy is employed when direct action on the source of the exposure is impractical or impossible. Two basic types of exposure circumstances are already present and emergency.

The idea of justification is utilised here to determine whether or not to take preventative measures. There will always be drawbacks to any decision to cut dosage, but the benefits should outweigh the costs.

In each case, governments or national authorities are tasked with deciding whether or not the strategy is justified to maximise the most excellent possible value to society as a whole rather than any one person in particular [23]. Users or other non-governmental organisations or individuals may provide valuable insight into many areas of the justification decision. Therefore, public consultation is typically used to inform justification judgments depending on factors such as the size of the source in question. Justification encompasses various topics, and numerous institutions may be responsible for its components. Here, thoughts on radiological safeguards will be considered with other factors.

Justification for medical procedures that put patients at risk necessitates a nuanced approach. Justification for the medical use of radiation should rest more with the profession than with the government or the competent regulatory authority. Yet, both types of planned exposure situations require justification. Due consideration must be given to the radioactive disadvantage from the exposure of the radiological crew and other individuals. However, the primary goal of medical exposure is to cause more good than harm to the patient. Medical professionals who operate question should have extensive training in radiological safety precautions because they are responsible for justifying the technique's usage [24]. Therefore, the Commission's Recommendations continue to include the need for justification prior to medical operations.

- **Unjustified Exposures**

The Commission believes that, absent special conditions, specific exposures should be automatically regarded as unjustified.

Some examples are as follows:

- Food, drink, cosmetics, toys, and personal jewellery or adornments can all boost their activity with the help of radioactive chemicals or activation.
- The use of radiation imaging or similar tools for artistic purposes is also unjustified.

A radiological examination is performed for occupational, health insurance, or legal purposes without consideration of clinical indications unless such an examination is predicted to yield substantial information about the examined person's health or to aid in significant forensic investigations. In most cases, this necessitates a clinical assessment of the captured image before the exposure may be considered appropriate.

For asymptomatic population groups, conducting a medical screening that exposes them to radiation should be avoided unless the benefits to the examined individuals or society as a whole are significant enough to outweigh the costs. Consideration must be given to the screening procedure's sensitivity, the effectiveness of therapy for recognised instances, and, for some diseases, the benefits to the community of disease control.

2. Optimisation: the requirement to minimise harm to society caused by such legitimate actions or practices.

The technique of protection optimisation is meant to be used in those cases where doing so is warranted. Whether it is a planned exposure, an emergency exposure, or an already existing exposure, the notion of optimisation of protection, with limits on the quantity of individual dose or risk, is at the heart of the protection system.

The process of minimising exposure risk (when exposures are not specific to be received), the number of exposed people, and the number of individual doses while also considering economic and societal considerations is what the Commission calls source-related optimisation [25]. Using decision support tools to arrive at an objectively optimal radiation protection plan requires using quantitative optimisation approaches like cost-benefit analyses. Over the past few decades, optimisation efforts have led to significant cuts in occupational and public exposures.

Optimisation is a continuing, iterative process that aims to achieve the highest possible level of security given the current conditions. Some ways of achieving this are listed below:

- a review of the context, including any potential risks (the process's framing);
- picking a good number to use as a ceiling or benchmark;
- the naming of potential safeguards;
- choose the most optimal action given current conditions, and
- actualisation of the decided-upon strategy.

Optimisation of protection has been found to increase radiation safety in predetermined conditions. The optimisation process can be guided to a more desirable endpoint with the help of constraints. Some sources and technologies can meet low-level limitations, while others can only meet high-level constraints. This is natural and should be reflected in regulatory bodies' and others' ability to pick suitable values for specific situations.

Planning protective activities and determining the optimum level of protection under the prevailing circumstances always involves the process of optimisation with the use of restrictions or reference levels. Only prospective doses, i.e., doses that may be received in the future, can be modified by decisions on preventive actions. Hence, only prospective doses are compared to the dose constraint or reference values [26]. They aren't meant to act as a dose cap after the fact.

The optimisation of protection is an iterative process that looks forward to avoiding or lessening potential risks. It involves qualitative and quantitative evaluations and considers both technological and socioeconomic progress.

All critical factors should be considered; thus, the procedure should be well-organised and methodical. The optimisation mindset constantly questions whether the best possible actions have been taken given the circumstances and whether every reasonable measure has been taken to limit exposure. In addition to sufficient resources and procedures, it necessitates top-down support from all relevant organisations.

The optimal course of action is context-dependent; it provides the highest possible level of safety under the given conditions. Therefore, setting an a priori dosage threshold at which optimisation efforts should cease is irrelevant. Regarding exposure, the optimal choice may lie either near or significantly below the relevant source-related limitation or reference level.

Maximising safety does not equate to minimising exposure. Protecting people to the greatest extent possible requires weighing the potential harm from exposure against the current means of doing so. As a result, the lowest-dose option is only sometimes the best [27].

It is important to consider reducing both the number of people exposed and the severity of their exposures. Optimisation of worker protection has always relied on the collective effective dose. The features of the individual exposure distribution within an exposed population must be carefully considered when comparing protective alternatives for optimisation.

Suppose an exposure affects a large number of people over a large geographic region or over a long period of time. In that case, the total collective effective dose may be a misleading aggregation of data that leads decision-makers astray. To overcome the limitations associated with collective effective dose, we must carefully analyse each relevant exposure situation to determine the individual characteristics and exposure parameters that best describe the exposure distribution among the concerned population for that situation.

By asking when, where, and from whom exposures occur, this type of analysis can identify distinct groups of people who share similar characteristics, whose effective collective doses can be calculated as part of the optimisation process, and for whom an optimal protection strategy can be defined (see Section 4.4). The difference between integrals defining the collective doses allotted to the individual groups is commonly used in practical optimisation assessments, which might lead to truncation of the collective doses.

It is impossible to codify every optimisation component; instead, there should be a shared commitment to the process [28]. The focus of the regulatory authority, when it comes to matters of optimisation, should be on methods, procedures, and judgments rather than on particular outcomes for a specific case.

The success of the optimisation process hinges heavily on the quality of communication established between the authorities and the operating management.

Societal values typically influence the ultimate decision on the level of radiation protection. Rather than relying just on radiological protection experts, involving important stakeholders in this decision-making process may be necessary.

3. Limitation: Individual dose restrictions must be applied to prevent justification and optimisation processes from increasing the danger to individuals or populations beyond what is considered safe.

- **Optimal Dose**

Dosage limits only apply in premeditated settings, not during actual medical procedures. Both the workforce and public nominal detriment coefficients are consistent with, if not slightly lower than, those published in 1990 [29]. These minor distinctions are irrelevant in practice. Dose limitations apply to the total exposure from sources previously justified within an exposure category, whether occupational or public.

In an emergency where an exposed person acts voluntarily to save lives or prevent a catastrophe, the individual is not subject to the dose restrictions. The standard dose limit may be waived for well-informed volunteers engaged in time-sensitive rescue operations. In contrast, later in emergency exposure situations, when recovery and restoration operations are underway, responders should be treated as occupationally exposed workers and afforded the same level of protection as other workers in the same industry, with exposures to radioactive materials kept well below the occupational dose limits recommended by the Commission. The Commission advises that women who have announced they are pregnant or are nursing not be employed as first responders undertaking life-saving or other urgent actions due to the inherent unpredictability of early response measures in an emergency exposure situation. The dose limits given by Commission in ICRP 103 are given in Table 13.2.

Table 13.2. The dose limits given by Commission in ICRP 103

Type of Limit	Occupational	Public
Effective Dose	20 mSv per year, averaged over defined period of 5 yrs and should not exceed 50 mSv in any single year.	1 mSv in a year
Annual Equivalent dose in:		
Lens of the eye	150 mSv	15 mSv
Skin	500 mSv	50 mSv
Hands and Feet	500 mSv	

Informed members of the public who are actively involved in caring for and comforting patients who have been discharged from the hospital after receiving therapy with unsealed radionuclides may be exempt from the public dose limit.

The comparable dosage limits for tissues are provided. This is because the Commission always expects wR values associated with stochastic effects to be lower than relevant RBE values associated with deterministic effects [30]. That is why we can confidently assume that the dosage limits offer at least as much safety from high-LET radiation as they do from low-LET. Therefore, the Commission concludes that using wR concerning deterministic effects is adequately conservative. It will be more appropriate to characterise the exposure regarding the absorbed dose and consider the relevant RBE in exceptional cases when high-LET radiation is the critical factor and where it mainly exposes a single tissue (such as the skin). In order to avoid misunderstandings, it is important to specify when an RBE-weighted absorbed dosage in Gy is being employed.

13.7. Dose Constraints and Reference Levels

Individual dosages are limited by combining the dose constraint and reference level ideas with protection maximisation. Dose limits or reference levels for individuals must be established at all times. The primary goal is to stay at or below these levels, and a secondary goal is to lower all doses to the lowest levels that can be achieved while still meeting societal and economic needs.

The Commission continues to use the term “dose constraint” for this exposure threshold in all planned exposure scenarios other than those involving patient medical exposure [31].

The Commission suggests using the term ‘reference level’ to denote this dose level in emergency and ongoing exposure circumstances. The Commission has maintained the distinction between the terms “planned exposure” and “other exposure” to emphasise the fact that in the former case, the limitation on individual doses can be applied during the planning stage, and the doses can be forecast to ensure that the constraint will not be exceeded. In other cases, there may be a broader variation in exposures, and the optimisation process may apply to initial individual doses higher than the reference level.

Medical diagnosis already uses diagnostic reference levels (i.e., planned exposure settings) to identify whether or not the levels of patient dose or given activity from a specific imaging procedure are abnormally high or low for those conditions. If this is the case, a regional review should be launched to assess whether or not the level of security has been optimised.

The specifics of the exposure under consideration will dictate the value selected for a constraint or reference level. Reference levels and dose restrictions do not mark a line between safe and dangerous, nor do they indicate a sharp increase or decrease in the health risk to individuals.

13.7.1. Dose Constraints

To put it another way, a dosage constraint is an upper bound on the expected dose in optimising protection for a prospective and source-related source (except medical exposure of patients). It is the dose above which it is implausible that protection is optimised for a specific source of exposure, necessitating intervention. Planned-situation dose restrictions will always be lower than the relevant dosage limit since they only provide a minimum degree of safety. It is essential to check that the doses implied by the source do not exceed the limit while making plans. A safe dose below the limit can be determined by protection optimisation. The intended result of the precautionary measures is then this optimised level.

If a dosage constraint is exceeded, it is required to assess whether or not the amount of protection is optimal, whether or not the correct dose constraint was chosen, and whether or not additional measures to lower doses to acceptable levels are warranted. The associated source-related limitation for potential exposures is a risk constraint [32]. Optimisation of protection is required to determine an acceptable level of exposure below the constraint rather than treating the constraint as a target value.

The dosage constraint is a dose value used to restrict the set of feasible optimisation targets such that only those choices with expected doses lower than the restriction are considered. The dosage constraint is an annual dose cap that any public member cannot exceed due to the scheduled operation of a designated controlled source. The Commission stresses that dose limitations should not be considered mandatory safety standards. The application of dose constraints and reference levels is given in Table 13.3.

Table 13.3. The Commission's system of protection applies dose constraint and reference levels under various situations

Type of Situation	Occupational Exposure	Public Exposure	Medical Exposure
Planned Exposure	Dose Limits Dose Constraints	Dose Limits Dose Constraints	Diagnostic reference level
Emergency exposure	Reference Level	Reference Level	N.A.
Existing Exposure	N.A.	Reference level	N.A.

13.7.2. Reference Levels

Reference levels are the dose or risk thresholds over which it is deemed improper to allow exposures to occur and, thus, for which preventive actions should be planned and optimised in an emergency or current controllable exposure circumstances. The current conditions of the exposure situation under consideration will determine the reference level value selected.

Doses to workers and members of the public can be measured or assessed after an emergency exposure scenario has arisen or after an existing exposure problem has been detected and protective steps have been adopted. In this case, the reference level can serve instead as a yardstick by which past protection measures were evaluated [33]. Whether or not exposures over the reference level are included in the dose distribution resulting from implementing a planned protective strategy depends on the efficacy of the approach. However, exposures over the reference level should be reduced to below the reference level.

Source-related dose limitations and reference values are affected by the following:

Doses above 100 mSv are associated with high cancer risk and an increased possibility of deterministic consequences. The Commission has determined that 100 mSv, whether experienced acutely or over a year, represents the upper limit for a reference level. Acute or annual exposures of more than 100 mSv would be justified only in extraordinary circumstances, such as saving life, preventing a catastrophic calamity, or because the exposure is inevitable. Extremely high exposures would have no positive consequences for anyone, individually or collectively.

Besides the restrictions, many numerical criteria established by the Commission in Publication 60 and later publications can be viewed as constraints or reference levels. Readers are encouraged to refer to Table 5 of ICRP 103 for details regarding the framework for source-related dose constraints and reference levels.

Choosing a reasonable dose limitation or reference level is crucial in optimising the protection principle into practice [34]. The first stage is to characterise the relevant exposure situation in terms of the nature of the exposure, the benefits from the exposure situation to both individuals and society, other societal factors, and the feasibility of reducing or preventing the exposures. You should be able to choose the proper constraint or reference level band by comparing its properties to those listed in the Table. Then, a general optimisation approach can determine a suitable value for the constraint or reference level by considering relevant factors such as national or regional characteristics and preferences and, where applicable, international standards and best practices.

13.8. As Low as Reasonably Achievable

All the previously mentioned dosage limits are maximum values subject to the ALARA principle. To ensure the safety of its employees, standard-setting committees prefer a "zero exposure" policy. However, this cannot happen if we want to see the great benefits of radiation and nuclear technology.

Since radiation can cause health problems, keeping tabs on how much people are exposed to it is essential. There should be no unwarranted exposure. The public and workers' exposure to facilities or equipment should be minimal. (ALARA is synonymous with the ICRP-preferred term "optimisation.") Risk should be taken by first weighing the rewards against other options' potential downsides [35].

Conclusion

This chapter presented a comprehensive overview of radiation safety principles, guidelines, and regulatory frameworks established to protect workers, patients, and the general public. It detailed the foundational principles of justification, optimization, and dose limitation, highlighting their application in planned, emergency, and existing exposure situations. The text explained the roles of organizations such as the ICRP and NCRP in shaping international standards and provided clear definitions of occupational, public, and medical exposures. Specific strategies, including dose constraints, reference levels, and the ALARA principle, were discussed to illustrate how radiation risk is managed in practice. By integrating these principles with careful monitoring and education, radiation safety programs help minimize harm while enabling the beneficial uses of ionizing radiation in medicine, industry, and research.

References

[1] Cousins C, Miller DL, Bernardi G, Rehani MM, Schofield P, Vañó E, Einstein AJ, Geiger B, Heintz P, Padovani RJ, Sim KH. *International commission on radiological protection.* ICRP publication. 2011 Apr 4;120:1-25.

[2] Sievert RM, Failla G. Recommendations of the international commission on radiological protection. *Health Physics* (England). 1959 Jul 1;2.

[3] Schauer DA, Linton OW. National Council on Radiation Protection and Measurements report shows substantial medical exposure increase. *Radiology.* 2009 Nov;253(2):293-6.

[4] Taylor LS. Brief history of the National Committee on Radiation Protection and Measurements (NCRP) covering the period 1929–1946. *Health Physics.* 1958 Jan 1;1(1):3-10.

[5] Wrixon AD. New ICRP recommendations. *Journal of radiological protection.* 2008 May 22;28(2):161.

[6] Källman P, Ågren A, Brahme A. Tumour and normal tissue responses to fractionated non-uniform dose delivery. *International journal of radiation biology.* 1992 Jan 1;62(2):249-62.

[7] Stewart FA, Akleyev AV, Hauer-Jensen M, Hendry JH, Kleiman NJ, Macvittie TJ, Aleman BM, Edgar AB, Mabuchi K, Muirhead CR, Shore RE. ICRP publication 118: ICRP statement on tissue reactions and early and late effects of radiation in normal tissues and organs–threshold doses for tissue reactions in a radiation protection context. *Annals of the ICRP.* 2012 Feb 1;41(1-2):1-322.

[8] Miller RW. Delayed effects of external radiation exposure: a brief history. *Radiation research.* 1995 Nov 1;144(2):160-9.

[9] Adams N. Dependence on age at intake of committed dose equivalents from radionuclides. *Physics in Medicine & Biology.* 1981 Nov 1;26(6):1019.

[10] Ritz B, Morgenstern H, Crawford-Brown D, Young B. The effects of internal radiation exposure on cancer mortality in nuclear workers at Rocketdyne/Atomics International. *Environmental Health Perspectives.* 2000 Aug;108(8):743-51.

[11] Venneri L, Rossi F, Botto N, Andreassi MG, Salcone N, Emad A, Lazzeri M, Gori C, Vano E, Picano E. Cancer risk from professional exposure in staff working in cardiac catheterization laboratory: insights from the National Research Council's Biological Effects of Ionizing Radiation VII Report. *American heart journal.* 2009 Jan 1;157(1):118-24.

[12] Thierry-Chef I, Marshall M, Fix JJ, Bermann F, Gilbert ES, Hacker C, Heinmiller B, Murray W, Pearce MS, Utterback D, Bernar K. The 15-country collaborative study of cancer risk among radiation workers in the nuclear industry: study of errors in dosimetry. *Radiation research.* 2007 Apr 1;167(4):380-95.

[13] Kong TY, Kim S, Lee Y, Son JK, Maeng SJ. Radioactive effluents released from Korean nuclear power plants and the resulting radiation doses to members of the public. *Nuclear Engineering and Technology*. 2017 Dec 1;49(8):1772-7.

[14] Martin CJ. Effective dose: how should it be applied to medical exposures?. *The British journal of radiology.* 2007 Aug;80(956):639-47.

[15] Fryer M, Collins CD, Ferrier H, Colvile RN, Nieuwenhuijsen MJ. Human exposure modelling for chemical risk assessment: a review of current approaches and research and policy implications. *Environmental science & policy.* 2006 May 1;9(3):261-74.

[16] International Commission on Non-Ionizing Radiation Protection. Guidelines for limiting exposure to time-varying electric and magnetic fields (1 Hz to 100 kHz). *Health physics*. 2010 Dec 1;99(6):818-36.

[17] Valentin J, Boice Jr JD, Clarke RH, Cousins C, Gonzalez AJ, Lee J, Lindell B, Meinhold CB, Mettler Jr FA, Pan Z, Pentreath RJ. Published on behalf of the International Commission on Radiological Protection.

[18] Protection R. ICRP publication 103. Ann ICRP. 2007;37(2.4):2.

[19] López PO, Dauer LT, Loose R, Martin CJ, Miller DL, Vañó E, Doruff M, Padovani R, Massera G, Yoder C. ICRP publication 139: occupational radiological protection in interventional procedures. *Annals of the ICRP*. 2018 Mar;47(2):1-18.

[20] Clarke RH, Valentin J. The History of ICRP and the Evolution of its Policies: Invited by the Commission in October 2008. *Annals of the ICRP*. 2009 Feb;39(1):75-110.

[21] Wagner LK, Eifel PJ, Geise RA. Potential biological effects following high X-ray dose interventional procedures. *Journal of Vascular and Interventional Radiology*. 1994 Jan 1;5(1):71-84.

[22] Vom J, Williams I. Justification of radiographic examinations: What are the key issues?. *Journal of medical radiation sciences*. 2017 Sep;64(3):212-9.

[23] Valentin J, Boice Jr JD, Clarke RH, Cousins C, Gonzalez AJ, Lee J, Lindell B, Meinhold CB, Mettler Jr FA, Pan Z, Pentreath RJ. Published on behalf of the International Commission on Radiological Protection.

[24] Khong PL, Ringertz H, Donoghue V, Frush D, Rehani M, Appelgate K, Sanchez R. ICRP publication 121: radiological protection in paediatric diagnostic and interventional radiology. *Annals of the ICRP.* 2013 Apr 1;42(2):1-63.

[25] Kalra MK, Maher MM, Toth TL, Hamberg LM, Blake MA, Shepard JA, Saini S. Strategies for CT radiation dose optimization. *Radiology*. 2004 Mar;230(3):619-28.

[26] Valentin J, Boice Jr JD, Clarke RH, Cousins C, Gonzalez AJ, Lee J, Lindell B, Meinhold CB, Mettler Jr FA, Pan Z, Pentreath RJ. Published on behalf of the International Commission on Radiological Protection.

[27] Khong PL, Ringertz H, Donoghue V, Frush D, Rehani M, Appelgate K, Sanchez R. ICRP publication 121: radiological protection in paediatric diagnostic and interventional radiology. *Annals of the ICRP.* 2013 Apr 1;42(2):1-63.

[28] Trattner S, Pearson GD, Chin C, Cody DD, Gupta R, Hess CP, Kalra MK, Kofler Jr JM, Krishnam MS, Einstein AJ. Standardization and optimization of CT protocols to achieve low dose. *Journal of the American College of Radiology*. 2014 Mar 1;11(3):271-8.

[29] Ramzaev PV, Tarasov SI, Troitskaya MN, Ermolaeva AP. Progress in basic principles of limitation in radiation protection. In Proceedings of the 4. *International congress of the International Radiation Protection Association.* Paris, 24-30 April 1977 1977.

[30] Wrixon AD. New ICRP recommendations. Journal of radiological protection. 2008 May 22;28(2):161.

[31] Thieke C, Bortfeld T, Niemierko A, Nill S. From physical dose constraints to equivalent uniform dose constraints in inverse radiotherapy planning. *Medical physics.* 2003 Sep;30(9):2332-9.

[32] Vetter RJ. ICRP Publication 103, *The recommendations of the international commission on radiological protection.*

[33] González AJ. Radiation safety standards and their application: international policies and current issues. *Health physics.* 2004 Sep 1;87(3):258-72.

[34] Kamdem EF, Samba ON, Manemo CT, Kouam BB, Abogo S, Tambe J, Amougou JC, Guegang E, Zeh OF, Moifo B, Nguemgne C. Establishment of Local Diagnostic Reference Level for Routine Paediatric Computed Tomography Examinations in Bafoussam West Cameroon. *Radiation Protection Dosimetry*. 2022 Aug;198(12):815-20.

[35] Hendee WR, Edwards FM. *ALARA and an integrated approach to radiation protection. In Seminars in nuclear medicine* 1986 Apr 1 (Vol. 16, No. 2, pp. 142-150). WB Saunders.

List of Contributors

Anurag Luharia, PhD
Department of Radio physics and Radio safety
Datta Meghe Institute of Higher Education and Research
Wardha, India

Ashish Uke, MD
Department of Radiotherapy
Datta Meghe Institute of Higher Education and Research
Wardha, India

Gaurav Mishra, MD, PhD
Department of Radiodiagnosis
Datta Meghe Institute of Higher Education and Research
Wardha, India

Sanjay Dhoble, PhD
Department of Physics
Nagpur University
Nagpur, India

Ignatius Komakech, PhD
Department of Oncology
Uganda Cancer Institute
Kampala, Uganda

Anchineyan Pichandi, PhD,
Department of Central Physics
Health Care Global Enterprise Ltd.
Banglore, India

Shweta Dahake, MSc
Department of Radio physics and Radio safety
Datta Meghe Institute of Higher Education and Research
Wardha, India

N. Gajendran, MSc
Department of Radiation Oncology
Regency Hospital Ltd.
Kanpur, India

Shreya Naik, MSc
School of Allied Health Science
Datta Meghe Institute of Higher Education and Research
Wardha, India

Albert Paul Varghese, MSc
School of Allied Health Science
Datta Meghe Institute of Higher Education and Research
Wardha, India

Maruf Ahmad, MSc
Department of Radiology
Centurion University of Technology and Management
Jatni, Bhubaneswar, Odisha, India

Nandini, MSc
Department of Radiology and Imaging Technology
Noida International University
Greater Noida (UP), India

Jayakrishnan Vaikkattil, MSc
Department of Nuclear Medicine
Manchester University NHS Trust
Manchester, UK

Saraswathula Bharadwaj, MD
Department of Radiodiagnosis
Datta Meghe Institute of Higher Education and Research
Wardha, India

Syed Asrar Ul Haq Andrabi, MSc
School of Allied Health Science
Datta Meghe Institute of Higher Education and Research
Wardha, India

Shrikant Chaudhary, MSc
Department of Nuclear Medicine
National Cancer Institute
Nagpur, India

Vaibhav Sonwani, MD
Department of Radiotherapy
HCG Cancer Centre
Nagpur, India

Suwarna Dangore, MDS
Department of Oral Medicine and Radiology
Datta Meghe Institute of Higher Education and Research
Wardha, India

Pratap Singh Parihar, MD, PhD
Department of Radiodiagnosis,
Datta Meghe Institute of Higher Education and Research
Wardha, India

Priyal Shrivastava MD
Department of Radio-diagnosis
Datta Meghe Institute of Higher Education and Research
Wardha, India

Jaishriram Rathored, PhD, Post Doc in Molecular Medicine
Department of Molecular Diagnostics
Datta Meghe Institute of Higher Education and Research
Wardha, India

Elangovan Doraisamy, MSc, DABR
Department of Radiation Oncology
UPMC Hillman Cancer Center
Pittsburgh, PA, USA

Shivali Kashikar, MD, PhD
Department of Radio-diagnosis
Datta Meghe Institute of Higher Education and Research
Wardha, India

Ravishankar Patil, MD
Department of Radiology
Datta Meghe Institute of Higher Education and Research
Wardha, India

Umang Jajoo, MD
Department of Radio-diagnosis,
Datta Meghe Institute of Higher Education and Research
Wardha, India

Gautam Kumar Sharan, MD
Department of Radiotherapy,
Jawaharlal Nehru Cancer Hospital and Research Centre
Bhopal, India

Manish Rathi, DMRE
Department of Radiology
Gode Medical College
Amravati, India

Swapnil Mohod, MDS, PhD
Department of Dentistry
Dr. Panjabrao Bhausaheb Deshmukh Memorial Medical College
Amravati, India

Mrunal Meshram, MDS, PhD
Department of Oral Medicine and Radiology
Datta Meghe Institute of Higher Education and Research
Wardha, India

Rajesh Amutha, MSc
Department of Radiotherapy
Rio Bravo Cancer Center
Bakersfield, CA, USA

Mary Joan, PhD
Dept of Radiation Oncology
Christian Medical College and Hospital
Ludhiana, India

Nilavarasu Shanmugam, MSc
Department of Radiotherapy
All India Institute of Medical Sciences
Nagpur, India

Index

S

T

U

V

W

X